MRCOG Part 1

550 SBAs and MCQs

MRCOG Part 1

550 SBAs and MCQs

Katherine Andersen MBBS BSc (Hons)
Specialist Trainee in Obstetrics and Gynaecology,
Barnet and Chase Farm Hospitals NHS Trust, London, UK

Tara Woodward MBBS BSc (Hons) PgDip Journalism
Specialist Trainee in Obstetrics and Gynaecology,
North Middlesex University Hospital NHS Trust, London, UK

Edited by
Maryam Parisaei MRCOG
Consultant Obstetrician and Gynaecologist,
Homerton University Hospital NHS Foundation Trust, London, UK

Amit Shah MD MRCOG
Consultant in Reproductive Medicine and Surgery,
Homerton University Hospital NHS Foundation Trust, London, UK

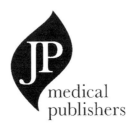

JP
medical
publishers

London • St Louis • Panama City • New Delhi

© 2013 JP Medical Ltd.
Published by JP Medical Ltd
83 Victoria Street, London, SW1H 0HW, UK
Tel: +44 (0)20 3170 8910   Fax: +44 (0)20 3008 6180
Email: info@jpmedpub.com   Web: www.jpmedpub.com

ISBN: 978-1-907816-36-9

British Library Cataloguing in Publication Data
A catalogue record for this book is available from the British Library

Library of Congress Cataloging in Publication Data
A catalog record for this book is available from the Library of Congress

JP Medical Ltd is a subsidiary of Jaypee Brothers Medical Publishers (P) Ltd, New Delhi, India

Commissioning Editor: Steffan Clements
Senior Editorial Assistant: Katrina Rimmer
Design: Designers Collective Ltd

Copy edited, typeset, printed and bound in India.

Foreword

The Membership of the Royal College of Obstetricians and Gynaecologists (MRCOG) remains the cornerstone for the assessment of knowledge required by trainee doctors in the UK. Passing the exam is a prerequisite for the progression through the structured training programme, towards the Certificate of Completion of Training (CCT) and entry on to the Specialist Register. The standard of the exam remains high and the curriculum is based on UK practice.

The MRCOG Part 1 exam can be taken at any time after graduation and must be passed before transition from ST2 to ST3 of the training programme. This book aims to provide an exam revision guide for trainee doctors in ST1 and ST2, and international candidates preparing to sit the exam. For international graduates often working outside of recognised training programmes it is a tough exam to pass. Yet many candidates continue to take the exam knowing that success will demonstrate the acquisition of knowledge to a high standard, which will enhance the treatment of the women and babies in their care.

The MRCOG Part 1 has changed in the last few years. It has always tested the knowledge-base in all the basic sciences as they pertain to obstetrics and gynaecology, but a new question format has been introduced to allow the syllabus to be tested in a more clinically relevant manner. Doctors planning to take the exam must now learn how to answer both multiple choice questions (MCQs) and the new single best answer (SBA) format, and for this they require exam technique and clinical knowledge.

This book contains 550 SBAs and MCQs arranged into individual chapters based on the exam syllabus. Covering all the basic sciences as well as current RCOG clinical recommended practice, it provides a comprehensive revision aid with helpful explanations after each question. The book also offers guidance on other information sources and a suggested reading list. At the back of the book there are two practice papers for readers to test their knowledge and practise exam technique.

Maggie Blott FRCOG
Consultant in Obstetrics and Maternal Medicine, University College London, London, UK
Former Vice President (Education) of the Royal College of Obstetricians and Gynaecologists, UK

Preface

Passing the MRCOG Part 1 is regarded as the first step in becoming an obstetrician and gynaecologist. For many candidates, it will be their first postgraduate exam and the task of passing at first sitting can seem daunting. However, we believe that with appropriate preparation candidates can feel confident in passing the exam first time.

The new curriculum now combines subject matters from everyday clinical practice as well as all the basic medical sciences and is much more clinically orientated than before. There is also a new format with the introduction of single best answer (SBA) questions, the removal of extended matching questions (EMQs) and the reduced proportion of multiple choice questions (MCQs). This book reflects both the new curriculum and format.

The 550 questions presented in this book cover the syllabus in a format which mimics the exam itself. Working through the book will allow trainees to gauge their level and breadth of knowledge and will highlight topics which need to be concentrated on further. Within the answer sections, references are made to the latest evidence-based practice, and tables and diagrams are used to aid in the assimilation of this information.

The philosophy of this book is to provide trainees with an insight into the new assessment technique of the MRCOG Part 1 and to build confidence by approaching the exam in a systematic manner. We hope you enjoy working through the questions in this book and wish you best of luck in the exam.

Katherine Andersen
Tara Woodward
Maryam Parisaei
Amit Shah
April 2012

Acknowledgements

We would like to thank Dr Helen Hammond for her eagerness to review all 550 questions and for her excellent advice regarding their content.

Thanks also to Dr Simon Tod from Sydney, Australia, who gave much appreciated advice regarding the book's statistical content.

Katherine Andersen
Tara Woodward

Exam revision advice

Exam format

The MRCOG Part 1 exam consists of Paper 1 and Paper 2. Each paper consists of 60 single best answer (SBA) questions and 30 multiple choice questions (MCQs). Each paper must be completed within two hours and thirty minutes. The SBA and MCQ sections are marked out of 150 marks each.

Single best answer (SBA) questions

A SBA comprises three components: a stem (most commonly a clinically relevant vignette), a lead in question and five answer options. The answer options are homogenous and are presented in alphabetical or numerical order for ease of reference. Candidates should read the question carefully then select the single most appropriate answer from the five options.

The nature of a SBA means that there are four distracters surrounding the correct answer. Of the four distracters, there may be one or two distracters which can reasonably be identified as incorrect. There are also likely to be one or two distracters that are plausible answers. At this point, candidates will need to read the stem and lead in question again, then make a judgement as to which answer fits best.

Multiple choice questions (MCQs)

A MCQ is made up of five stems, which must each be answered true or false. Marks are given for answering stems correctly. All the questions need to be answered and there is no negative marking for answering stems incorrectly.

How to use this book

We believe that one of the best ways to revise for the exam, and crucial to passing at first attempt, is to work through practice questions again and again. In this way, confidence will be gained with the new question format and the full curriculum will be covered.

Further reading suggestions are provided to accompany explanations in this book to direct further learning. We feel that this is a more appropriate way for trainee doctors to improve knowledge in certain topics in obstetrics and gynaecology than by memorising sections from large textbooks. We hope that directed learning will enable trainees to concentrate on areas of weakness.

We have included two mock exam papers at the end, which can be tested under timed conditions to provide a good sense of the time restraints of the real exam. Allow two and a half hours to sit each paper, and remember that in the new format there are 60 SBAs and only 30 MCQs.

Finally, having a study buddy is good way to maximise exam preparation. In addition to keeping each other on track, you will be able assist each other with areas of the curriculum that the other may be struggling with. We both studied for the exam together, which gave us focus, a timetable to keep to and some friendly competiveness to make sure we took our exam preparation seriously.

Katherine Andersen
Tara Woodward

Contents

Recommended reading

Bennett P, Williamson C (eds). Basic Sciences in Obstetrics and Gynaecology: A Textbook for MRCOG Part 1, 4th edn. Edinburgh: Churchill Livingstone, 2010.

Chamberlain G, Steer P (eds). Turnbull's Obstetrics, 3rd edn. London: Churchill Livingstone, 2001.

Collins S, Arulkumaran S, Hayes K, et al. Oxford Handbook of Obstetrics and Gynaecology, 2nd edn. Oxford: Oxford University Press, 2010.

Connor JM. Medical Genetics for the MRCOG and Beyond. London: RCOG Press, 2005.

Fiander A, Thilganathan B (eds). Your Essential Revision Guide MRCOG Part 1. London: RCOG Press, 2010.

Kumar V, Abbas A, Fausto N, Aster J. Robbins and Cotran Pathologic Basis of Disease, 8th edn. Philadephia: Saunders Elsevier, 2009.

Nelson-Piercy C. Handbook of Obstetric Medicine, 4th edn. London: Informa Healthcare, 2010.

Royal College of Obstetricians and Gynaecologists, Green-top Guidelines. London: RCOG. www.rcog.org.uk/guidelines.

Chapter 1

Anatomy

Questions: MCQs

Answer each stem 'True' or 'False'.

1. **The following form part of the superior anatomical boundary (pelvic inlet) of the true pelvis:**
   A Linea alba
   B Sacroiliac joint
   C Ischial fossa
   D Iliac crest
   E Iliopectineal line

2. **The diameters of the pelvis:**
   A The anatomical anteroposterior diameter (true conjugate) is approximately 11 cm
   B The obstetric conjugate is larger than the true conjugate
   C The anatomical transverse diameter forms the largest pelvic diameter (approximately 13 cm)
   D The obstetric transverse diameter bisects the true conjugate
   E The external conjugate has no true obstetric importance

3. **The pudendal nerve:**
   A Arises from the posterior rami of S2, S3 and S4
   B Supplies the levator ani
   C Leaves the pelvis through the greater sciatic foramen
   D Supplies the clitoris
   E Crosses over the ischial tuberosity, lateral to the internal pudendal artery

4. **Pelvic nerve supply:**
   A Pelvic splanchnic nerves are derived from the dorsal primary rami of spinal nerves S2–S4
   B The inferior rectal nerve is a branch of the pudendal nerve
   C The rectal plexus is derived from the anterior part of the inferior hypogastric plexus
   D The external anal sphincter is supplied by the inferior rectal nerve
   E The anterior labial nerve is a branch of the ilioinguinal nerve

5. **With regard to veins of the pelvis:**
    A The left ovarian vein drains directly into the inferior vena cava
    B The internal pudendal vein passes through the pudendal canal
    C The uterine venous plexus connects the ovarian vein and the vaginal venous plexus
    D The internal pudendal vein drains into the great saphenous vein
    E The rectal venous plexus is a site of portocaval anastomosis

6. **With regard to innervation of the lower limb:**
    A The tibial nerve is derived from L4–S1
    B Damage to the common peroneal nerve typically results in foot drop
    C The femoral nerve divides into an anterior and posterior branch before passing beneath the inguinal ligament
    D The femoral nerve is derived from the posterior division of L2–L4
    E The sciatic nerve is derived from L4–S3

7. **The anal canal:**
    A The upper half is lined with cuboidal epithelium
    B The lower half is lined with non-keratinised stratified squamous epithelium
    C The fibres of ischiococcygeus form part of the internal anal sphincter
    D The dentate line lies at the border of the upper one-third and lower two-thirds of the anal canal
    E Hilton's line indicates the junction between keratinised and non-keratinised stratified squamous epithelium

8. **Rectus sheath:**
    A The rectus sheath is made up of the aponeuroses of transversus abdominis and internal oblique
    B Below the arcuate line, the posterior rectus abdominis is separated from the peritoneum by transversalis fascia and connective tissue
    C Pyramidalis is external to the rectus sheath
    D The rectus sheath contains the ventral rami of lower eight thoracic nerves
    E Contains an anastomosis between the internal thoracic artery and superior epigastric artery

9. **The pudendal canal:**
    A Contains the pudendal nerve, artery and vein
    B The pudendal nerve is not located in the pudendal canal
    C Runs superiorly to the sacrotuberous ligament
    D Runs laterally to obturator internus
    E Passes medial to the ischial spines

10. **The bladder:**
    A The pudendal nerve plays no part in innervation of the bladder
    B The sympathetic nervous system has no motor function in the bladder
    C The main blood supply to the bladder is from the branches of the posterior trunk of the internal iliac artery

D   Lymphatic drainage of the bladder is to the internal iliac nodes
E   It is derived embryologically from the mesonephric duct

11. The human testis:

A   Has an average length of 2–3 cm
B   Descends through the inguinal ring after birth to reside in the scrotum
C   Are surrounded by the tunica vaginalis
D   The tunica albuginea is covered by tunica vaginalis
E   The hydatid of Morgagni is a remnant of the müllerian duct

12. The ureters:

A   Are retroperitoneal structures
B   Are 35 cm long
C   Cross in front of the uterine arteries
D   Originate embryonically from the ureteric buds
E   Insert into the bladder posteromedially

13. The vagina:

A   Is lined with striated squamous epithelium
B   Has an acidic pH
C   Has secretory glands which provide lubrication
D   Is approximately 7 cm long anteriorly
E   Is covered anteriorly by visceral peritoneum

14. The vagina:

A   Has its venous drainage supplied by the external iliac vein
B   Is derived from the embryonic mesonephros
C   Originates from mesoderm
D   Has a shorter anterior wall than posterior wall
E   Has superiorly supplied by the uterine artery

15. Superiorly, the vagina:

A   Receives its arterial blood supply from the uterine arteries
B   Receives its lymphatic drainage via the inguinal lymph nodes
C   Receives its venous supply from the uterine vein
D   Receives somatic innervation via the pudendal nerve
E   Is lined with secretory columnar epithelium

16. The uterus:

A   In non-gravid state weighs approximately 90 g
B   Consists of the three muscle layers: the perimetrium, the myometrium and the endometrium
C   Is related anteriorly to the pouch of Douglas
D   Is 10 cm long
E   Receives its main arterial supply from the uterine arteries

17. The female urethra:

A   Is directly related to the anterior vaginal wall

B   Is surrounded by Bartholin's glands at the urethral orifice in the vestibule
C   In its upper two-thirds, it has the same blood supply as the bladder
D   Is innervated by the pudendal nerve
E   Is lined with transitional epithelium at its origin proximal to the bladder

18. The average female pelvis:

A   Is gynaecoid in shape
B   Has a round obturator foramen
C   Has a heart-shaped inlet
D   Has a wide pubic arch
E   Has a subpubic angle of 60°

19. The adrenal glands:

A   Sit superiorly to the kidneys
B   The medulla originates from the embryonic endoderm
C   The cortex develops from coelomic mesothelium
D   Lymphatic drainage is from the lumbar lymph nodes
E   The right adrenal gland sits anterior to the diaphragm

20. The adrenal glands:

A   The left adrenal gland is triangular-shaped
B   The adrenal medulla consists of chromaffin cells
C   The right adrenal vein drains into the right renal vein
D   Have part of their nerve supply provided by the thoracic splanchnic nerves
E   The left adrenal gland is in contact with the spleen

21. The inguinal canal:

A   Part of the external oblique forms the anterior wall of the canal
B   Contains the ilioinguinal nerve
C   The internal oblique originates from the lateral third of the inguinal ligament
D   Contains the male spermatic cord
E   The superficial inguinal ring lies superiorly and lateral to the pubic tubercle

22. The femoral triangle:

A   The inguinal ligament provides the superior boundary
B   The medial border is formed from the gracilis
C   The lateral border is formed from both sartorius and iliacus
D   The femoral artery lies medial to the femoral vein
E   The femoral nerve lies lateral to the femoral artery

23. The femoral region:

A   The femoral ring is bounded medially by the lacunar ligament
B   The femoral artery is a continuation of the internal iliac artery
C   The femoral septum is covered by parietal peritoneum
D   The femoral canal often contain Cloquet's node
E   The femoral sheath covers the femoral nerve

24. **The muscles of the posterior abdominal wall:**
    A   Iliacus is innervated by the femoral nerve
    B   Iliopsoas acts to extend the thigh
    C   Arterial supply is predominantly from the abdominal aorta
    D   Quadratus lumborum is innervated by the subcostal nerve
    E   Psoas minor is absent in females

Questions: SBAs

For each question, select the single best answer from the five options listed.

25. Which of the following structures does not pass through the diaphragm?

    A   Azygos vein
    B   Cisterna chyli
    C   Inferior vena cava
    D   Oesophagus
    E   Thoracic duct

26. Which vessel provides blood supply to the intestine from the splenic flexure of the transverse colon to the rectum?

    A   Inferior mesenteric artery
    B   Median sacral artery
    C   Middle colic artery
    D   Rectal artery
    E   Superior mesenteric artery

27. A 21-year-old woman undergoes a laparoscopic ovarian cystectomy to remove a dermoid cyst. Three days after the operation, she presents to the emergency department feeling unwell and her haemoglobin level is found to be 6 g/dL. Damage to a blood vessel is suspected from the laparoscopic procedure.

    Which vessel crosses the common and external iliac artery in the infundibulopelvic fold?

    A   Femoral artery
    B   Inferior mesenteric artery
    C   Median sacral artery
    D   Ovarian artery
    E   Renal artery

28. What is the nerve root of the ilioinguinal nerve?

    A   T12 and L1
    B   L1
    C   L1 and L2
    D   L2
    E   L2 and L3

29. A 27-year-old woman has a cervical smear result which shows 'borderline' changes.

    Which cells line the ectocervix?

    A   Ciliated cells
    B   Columnar epithelium
    C   Cuboidal epithelium

D Smooth muscle cells
E Stratified squamous epithelium

30. A 32-year-old woman undergoes an emergency caesarean section for failure to progress at 9 cm cervical dilatation.

    Which of the following correctly describes the pelvic shape which has an anteroposterior diameter of the inlet, greater than the transverse diameter?

    A Android
    B Anthropoid
    C Gynaecoid
    D Male
    E Platypelloid

31. An 18-year-old woman attends the gynaecology clinic complaining of urinary incontinence, 3 months after suffering a third degree perineal tear during a normal vaginal delivery.

    Which muscle forms the main bulk of the levator ani muscle?

    A Bulbocavernosus
    B Iliococcygeus
    C Ischiococcygeus
    D Pubococcygeus
    E Urogenital diaphragm

32. Which of the following organs is derived from ectodermal neural crest cells?

    A Adrenal gland inner medulla
    B Adrenal gland outer cortex
    C Liver
    D Pancreas
    E Spleen

33. A 63-year-old woman complains of numbness over her thigh following a radical hysterectomy for stage IV endometrial carcinoma.

    What is the nerve root of the obturator nerve?

    A Anterior division L1–L4
    B Anterior division L2–L4
    C Anterior division L3–L4
    D Posterior division L2–L4
    E Posterior division L3–L4

34. An 82-year-old woman attends her general practitioner's surgery complaining of a painful lump in the groin.

    Which of the following does not form a boundary of the femoral triangle?

    A Adductor longus

    B   Inguinal ligament
    C   Obturator internus
    D   Pectineus
    E   Sartorius

35. A 32-year-old woman complains of pain in the right buttock. She is 36 weeks pregnant and has a history of chronic back pain.

Which nerve supplies the gluteus maximus muscle?

    A   Inferior gluteal
    B   Internal obturator
    C   Internal obturator (lateral cutaneous nerve of the thigh)
    D   Sciatic
    E   Superior gluteal

36. Following a routine elective caesarean section, the rectus sheath is being sutured.

With regards to the rectus sheath which of the following is correct?

    A   Arcuate line demarcates the upper limit of the posterior layer of rectus sheath
    B   External oblique aponeurosis forms the posterior aspect of the sheath
    C   Internal oblique aponeurosis always passes in front of rectus abdominis
    D   Scarpa's fascia is superficial to Camper's fascia and the external oblique
    E   Transversalis fascia lies directly below the rectus sheath

37. A 47-year-old woman undergoes a routine transabdominal hysterectomy to remove a large fibroid uterus. She is found to have a fibroid in the broad ligament and there is concern that her ureter may have been damaged due to the difficult operation.

With regards to the path of the ureter, which of the following is correct?

    A   In the broad ligament, both ureters pass over their respective uterine artery
    B   Runs lateral to the internal iliac artery
    C   Ovarian vessels enter the pelvis posterior to the ureters
    D   Upper one-third of the ureters lie in the abdomen
    E   Ureters cross close to the bifurcation of the common iliac vessels

38. What structure does the right ovarian vein empty into?

    A   Azygos vein
    B   Inferior vena cava
    C   Internal iliac vein
    D   Right renal vein
    E   Right pudendal vein

39. A 27-year-old woman has a forceps delivery under regional block. She suffers multiple second degree tears to the lateral vaginal wall.

Sensory innervation of the vagina is provided by which nerve?

A Dorsal nerve of the clitoris
B Inferior hypogastric plexus
C Inferior rectal nerve
D Obturator nerve
E Pudendal nerve

40. Which artery supplies the structures derived from the foregut of the embryo?

A Coeliac trunk
B Inferior mesenteric
C Middle rectal
D Renal
E Superior mesenteric

41. A 73-year-old woman undergoes a laparoscopic assisted vaginal hysterectomy and oophorectomy. There is a large bleed during the procedure and it is converted to a laparotomy.

Which of the following provides the arterial blood supply of the left ovary?

A Abdominal aorta
B External iliac artery
C Internal iliac artery
D Left ovarian artery
E Obturator artery

42. During a laparoscopic-assisted vaginal hysterectomy the surgeon accidentally damages the ovarian artery.

Regarding the left ovarian artery, which of the following is correct?

A Anastomoses with the vaginal artery
B Is a branch of the abdominal aorta
C Follows the course of the left ovarian artery
D Lies inferiorly to the inferior mesenteric artery
E Supplies both left and right ovaries

43. Which of the following arteries is a terminal branch (not paired) of the abdominal aorta?

A Gonadal
B Median sacral
C Phrenic
D Renal
E Suprarenal

44. A 32-year-old woman has an episiotomy repaired following a forceps delivery.

Which of the following does not insert into the perineal body?

A   Bulbocavernosus
B   External anal sphincter
C   Ischiocavernosus
D   Levator ani
E   Transverse perineal

45. A woman undergoes an emergency caesarean section at full dilatation following a failed trial of instrumental delivery. There is a lateral extension to the uterine excision which is bleeding.

Identify which of the following gives the correct pairing of artery and its origin.

	Artery	Origin
A	Internal pudendal	Posterior division of internal iliac
B	Ovarian artery	Common Iliac
C	Testicular artery	Abdominal aorta
D	Uterine artery	Abdominal aorta
E	Uterine artery	Anterior division of the internal iliac

46. Which of the following is not part of the bony pelvis?

A   Fourth lumbar vertebrae
B   Ilium
C   Ischium
D   Pubis
E   Sacrum

47. Which of the following describes the anatomy of the inguinal region?

A   The deep inguinal ring lies at the lateral two-thirds of the inguinal ligament
B   The deep inguinal ring transmits the ilioinguinal nerve
C   The superficial inguinal ring lies below the pubic tubercle
D   The superficial inguinal ring transmits the genitofemoral nerve
E   The superficial inguinal ring transmits the round ligament

48. Which of the following nerves is transmitted by the superficial inguinal ring?

A   Femoral nerve
B   Genitofemoral nerve
C   Ilioinguinal nerve
D   Peroneal nerve
E   Sciatic nerve

Answers

1. A False

   B True

   C False

   D False

   E True

   The female pelvis can be divided anatomically into two broad areas: the false pelvis and the true pelvis. The false pelvis lies above the pelvic brim and has no obstetric importance. The true pelvis lies below the pelvic brim and is related to child birth.

   The true pelvis comprises an inlet, outlet and cavity. The pelvic inlet (brim) has the following boundaries: sacral promontory, sacroiliac joints, alae of sacrum, iliopectineal line, upper border of superior pubic rami and upper border of pubic symphysis.

2. A True

   B False

   C True

   D True

   E True

   The diameters of the pelvis can be broadly categorised into transverse, anteroposterior and oblique (**Figure 1.1**).

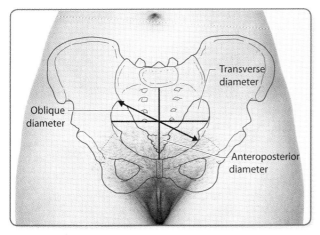

Figure 1.1 Anterior view of the female bony pelvis. (Reproduced from Tunstall R and Shah N. Pocket Tutor Surface Anatomy. London: JP Medical Ltd, 2012 and courtesy of Sam Scott-Hunter, London.)

3. A False

   B True

   C True

D True

E False

The pudendal nerve originates from the anterior (ventral) rami of S2, S3 and S4. After passing between piriformis and coccygeus, it leaves the pelvis through the greater sciatic foramen. It then crosses the ischial spine with the internal pudendal artery and re-enters the pelvis through the lesser sciatic foramen. The pudendal nerve passes medially to the internal pudendal artery (**Figure 1.2**).

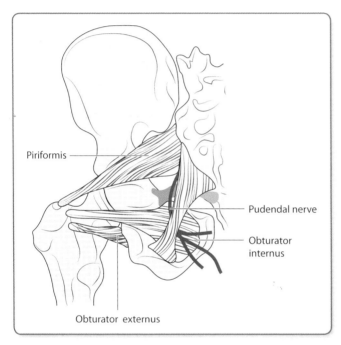

Figure 1.2 Anatomy of the pudendal nerve.

Piriformis

Pudendal nerve

Obturator internus

Obturator externus

4. **A** False

   B True

   C False

   D True

   E True

Pelvic splanchnic nerves provide parasympathetic innervation to the pelvis and are derived from the ventral primary rami of S2–S4. They control micturition, defaecation and erection. The inferior hypogastric plexus is formed from fibres of the sacral splanchnic nerves, pelvic splanchnic nerves and hypogastric nerves, and supplies the viscera of the pelvis. The rectal plexus is a posterior division of the inferior hypogastric plexus. The pudendal nerve gives off the inferior rectal nerves, before dividing into two terminal branches: the dorsal nerve of the penis/clitoris and the perineal nerve.

The ilioinguinal nerve is derived from L1 and one of its terminal divisions is the anterior labial nerve, which supplies the skin of the mons pubis and labia majora.

5. A False

    B True

    C True

    D False

    E True

The right ovarian vein drains directly into the inferior vena cava. The left ovarian vein drains into the left renal vein. The internal pudendal vein drains into the internal iliac vein and the external pudendal vein drains into the great saphenous vein. The internal pudendal vein passes through the pudendal canal with the pudendal artery and nerve. The uterine plexuses lie in the superior angles of the uterus, between the two layers of the broad ligament. They connect the ovarian and vaginal plexuses and drain directly into the hypogastric vein. The two other sites of portocaval anastomosis are in the oesophagus and hepatic circulation.

6. A False

    B True

    C False

    D True

    E True

Innervation of the lower limb is from the lumbosacral plexus, which is formed from the ventral rami of spinal nerves T12–S4. The sciatic nerve is a nerve of the posterior leg, derived from L4–S3 and contains fibres from anterior and posterior aspects of the lumbosacral plexus. The tibial nerve is derived from the anterior division of L4–S3 and is a branch of the sciatic nerve. The tibial nerve passes through the popliteal fossa and provides branches to the posterior aspect of the calf, as well as the knee joint. The femoral nerve arises from the dorsal division of the ventral rami of L2–L4. It passes beneath the inguinal ligament to enter the thigh, where it then divides into an anterior and posterior division. It provides innervation to the quadriceps muscle and sartorius, as well as anterior cutaneous branches.

7. A False

    B True

    C False

    D False

    E True

The anal canal is approximately 3 cm long and lies between the anorectal junction and the anal orifice. The upper two-thirds is lined with cuboidal epithelium and is supplied by the superior rectal artery. The lower one-third is lined with non- keratinised stratified squamous epithelium and is supplied by the inferior rectal artery. At the anal orifice there is a transition to keratinised stratified squamous epithelium with the presence of sweat glands and hair. Hilton's line is a white line which indicates the junction of the keratinised from the non-keratinised epithelium. The pectinate line is an important landmark embryologically which lies at the junction of the upper two-thirds and lower one-third. The fibres of pubococcygeus blend with the internal anal sphincter.

8. A False

    B True

    C False

    D False

    E False

The rectus sheath is formed from the aponeurosis of the transversus abdominis, internal and external oblique muscles. At the lateral margin of the rectus abdominis, the internal oblique splits into an anterior and posterior layer, passing in front and behind. In front of the rectus abdominis runs the external oblique aponeurosis and the anterior layer of internal oblique. Behind the rectus runs the posterior layer of internal oblique and the transversus abdominis. The aponeuroses of each side meet at the central linea alba. Below the arcuate line, all aponeuroses pass in front of the rectus abdominis, meaning that the posterior aspect of the lower third of rectus is separated from the peritoneum by transversalis fascia and extraperitoneal connective tissue. The ventral rami of the lower seven thoracic nerves and anastomosis between the superior and inferior epigastric vessels occurs within the rectus sheath. Where pyramidalis is present, it lies within the rectus sheath anterior to rectus abdominis.

9. A True

    B False

    C True

    D False

    E False

The pudendal canal contains the pudendal nerve, artery and vein. It runs medially to the obturator internus and is in close contact with the obturator fascia. It runs out through the greater sciatic foramen and passes laterally to the ischial spines before passing back in through the lesser sciatic foramen.

10. A True

    B True

    C False

    D True

    E False

The urinary bladder is a muscular distensible organ that is located in the pelvis. The main blood supply to the bladder comes from the superior and inferior vesical arteries, which are branches of the anterior trunk of the internal iliac artery. There is also some contribution from the uterine and vaginal arteries. The detrusor muscle is innervated from the S2–S4 nerve root, but the main contribution is from S3. The bladder is predominantly under parasympathetic control, from the inferior hypogastric plexus and the pelvic splanchnic nerves. The sympathetic nervous system only affects blood vessels in the bladder and has no motor function. The human bladder is derived in the embryo from the urogenital sinus.

11. A False

B False

C True

D True

E True

The testes are oval glands that have an average length of 4–5 cm and a diameter of 2–3 cm. They originate embryologically in the abdomen, but descend through the inguinal canal prior to birth. Each testis is surrounded by the tunica vaginalis, which is a serous membrane, derived from the peritoneum. Underneath the tunica vaginalis is a fibrous layer that encapsulates the testis, called the tunica albuginea. It forms septa that divide each testis internally to form 200–300 lobules. It is within each of these lobules that the seminiferous tubules are located.

12. A True

B False

C False

D True

E False

Ureters are muscular tubular structures, approximately 25 cm long, which run along the posterior abdominal wall. They are retroperitoneal through their entire course and carry urine from the kidneys to the bladder. The ureter begins at the kidney and descends from the renal pelvis along the medial border of the psoas muscle. From there, it enters the pelvis and crosses the common iliac artery. In females the ureters travel in the broad ligament and run under the uterine artery eventually inserting into the bladder posterolaterally. The openings of the ureters into the bladder are approximately 2–3 cm apart.

13. A True

B True

C False

D True

E False

The vagina is a muscular elastic tube that extends from the cervix to the vulva. It is a tubular structure, is approximately 10 cm in length, and lies in a superior and posterior direction. The anterior wall is shorter than the posterior wall; the anterior wall is 6.0–7.5 cm and the posterior wall up to 9 cm long. Vaginal lubrication is provided by the Bartholin's glands, which are situated at the 5 and 11 o'clock position near the vaginal opening. The vagina itself does not contain any glands. The epithelium of the vagina is non-keratinised stratified squamous. The overall pH of the vagina is acidic and this is caused in part from the degradation of glycogen which is stored in the vaginal mucosa.

14. A True

    B False

    C True

    D True

    E True

The superior aspect of the vagina is supplied by the uterine artery and the middle to inferior aspect of the vagina supplied by the vaginal artery. The vaginal artery is a branch of the uterine artery. The vagina originates from the paramesonephric duct and urogenital sinus, which are mesodermal.

15. A True

    B False

    C True

    D False

    E False

In outline, the blood and nerve supply to the vagina are:

- Artery: superior – uterine artery
            inferior – vaginal artery
- Vein: vaginal vein
- Lymph: superior – internal iliac nodes
            inferior – superficial inguinal nodes
- Nerve: sympathetic – lumbar splanchnic plexus
            parasympathetic – pelvic splanchnic nerves

16. A True

    B True

    C False

    D False

    E True

The average uterus weighs around 90 g and is approximately 7.5 cm long. This muscular organ has three layers: perimetrium, myometrium and endometrium. The major part of the uterus is the body: the fundus forms the superior portion of the uterus and sits above the openings to the fallopian tubes; and the cervix forms the base of the uterus, which partially projects into the vagina. The uterus sits between the bladder (anteriorly) and the rectum (posteriorly). A covering of peritoneum extends over the anterior and superiors aspects of the uterus. Anteriorly, the peritoneum also covers the bladder, the area between both organs forming the vesicouterine pouch. Posteriorly, the peritoneum reflects down over the body of the uterus, over the posterior fornix of the vagina and then over the front and lateral aspects of the rectum to form the rectouterine pouch, also known as the pouch of Douglas.

17. A True

B False

C False

D True

E True

The female urethra has the same blood supply as the bladder in its upper third, which is the pudendal artery. The lower two-thirds has the same supply as the clitoris and anterior vaginal wall, namely the vaginal artery. The ureter nerves running to the urethra come from the pudendal nerve, with afferents going to the pelvic splanchnic nerves.

18. A True

B False

C False

D True

E True

The typical female, gynaecoid pelvis has an oval-shaped inlet (heart-shaped in males), a large pelvic outlet in comparison to males, a wide pubic arch and a subpubic arch of around 90°; the female obturator foramens are oval. The male pelvis is thicker and generally heavier than the female pelvis. The male pelvic inlet is heart-shaped with a small outlet; the subpubic angle is around 60°. The female pelvis may have male characteristics and be described as an android pelvis. Two further types of pelvis have been described: platypelloid and anthropoid.

19. A True

B False

C True

D True

E True

The adrenal glands are paired retroperitoneal organs, found superiorly to the kidneys. Each is approximately 3–5 cm long and weighs 5 g. The adrenal gland is divided into two different functional regions: the peripheral cortex, which makes up about 80% of the gland and the central medulla. The adrenal cortex has embryological origin from mesoderm and the adrenal medulla is derived from neural crest cells. Each adrenal gland has a corresponding vein. The right adrenal vein drains directly into the inferior vena cava and the left adrenal vein into the renal vein.

20. A False

    B True

    C False

    D True

    E True

The adrenal (or suprarenal glands) sit below the diaphragm and above the kidneys. The left gland has a semi-lunar shape and sits snug proximal to the spleen, pancreas and stomach. The right triangular adrenal gland sits slightly lower than its counterpart, making contact with the liver and inferior vena cava (IVC). The outer cortex of the glands originates from mesoderm and is responsible for corticosteroid and androgen production. The inner medulla derives from neural crest cells and its chromaffin cells secrete catecholamines. The glands receive their blood supply from the suprarenal arteries (superior, middle and inferior). The left suprarenal vein drains into the left renal vein and the right suprarenal vein drains into the IVC.

21. A True

    B True

    C False

    D True

    E True

The inguinal ligament is formed in part from the external oblique aponeurosis. The inguinal canal passes between the deep inguinal ring and the superficial inguinal ring. Contents of the inguinal canal include the round ligament, a branch of the genitofemoral nerve and the ilioinguinal nerve.

22. A True

    B False

    C False

    D True

    E False

The boundaries of the femoral triangle are:

- **Superiorly**: the inguinal ligament
- **Laterally**: sartorius muscle
- **Medially**: adductor longus muscle (medial border)
- **Floor**: adductor longus, pectineus, iliacus and psoas major
- **Contents**: femoral nerve, femoral vein, femoral artery, lymph nodes and fat

23. A True

    B False

C True

D True

E False

The femoral vessels pass beneath the inguinal ligament. The femoral sheath is produced from the transversalis as the vessels pass inferiorly into the thigh region. The femoral sheath has the femoral nerve laterally to it. The node of Cloquet is a lymph node that drains the clitoris and glans penis and it is located in the femoral canal, which is also situated within the femoral sheath.

24. A True

B False

C True

D True

E False

The major muscles of the posterior abdominal wall are the psoas major, iliacus and quadratus lumborum. The psoas major originates at the lateral aspects of all five of the lumbar vertebrae, passing downwards and laterally where it attaches to the lesser trochanter of the femur. It allows for lateral flexion of the trunk ipsilaterally. It is innervated by the ventral rami of the lumbar nerves L1–L3 (or L2–L4). Iliacus originates from the anterior superior iliac spine and also the sacrum. It joins the psoas major (also inserting at the lesser trochanter of the femur) and they form iliopsoas, which is the major flexor of the thigh. Iliacus is innervated by the femoral nerve (L2–L4). Quadratus lumborum originates at the 12th rib and as it descends becomes broader. It inserts into the aponeurosis of the iliolumbar ligament and the iliac crest. It flexes laterally and also extends the spinal column, as well as fixing the 12th rib during inspiration. Psoas minor is only present of 50% of humans, irrespective of gender.

25. B Cisterna chyli

The cisterna chyli is a dilated sac at the base of the thoracic duct, which forms part of the lymphatic drainage of the pelvis and abdomen. The lymph passes to the thoracic duct which, after passing through the aortic hiatus, opens into the junction of the left subclavian vein and internal jugular vein (**Table 1.1**).

26. A Inferior mesenteric artery

The inferior mesenteric artery arises just behind the horizontal part of duodenum (part 4). It lies retroperitoneally and crosses the left common iliac artery, medial to the ureter. The distribution of blood supply extends from the splenic flexure to the upper part of the rectum, which includes the descending colon and sigmoid colon. The distribution of blood supply of the inferior mesenteric artery corresponds to the embryonic hindgut. Branches include the left colic artery and the superior rectal artery.

Table 1.1 Apertures of the diaphragm

	Level	Structure
Caval opening	T8	Inferior vena cava
		Branches phrenic nerve
Oesophageal opening	T10	Oesophagus
Aortic hiatus	T12	Aorta
		Thoracic duct
		Azygos vein

27. D Ovarian artery

Ovarian arteries are a branch of the abdominal aorta. They run retroperitoneally, leaving the abdomen by crossing the common or external iliac arteries in the infundibulopelvic fold. They are medial to the ureter in the upper abdomen and cross obliquely anterior to the ureter in the middle to lower lumbar region, lying lateral to the ureter in the lower abdomen and pelvis. The infundibulopelvic ligament is a fold of the peritoneum, also known as the suspensory ligament of the ovary. It passes laterally from the ovary to the wall of the pelvis. See **Figure 1.3** for the abdominal aorta and its branches.

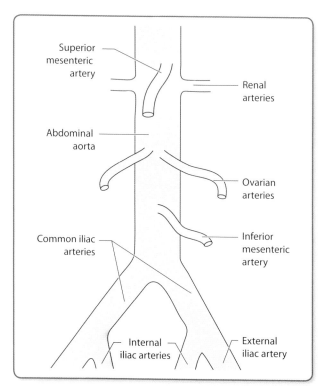

Figure 1.3 Abdominal aorta and its branches.

28. B L1

The ilioinguinal nerve arises from the L1 nerve root along with the larger iliohypogastric nerve. It travels obliquely across the quadratus lumborum and perforates the transversus abdominis near the anterior part of the iliac crest. It travels through part of the inguinal canal, passing through the superficial inguinal ring. It supplies the mons pubis and labium majus.

29. E Stratified squamous epithelium

The cervix has a conical shape with a varied epithelium. The ectocervix is the lower intravaginal portion of the cervix and is lined by non-keratinised stratified squamous epithelium. The endocervix is the cavity of the cervix, linking the external and the internal os. It is lined by mucin-secreting simple columnar epithelium. The border between these two types of epithelium is the squamocolumnar junction, or transformation zone. The transformation zone is the area where metaplasia frequently takes place and it is from here that the cervical smear test is taken .There are certain times when metaplasia is physiological, such as during puberty when the endocervix everts and postmenopause when the transformation moves upwards.

30. B Anthropoid

The basic shapes of the pelvis are as follows:

- **Gynaecoid pelvis (50%):** normal female type, inlet is slightly transverse oval; sacrum is wide with average concavity and inclination; subpubic angle is 90–100°.
- **Anthropoid pelvis (25%):** ape-like; anteroposterior (AP) diameters are long; transverse diameter short; sacrum long and narrow, subpubic angle is narrow.
- **Android pelvis (20%):** male type, inlet is triangular or heart-shaped with anterior narrow apex, subpubic angle is narrow < 90°.
- **Platypelloid pelvis (5%):** flat female type, AP diameter is short, transverse diameter is long, subpubic angle is wide.

31. D Pubococcygeus

The levator ani muscle is formed by the pubococcygeus, iliococcygeus and ischiococcygeus. Although considered in three parts, the muscle forms a continuous sheet, which provides significant support to the pelvic organs.

Pubococcygeus forms the bulk of the levator ani muscle, arising from the back of the pubis and the white line that runs in front of the obturator canal. Its fibres form a U-shaped loop which runs around the urethra, vagina and anorectal junction, with the medial fibres blending with the upper urethra. Intermediate fibres loop around the vagina, closing the lower end on contraction. Lateral fibres run around the anus, inserting into the lateral and posterior walls of the anal canal between the internal and external sphincters.

Iliococcygeus arises from the white line behind the obturator canal and inserts into the lateral margins of the coccyx.

Ischiococcygeus arises from ischial spine and inserts into the coccyx.

32. A Adrenal gland inner medulla

The adrenal glands are retroperitoneal endocrine organs and are situated near the kidneys. They are surrounded by adipose tissue and renal fascia and are usually found at the level of the 12th thoracic vertebra. The outer cortex is mainly responsible for the synthesis of corticosteroid hormones and aldosterone and is derived from coelomic mesothelium. The inner medulla chromaffin cells are the source of catecholamines and these cells are derived from ectodermal neural crest cells.

33. B Anterior division L2–L4

The obturator nerve arises from the anterior division of L2–L4. It emerges from the medial border of the psoas major and descends along the muscle. It runs above and in front of the obturator vessels. It passes through the obturator foramen and enters the thigh through the obturator canal. After passing through the obturator canal, it divides into the anterior and a posterior branch. The anterior branch provides an articular branch to the hip and anterior adductor muscles. The obturator nerve provides sensory innervation to the skin on the medial surface of the thigh. The posterior branch innervates the deeper adductor muscles. The femoral nerve is formed from the posterior division of L2–L4.

34. C Obturator internus

The femoral triangle is an anatomical area in the upper thigh. The borders of the femoral triangle can be remembered by the mnemonic, **SAIL: S**artorius (laterally), **A**dductor longus (medially) and **I**nguinal **L**igament (superiorly). The floor of the femoral triangle is formed by the iliopsoas laterally and pectineus medially. Important structures passing through the femoral triangle include the femoral nerve, artery and vein (**Figure 1.4**).

35. A Inferior gluteal

Gluteus maximus:

- **Origin**: posterior gluteal line of inner upper ilium, posterior surface of lower sacrum, lumbodorsal fascia and sacrotuberous ligament
- **Insertion**: iliotibial band, ischial tuberosity
- **Nerve**: inferior gluteal
- **Artery**: superior and inferior gluteal arteries
- **Action**: extension and external rotation of hip

36. E Transversalis fascia lies directly below the rectus sheath

The rectus sheath is formed from the aponeuroses of three muscles: transversus abdominis, external and internal oblique muscles. Above the arcuate line, the aponeurosis of the external oblique passes in front of the rectus abdominis and

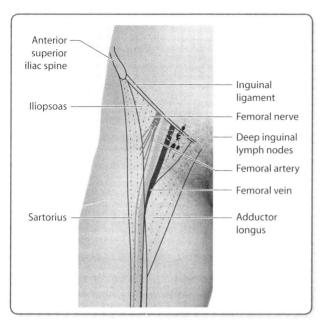

Figure 1.4 Anatomy of the femoral triangle. (Reproduced from Tunstall R and Shah N. Pocket Tutor Surface Anatomy. London: JP Medical Ltd, 2012 and courtesy of Sam Scott-Hunter, London.)

the transversus abdominis passes behind; the aponeurosis of the internal oblique divides into two at the lateral margin, with the anterior lamellae passing in front of the rectus abdominis and the posterior lamellae passing behind. Scarpa's fascia is deep to the Camper's fascia and superficial to external oblique muscle. See **Figure 1.5** for the anatomy of the rectus sheath above and below the arcuate line. The transversalis fascia forms the layer below the rectus sheath.

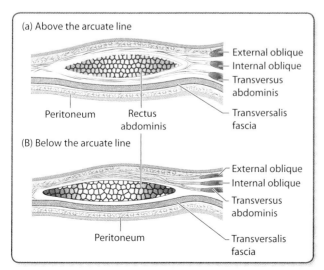

Figure 1.5 Anatomy of the rectus sheath.

37. E Ureters cross close to the bifurcation of the common iliac vessels

The ureters leave the kidney and travel inferiorly and medially along the psoas muscle. They run along the posterior pelvic brim and cross anteriorly to the bifurcation of the common iliac vessels. They continue posteroinferiorly and turn medially at the ischial spines. They then run in the base of the broad ligament where they are crossed by the uterine artery (water under the bridge). The ureter passes the lateral vaginal fornix and enters the bladder.

38. B Inferior vena cava

The right ovarian vein empties directly into the inferior vena cava. The left ovarian vein empties into the left renal vein before reaching the inferior vena cava.

39. E Pudendal nerve

The pudendal nerve provides sensory innervation to the vagina. The pudendal nerve passes into the urogenital region at the end of its course and gives off the perineal branches, which supply the vagina and posterior two-thirds of the vulva. It also branches off the dorsal nerve to the clitoris.

40. A Coeliac trunk

The embryonic foregut is the part which forms the mouth to the duodenum. The coeliac trunk is the first branch of the aorta once it has passed through the diaphragm. The coeliac trunk then branches into three: to the left gastric artery, the splenic artery and the common hepatic arteries.

The superior mesenteric artery provides blood supply to the embryonic midgut and the inferior mesenteric to the embryonic hindgut.

41. D Left ovarian artery

Both ovaries receive their arterial supply from the ovarian arteries, which are direct branches of the abdominal aorta. Venous drainage of the right ovary is supplied by the right ovarian vein, a branch of the inferior vena cava (IVC). The left ovary's venous supply is from the left renal vein, which then drains into the IVC. The differing blood supply of the ovaries, in comparison to the other pelvic viscera, reflects the embryonic origin and subsequent descent of the ovaries from near the kidneys, down into the pelvis.

42. B Is a branch of the abdominal aorta

The ovarian arteries both arise from the abdominal aorta. The paired arteries, which sit below the renal arteries and above the inferior mesenteric artery, descend along the posterior abdominal wall. These arteries cross the external iliac vessels at the level of the pelvic brim. Each artery supplies its respective ovary and fallopian tube, anastomosing with the uterine arteries. Arterial and venous supply to the ovaries follow a similar course, however, the right ovary receives its venous supply from the right ovarian vein, which reaches the inferior vena cava and the left ovary is supplied by the left renal vein.

43. B Median sacral

The aorta enters the abdomen through the aortic hiatus of the diaphragm at the level of T12. At the level of L4 the abdominal aorta bifurcates into the common iliac vessels, which in turn divide to form the external and iliac vessels. The abdominal aorta has three terminal branches which are: right and left common iliac arteries and the median sacral artery. There are another four paired branches which are: phrenic, suprarenal, renal and gonadal arteries.

44. C Ischiocavernosus

The perineal body (or central tendon of the perineum) is a midline structure formed of fibromuscular tissue found between the vagina and the anus in females. The external anal sphincter, transverse perineal muscles, bulbocavernosus muscle and the levator ani muscles all insert into the perineal body. The ischiocavernosus muscle is a muscle of the superficial pouch of the perineum. Lying between the perineal membrane and the subcutaneous tissue, it arises from the inferior ischial ramus and compresses the crus clitoris, hence promoting clitoral erection. See **Figure 1.6** for the anatomy of the perineum.

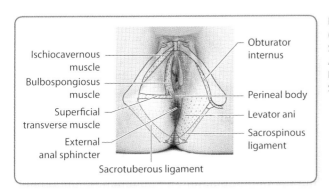

Ischiocavernous muscle
Bulbospongiosus muscle
Superficial transverse muscle
External anal sphincter
Sacrotuberous ligament
Obturator internus
Perineal body
Levator ani
Sacrospinous ligament

Figure 1.6 Perineal body. (Reproduced from Tunstall R and Shah N. Pocket Tutor Surface Anatomy. London: JP Medical Ltd, 2012 and courtesy of Sam Scott-Hunter, London.)

45. E Uterine artery, anterior division of the internal iliac

The uterine artery is a branch of the anterior division of internal iliac artery (the main artery to supply the pelvic viscera). Ovarian arterial supply comes from the ovary arteries which are direct branches of the abdominal arteries. Equivalent to the female ovarian arteries is the testicular artery, which is a branch of the abdominal aorta and supplies the testes. The internal pudendal artery, which supplies the perineum, is a branch of the anterior division of the internal iliac artery.

46. A Fourth lumbar vertebrae

The bony pelvis consists of the innominate bone, which is formed from the ilium, ischium and the pubis, together with the sacrum and the fifth lumbar vertebrae. The sacrum is actually formed from the five sacral vertebrae. The sacrum articulates with the fifth lumbar vertebrae. **Figure 1.7** shows the structure of the bony pelvis.

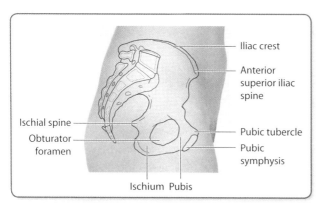

Iliac crest

Anterior superior iliac spine

Ischial spine

Obturator foramen

Pubic tubercle

Pubic symphysis

Ischium Pubis

Figure 1.7 Bony pelvis. (Reproduced from Tunstall R and Shah N. Pocket Tutor Surface Anatomy. London: JP Medical Ltd, 2012 and courtesy of Sam Scott-Hunter, London.)

47. E The superficial inguinal ring transmits the round ligament

The deep inguinal ring is situated at the midpoint of the inguinal ligament. It can be located by finding the midpoint between the anterior superior iliac spine and the pubic tubercle. The superficial inguinal ring lies just above, and lateral to the pubic tubercle. The deep and superficial rings mark the entrance (deep ring) and exit (superficial ring) to the inguinal canal.

The canal's boundaries are:

- **Anterior wall**: external oblique aponeurosis, with lateral reinforcement from the internal oblique
- **Posterior wall**: transversalis fascia, with the conjoint tendon (internal oblique and transversus abdominis) providing medially
- **Superiorly**: internal oblique
- **Inferiorly**: inguinal ligament

Running through the canal is the round ligament in females and the spermatic cord in males. The ilioinguinal nerve passes through the superficial inguinal ring only, having travelled down the lateral abdominal wall between the internal and external oblique muscles. See **Figure 1.8** for the anatomy of the inguinal canal.

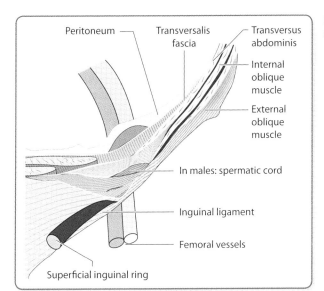

Figure 1.8 Anatomy of inguinal canal.

Peritoneum — Transversalis fascia — Transversus abdominis — Internal oblique muscle — External oblique muscle — In males: spermatic cord — Inguinal ligament — Femoral vessels — Superficial inguinal ring

48. C Ilioinguinal nerve

Only the ilioinguinal nerve passes through the superficial inguinal ring; it is not carried through the deep inguinal ring, having travelled down the lateral abdominal wall between the internal and external oblique muscles.

Chapter 2

Biochemistry

Questions: MCQs

Answer each stem 'True' or 'False'.

1. **With regard to glycolysis:**
    A   Net yield per glucose is one NADH molecule and one ATP molecule
    B   Takes place in the cytoplasm of the cell
    C   Glucokinase is an isoenzyme of hexokinase
    D   Is controlled by allosteric inhibition
    E   Only operates in aerobic conditions

2. **Glycogen:**
    A   Is a branched polymer of glucose
    B   Has its main stores in muscle
    C   Is broken down by glucose-6-phosphatase
    D   Its synthesis (i.e. glycogen synthase) is inhibited by adrenaline
    E   Levels in the blood stream are highest in the evening

3. **Tricarboxylic acid cycle:**
    A   Produces four NADH molecules per turn
    B   Uses acetyl coenzyme A as its substrate
    C   Takes place in the matrix of mitochondria
    D   Is regulated by substrate availability
    E   Each H_2 molecule produces three molecules of ATP

4. **Fat metabolism:**
    A   Fat can be metabolised anaerobically
    B   Fat can be used by the brain as a source of fuel
    C   Oxidation of fatty acids takes place in the mitochondria
    D   Beta-oxidation of fatty acids is controlled by supply of substrate
    E   The liver can synthesise fatty acids to ketone bodies

5. **Arachidonic acid:**
    A   Is a second messenger
    B   Is an amino acid
    C   Is a precursor of thromboxane
    D   Is inhibited by aspirin
    E   Is converted to prostaglandins

6. **Concerning ribonucleic acid (RNA):**
    A   Contains deoxyribose
    B   Uracil pairs with thymine
    C   Each nucleotide contains a phosphate group
    D   Is always single-stranded
    E   Is made by RNA polymerases

7. **The following are tumour suppressors:**
    A   *pRb*
    B   *p53*
    C   *BRCA1*
    D   Ras
    E   Myc

8. **Phenylketonuria:**
    A   Is an autosomal dominant condition
    B   Is caused by a defect in the metabolism of tyrosine
    C   Is detected using the Kleihauer–Betke test in newborns
    D   Untreated, results in severe intellectual impairment
    E   Can be managed using a protein-rich diet

9. **Regarding steroidogenesis:**
    A   Progesterone is the precursor of pregnenolone
    B   Cholesterol is the precursor of all other steroids
    C   Corticosterone is converted to aldosterone
    D   Pregnenolone is formed in cellular mitochondria
    E   Testosterone is a precursor of oestradiol

10. **Prostaglandins:**
    A   Are hydrophilic
    B   Are synthesised from arachidonic acid
    C   Are antagonised by non-steroidal anti-inflammatory drugs
    D   Consist of 18 carbon atoms
    E   Bind to G protein-coupled receptors

Questions: SBAs

For each question, select the single best answer from the five options listed.

11. Which condition is caused by the failure to mineralise newly formed osteoid?

   A Osteomalacia
   B Osteopaenia
   C Osteopetrosis
   D Osteoporosis
   E Paget's disease of bone

12. A 50-year-old woman presents to her general practitioner complaining of fatigue and upper abdominal pain, 6 weeks after sustaining a distal radial fracture. Her blood tests indicate hypercalcaemia and hypophosphataemia.

   What is the most likely diagnosis?

   A Bone metastases
   B Increased parathyroid hormone-related protein production
   C Primary hyperparathyroidism
   D Sarcoidosis
   E Secondary hyperparathyroidism

13. Which enzyme is involved in the rate-limiting step of the glycolysis pathway?

   A Glucokinase
   B Glucose 6-phosphate
   C Hexokinase
   D Phosphofructokinase
   E Phosphoglucose isomerase

14. What is the overall product of the glycolysis pathway?

   A Glucose
   B Pyruvate
   C 1 NADH + 1 ATP
   D 2 NADH + 2 ATP
   E 4 NADH + 4 ATP

15. A 28-year-old primiparous woman attends her booking appointment at 10 weeks' gestation. She is keen to maintain a healthy diet during her pregnancy and asks her midwife to explain the difference between essential and non-essential amino acids.

   Which of the following is a non-essential amino acid?

   A Arginine
   B Leucine
   C Methionine

    D Tryptophan
    E Tyrosine

16. A 24-year-old woman is admitted via the emergency department with persistent hyperemesis of pregnancy. She is now feeling very unwell and appears dehydrated. Her blood pressure is 110/60 mmHg, heart rate 100 beats per minute, SpO_2 98% on room air and a respiratory rate of 20 breaths per minute.

    Which is the most likely acid-base disorder in this patient?

    A Metabolic acidosis
    B Metabolic alkalosis
    C Mixed metabolic alkalosis and respiratory acidosis
    D Respiratory acidosis
    E Respiratory alkalosis

17. Following the birth of their second child with severe developmental delay, a couple is seen by a clinical geneticist. Genotyping suggests a rare autosomal recessive condition caused by a defect in the normal functioning of the citric acid cycle.

    Which of the following is not an intermediate of the citric acid cycle?

    A Alpha-ketoglutarate
    B Acetyl coenzyme A
    C Citrate
    D Oxaloacetate
    E Succinyl coenzyme A

18. Which of the following describes the appearance of sister chromatids during the anaphase of mitosis?

    A Alignment along the cell's horizontal plane
    B Alignment along the cell's vertical plane
    C Alignment at one pole
    D Separation to diagonal poles
    E Separation to opposite poles

19. A 12-year-old boy has gross developmental delay of unknown cause. On physical examination, he is noted to have macro-orchidism, prominent ears and a large forehead. He is seen by a clinical geneticist who suspects Fragile X syndrome and wishes to perform genotyping.

    Which of the following laboratory techniques is used to detect DNA sequences?

    A Eastern blotting
    B Northern blotting
    C Northwestern blotting
    D Southern blotting
    E Western blotting

20. A 58-year-old woman has recently been diagnosed with type 2 diabetes mellitus. As part of her routine care, her general practitioner checks and her fasting cholesterol levels. She is found to have a mildly raised total cholesterol level with a raised serum low-density lipoprotein level.

   Which of the following describes the function of low-density lipoproteins?

   A   Transport of cholesterol from the body's tissues to the liver
   B   Transport of cholesterol from the liver to tissues around the body
   C   Transport of chylomicrons from the liver to elsewhere in the body
   D   Transport of triglycerides from the intestine to other tissues for storage
   E   Transport of triglycerides from the liver to elsewhere in the body for oxidation

21. An infant is born at term by normal vaginal delivery. When the baby is 18 days old, he is brought to the emergency department by his parents. He is vomiting, severely dehydrated and appears to be underweight. The paediatricians diagnose a salt-wasting crisis and are concerned that he has a form of congenital adrenal hyperplasia.

   What hormone deficiency is characteristic of this disorder?

   A   Cholesterol
   B   Cortisol
   C   Dihydrotestosterone
   D   Oestradiol
   E   Testosterone

Answers

1. A False

    B True

    C True

    D True

    E False

    The net yield of the glycolytic pathway (**Figure 2.1**) per molecule of glucose is 2 molecules of nicotinamide adenine dinucleotide (NADH) and 2 molecules of adenosine triphosphate (ATP). The first step of glycolysis involves phosphorylation of glucose to glucose 6-phosphate by hexokinase. An isoenzyme of hexokinase, glucokinase is used in the liver, but has a lower affinity

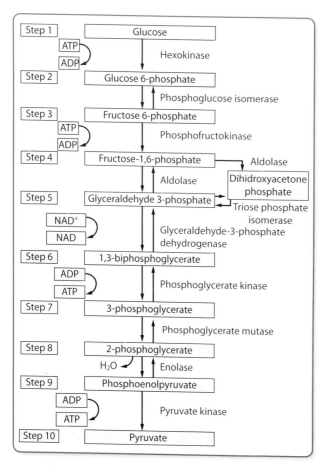

Figure 2.1 The glycolysis pathway.

for glucose. This reflects the liver's role in maintaining blood sugar levels. In allosteric inhibition, the shape of the enzyme is altered by the substrate binding to a site separate from the usual binding site. This leads to a reduction in the usual substrate binding and therefore the activity of the enzyme. The ATP allosterically inhibits phosphofructokinase.

2. A True

    B False

    C False

    D True

    E False

Glucose is stored in the body in the form of glycogen. It is stored in the liver and to a lesser degree, in muscles. Glycogen stores can be mobilised if glucose levels in the bloodstream are low and the main enzyme of glycogen breakdown is glycogen phosphorylase. Levels of glycogen do fluctuate, however, there is no diurnal pattern and levels reflect oral intake.

3. A False

    B True

    C True

    D True

    E True

The tricarboxylic acid (TCA) cycle takes place in the mitochondria of eukaryotic cells. One of the regulating factors is the availability of substrate.

Each turn of the TCA cycle produces:

- 3 NADH + 1 $FADH_2$
- 1 Guanosine-triphosphate (GTP)
- 2 CO_2

where NADH is nicotinamide adenine dinucleotide and $FADH_2$ is flavin adenine dinucleotide.

The GTP can be converted to adenosine triphosphate (ATP). The NADH and $FADH_2$ donate their electrons to the electron transport chain, which produces ATP.

Acetyl coenzyme A is produced from the metabolism of carbohydrates, proteins and fats and is converted into energy through the tricarboxylic acid cycle. Four pairs of hydrogen atoms are released per turn of the cycle, which then feed into the electron transport chain. Each hydrogen pair then reduces one atom of oxygen and by doing so releases three molecules of ATP. See **Figure 2.2** for the TCA cycle (or Krebs cycle).

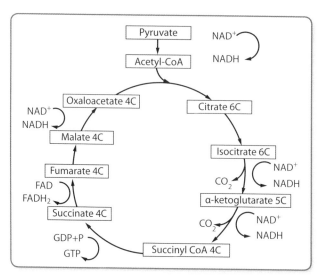

Figure 2.2 Krebs cycle.

4. A False

    B False

    C True

    D True

    E True

Metabolism of fats can only occur in the presence of oxygen and never occurs under anaerobic conditions. The brain has an absolute requirement for glucose as a fuel and, in the presence of starvation, ketone bodies may provide 75% of the energy supply. Oxidation of fatty acids occurs in the mitochondria. Fatty acids freely diffuse over the cell membrane and use the enzyme carnitine palmitoyltransferase to access the mitochondria. The β-oxidation of fatty acids produces acetyl coenzyme A, which may then be used as a substrate in the tricarboxylic acid cycle. Synthesis of ketone bodies may occur in the liver in the presence of starvation. During starvation, the acetyl coenzyme A produced by the oxidation of fatty acids may be channelled into ketogenesis, rather than into the tricarboxylic acid cycle.

5. A True

    B False

    C True

    D False

    E True

Arachidonic acid is a fatty acid attached to cellular membrane phospholipids by esterification. Freed from the phospholipids by the action of phospholipase A2, arachidonic acid has a series of roles. It is the precursor of the eicosanoids, i.e. prostaglandins, procyclins, and the thromboxanes, which have a wide variety of biological roles. The conversion of arachidonic acid to prostaglandin H_2 (the precursor of the eicosanoids) requires the action of the cyclooxygenase (COX) enzymes, COX-1 and COX-2. The formation of the eicosanoids, not arachidonic acid itself, is inhibited by the action of COX-inhibitors such as ibuprofen and aspirin. Arachidonic acid also acts a second messenger, whereby it transmits a signal from a cellular receptor, in response to stimulation by first messengers such as histamine.

6. A False

    B False

    C True

    D False

    E True

Ribonucleic acid (RNA), alongside its counterpart deoxyribonucleic acid (DNA), forms the basis of the genetic code of all living things. Each RNA nucleotide consists of a five carbon ribose sugar ring, a phosphate group linked to the ribose and a base. The bases found in RNA are uracil (U), cytosine (C), adenine (A) and guanine (G); this differs from DNA where instead of uracil there is thymine. Each of the bases links with its appropriate base pair from another nucleotide of RNA in order to form complementary strands of RNA.

Linked by hydrogen bonds uracil pairs with adenine and guanine pairs with cytosine. Codons are formed from each three adjacent RNA nucleotides in a chain of RNA and are described according to the sequence of each molecule's base, e.g. CCA refers to three RNA nucleotides adjacent to each other with the bases cytosine, followed by cytosine, followed by adenine. RNA is typically single-stranded, allowing it to form complex structures; however, it may be double-stranded (ds), e.g. rotavirus is one of a number of dsRNA viruses. The formation of RNA is catalysed by RNA polymerase, which links together RNA nucleotides using a DNA template in a process called transcription.

7. A True

    B True

    C True

    D False

    E False

During the cell cycle a series of checkpoints occur aiming to assess for imperfections within the cell, such as DNA damage. Should cellular imperfections be detected and are not fixable the cell typically will undergo apoptosis. Typically checkpoints for errors occur at critical periods in the cell cycle, e.g. a DNA damage check just prior to the 'S' phase, where DNA is replicated, a further DNA damage check just prior to mitosis, with a check to confirm spindle attachment occurring during mitosis itself. A series of proteins are used to perform these checks and facilitate either the ongoing cell cycle or apoptosis. *p53* is such a protein and in addition to checking for DNA damage can either hold a cell in an arrested state to allow for DNA repair, or in irreparable cases induce apoptosis. Genetic mutations involving both *p53* alleles are associated with the development of cancer. *BRCA1* is a DNA repair protein that repairs breaks in DNA's double strands. *pRb*, the retinoblastoma protein, is another tumour suppressor protein that inhibits cells from entering the 'S' phase. Ras proteins are involved in regulation of cell signalling and are considered a proto-oncoprotein. Myc is a transcription factor which facilitates the progression of the cell cycle. Over expression of both Ras and Myc is associated with cancer development.

8. A False

    B True

    C False

    D True

    E False

Phenylketonuria is a congenital autosomal recessive disorder, associated with a mutation of a gene found on chromosome 12. It results in the inability to metabolise the essential amino acid phenylalanine into tyrosine, owing to a deficiency of the enzyme phenylalanine hydroxylase. Elevated levels of phenylalanine lead to an accumulation of its by-products, such as phenylacetate and phenylpyruvate, with devastating consequences. Further metabolic disturbance is caused by the deficiency in tyrosine. Phenylketonuria is associated with severe intellectual impairment if untreated, and therefore all newborns in the UK are screened for the condition in the first week of life.

The Guthrie test involves taking a spot of blood, which is placed on a paper disc. The disc is then placed with bacteria, which overgrows in the presence of the high levels of phenylalanine. Treatment strategies for individuals with phenylketonuria include a lifelong diet of foods low in phenylalanine and pharmaceuticals, which aim to reduce phenylalanine.

9. A False

    B True

    C True

    D True

    E True

Steroids are organic compounds, which all consist of a common core of 20 carbon atoms arranged into four rings with varying side-chains. Three of these carbon rings are cyclohexanes and contain six carbon atoms, whereas the remaining ring consists of five carbon atoms and is cyclopentane.

Steroidogenesis is the synthesis of steroids from the common precursor cholesterol into other forms of steroids. The conversion of cholesterol, which itself contains 27 carbon atoms, to other steroids is catalysed by a series of enzymes. The first product of steroidogenesis is pregnenolone, which is produced in cellular mitochondria via the action of cytochrome P450, which cleaves a side-chain from cholesterol. This first product can then be converted into progesterone with further conversion to the mineralocorticoids, i.e. aldosterone, or into 17α-hydroxyprogestrone pregenolone with subsequent pathways facilitating either the production of the glucocorticoids, or the androgens and oestrogens. Testosterone is formed from androstenedione and may be converted to either dihydrotestosterone or oestradiol (E2).

10. A False

    B True

    C True

    D False

    E True

Prostaglandins are a form of eicosanoid and are derived from fatty acids, hence the hydrophobic nature. Produced by most nucleated cells, they are synthesised predominantly from the oxidation of arachidonic acid by the action of cyclooxygenases (COXs), i.e. COX-1 and COX-2. All prostaglandins consist of 20 carbon atoms, which include a five carbon ring. Prostaglandins have a wide range of functions, including vasoconstriction and dilation, bronchoconstriction and dilation, uterine contraction, platelet inhibition and aggregation, as well as pyogenic properties.

NSAIDs such as ibuprofen are COX inhibitors and therefore antagonise the formation of prostaglandins. There are a variety of prostaglandin receptors corresponding to different prostaglandins found on many cell types, all of which are G protein-coupled receptors (GPCRs). Major prostaglandins include prostaglandin E2 (PGE2), which is also the constituent of dinoprostone-based induction agents; prostaglandin I2 (PGI2 or prostacyclin), whose major functions include inhibition of platelet aggregation; and prostaglandin F2 alpha (PGFα), which is involved in uterine contraction amongst other properties.

11. A Osteomalacia

Pregnancy is associated with increased levels of parathyroid hormone, calcitriol and calcium. Higher concentrations of calcium are absorbed from the gut. Calcium and phosphate are transferred to fetal circulation by active transport. See **Table 2.1** for conditions associated with abnormalities of bone.

12. C Primary hyperparathyroidism

Parathyroid hormone (PTH) leads to an increase in blood calcium and a reduction in phosphate. Primary hyperparathyroidism causes hypercalcaemia by increased secretion of parathyroid hormone, in 80% of cases from an adenoma of the parathyroid gland. Other causes include hyperplasia or multiple adenomas. It is the third most common endocrine condition, with a population frequency

Table 2.1 Disorders of the bone and their typical serum biochemistry

Condition	Calcium	Phosphate	Alkaline phosphatase	Parathyroid hormone	Comment
Osteoporosis	Normal	Normal	Normal	Normal	Decreased bone mass
Osteopetrosis	Normal	Normal	Normal	Normal	Marble bone disease
Osteomalacia Rickets	Reduced	Reduced	Increased	Increased	Soft bones
Osteitis fibrosa cystica	Increased	Reduced	Increased	Increased	Brown tumour
Paget's disease of bone	Normal	Normal	Increased	Normal	Abnormal architecture of bone

of 1:500–1:1000. Symptoms are usually those of hypercalcaemia. Blood tests usually show increased calcium and PTH and low phosphate. Treatment involves surgical removal of the adenoma. Secondary hyperparathyroidism consists of high PTH, but low calcium. Bone metastases would lead to hypercalcaemia, but not hypophosphataemia.

13. D Phosphofructokinase

Glycolysis is the metabolic process that occurs within all aerobic and anaerobic cells and produces two molecules of pyruvate from one molecule of glucose. This process of glucose oxidation also generates a gain of two molecules of ATP and two molecules of NADH. Phosphofructokinase is the enzyme that converts fructose 6-phosphate to fructose 1,6-biphosphate. This irreversible step is considered the rate-limiting step of glycolysis. In aerobic conditions the generated pyruvate then enters the tricarboxylic acid cycle (**Figure 2.2**) within the mitochondria and subsequently generates ATP in a process of oxidative metabolism.

14. B Pyruvate

Glycolysis is the metabolic pathway that converts glucose into pyruvate and takes place in the cytoplasm of the cell. Glycolysis forms a sequence of 10 reactions, involving intermediary compounds at each step, which can provide entry points into the pathway. This metabolic pathway is common to both aerobic and anaerobic forms of respiration. In aerobic respiration, pyruvate then enters the tricarboxylic acid cycle, which takes place within the mitochondria. In anaerobic conditions, the pyruvate obtained from glycolysis is reduced to lactate via the action of lactate dehydrogenase.

15. E Tyrosine

Essential amino acids are those that cannot be synthesised directly and therefore must be obtained through dietary intake. Non-essential amino acids are those that can be synthesised without the need for dietary supplementation (**Table 2.2**).

Table 2.2 Essential and non-essential amino acids			
Essential amino acids		**Non-essential amino acids**	
Arginine	Methionine	Alanine	Glutamic acid
Histidine	Phenylalanine	Aspartic acid	Glycine
Isoleucine	Threonine	Asparagine	Proline
Leucine	Tryptophan	Cysteine	Serine
Lysine	Valine	Glutamine	Tyrosine

16. B Metabolic alkalosis

This patient has developed a metabolic alkalosis secondary to persistent vomiting and loss of hydrochloric acid from the stomach contents. Compensation occurs in the lungs by trying to retain carbon dioxide through hypoventilation. Carbon dioxide is then used for the formation of carbonic acid, reducing pH. Peripheral chemoreceptors are sensitive to pH and are stimulated by the decrease in H^+ concentration. The increase in pCO_2 leads to activation of central chemoreceptors, which are sensitive to partial pressure of carbon dioxide in the blood. This then leads to a rise in respiration rate.

17. B Acetyl coenzyme A

Acetyl coenzyme A (acetyl-CoA) is not an intermediate of the citric acid cycle [also known as the tricarboxylic acid cycle (TCA cycle) or the Krebs cycle]. The final product of glycolysis, pyruvate, is converted to acetyl-CoA via a process of pyruvate decarboxylation by the action of pyruvate dehydrogenase. Acetyl-CoA then enters the citric acid cycle. All of the other possible answers given are actually different intermediates produced by the citric acid cycle (**Figure 2.2**).

18. E Separation of sister chromatids to opposite poles

Mitosis describes the process by which cells are able to duplicate and then separate their chromosomes in order to produce identical copies of the original cell. This form of cell replication only occurs in eukaryotic cells. Erroneously thought of as a time of cellular quiescence the cell spends most of its time in 'interphase' a period divided into two growth periods G1 and G2, which are separated by the 'S' phase during which the cell experiences Swanson DNA duplication in preparation for mitosis.

Mitosis truly commences as prophase during which there is condensation of chromatin into chromosomes. This stage is followed by metaphase where sister chromatids are produced by DNA replication during the 'S' phase of interphase and then align at the cell's equatorial plane, also known as the metaphase plane. Anaphase describes subsequent separation of the sister chromatids to opposite poles of the cell. Following this separation there is breakdown of the parent cell's nuclear membrane, which then reforms around each separate set of chromosomes. Cytokinesis describes the separation of the cytoplasm and marks the final step in the formation of the daughter cells.

19. D Southern blotting

The Southern blot is a technique used to identify specific sequences of DNA amongst material containing many other DNA sequences. Developed by the microbiologist Edward Southern in the 1970s, it uses electrophoresis techniques to identify target DNA sequences. Techniques that use principles identified by Southern have been given similar nomenclature in tribute to his original methods.

Northern blotting is used to identify specific RNA sequences in RNA-rich matter. Western blotting identifies specific proteins in samples using both gel electrophoresis and also immunoblotting, whereby antibodies mark the 'target' protein of interest. Eastern blotting can be considered as an extension of the Western blotting technique and detects protein post-translational modifications. Northwestern blotting is a fictional technique.

20. B Transport of cholesterol from the liver to tissues around the body

Lipoproteins form the basis of the transport of fats around the body. All lipoproteins consist of both fats and proteins in a complex consisting of a hydrophilic outer surface and a hydrophobic core. Low-density lipoproteins (LDLs) predominantly consist of cholesterol and cholesterol esters and they transport cholesterol from the liver to tissues around the body whose cells are expressing the LDL receptor. LDLs are often referred to as 'the bad cholesterol' due to their association with atheromatous change (blood vessels may also express LDL receptors).

High-density lipoproteins (HDLs) are the smallest of the lipoproteins and are protein and cholesterol-rich. HDLs 'collect' cholesterol from cells which are then sequestered into its hydrophobic core and are carried to the liver (and steroid producing organs such as the ovaries), where their cholesterol is released through the action of HDL receptors. Very low-density lipoproteins (VLDLs) are produced in the liver and comprise of predominantly triglycerides and cholesterol; in the blood these VLDLs are converted to LDLs. Chylomicrons are responsible for transporting dietary fats, predominantly in the form of triglycerides from the small intestine to tissues, such as the liver and skeletal muscle for usage.

21. B Cortisol

Congenital adrenal hyperplasia (CAH) is used to describe a series of autosomal recessive conditions characterised by a deficiency in cortisol production (and in some forms, aldosterone). Altered steroidogenesis results primarily in both cortisol deficiency and excess of its steroid precursors such as testosterone. In males, CAH may not be detected until after the first weeks of birth, when they may present with symptoms of a salt-wasting crisis such as severe vomiting, dehydration and appear to be shocked. This presentation is due to aldosterone and cortisol deficiency leading to biochemical imbalances such hyperkalaemia, and hyponatraemia.

In females CAH, in its most common form, is typically diagnosed at the birth of a genetically female infant with ambiguous genitalia caused by fetal exposure to excessive levels of androgens in utero. The most common form of CAH is caused by a deficiency in 21-hydroxylase, an enzyme involved in the conversion of progesterone and 17α-hydroxyprogesterone to the precursors of cortisol. Other forms of CAH include 11β-hydroxylase deficient CAH, which results in cortisol deficiency alongside excessive aldosterone, leading to hypertension; and 17-hydroxylase deficient CAH, which alongside excessive aldosterone is also associated with deficiency in the oestrogens leading to oligomenorrhoea and infertility.

Speiser PW, Perrin C, White MD. Congenital Adrenal Hyperplasia. N Engl J Med 2003; 349:776-788

Chapter 3

Embryology

Questions: MCQs

Answer each stem 'True' or 'False'.

1. **With regard to early embryonic development:**
    A The trilaminar disc forms during the second week of development
    B The notochord forms around 18 days
    C The primitive streak is formed by day 15
    D The anterior neuropore closes by day 24
    E Upper limb buds appear around day 32

2. **With regard to pharyngeal arches:**
    A 1st arch: eustachian tube and middle ear
    B 2nd arch: muscles of facial expression, served by 7th cranial nerve
    C 3rd arch: common carotid artery
    D 4th arch: glossopharyngeal nerve (IX cranial nerve)
    E 5th arch: laryngeal cartilages

3. **Functions of the metanephros include:**
    A Production of urine
    B Electrolyte balance of the fetus
    C Production of amniotic fluid
    D Begin functioning during the 8th week
    E Production of fetal haemoglobin

4. **With regard to development of the alimentary system:**
    A Embryonic foregut is supplied by the coeliac artery
    B Midgut includes the second part of the duodenum
    C Hindgut incorporates the appendix
    D Meckel's diverticulum is a remnant of the vitelline duct
    E Gut is derived from endoderm

5. **With regard to amniotic fluid:**
    A Prior to keratinisation, it is formed from fluid passing across fetal skin
    B Consists mainly of water during the first trimester
    C Fetal renal function begins during the 6th week
    D Compared with blood, amniotic fluid is slightly alkalotic
    E Albumin is the main protein

Questions: SBAs

For each question, select the single most appropriate answer from the five options listed.

6.   Which one of the following constitutes the parameters for a normal sperm count?

	Volume (mL)	Motility (% progressive)	Count (million/mL)	Morphology (% normal forms)
A	2.0–5.0	20	20	<10
B	1.5–5.0	90	20	<20
C	1.5–5.0	40	15	<5
D	1.0–3.0	80	60	<10
E	1.0–3.0	90	20	<5

7.   Which of the following best describes the process of compaction?

   A   It leads to the formation of the trophoblast
   B   It leads to the formation of the cytotrophoblast
   C   It is a reaction of the chromosomes during meiosis
   D   It leads to the formation of the morula after the 16 cell stage
   E   It refers to the reaction of the sperm head on penetration of the ovum

8.   Which of the following is correct regarding germ cell layers?

   A   Endoderm: endocrine glands
   B   Endoderm: nervous system
   C   Ectoderm: most proximal layer
   D   Mesoderm: lung cells
   E   Mesoderm: skin epidermis

9.   The cells of which structure form the chorionic villi?

   A   Neural crest
   B   Endoderm
   C   Primitive streak
   D   Hypoblast
   E   Extraembryonic mesoderm

10. Which of the following has the correct association regarding development of urogenital system?

   A   Genital fold – clitoris
   B   Genital tubercle – labia minora
   C   Ureteric bud – urinary bladder
   D   Mesonephric ducts – vagina
   E   Metanephros – kidney

11. Which of the following statements best describes the development of the cardiac system?

    A   Fetal circulation includes two umbilical veins
    B   The ligamentum venosum is a remnant of the umbilical vein
    C   The heart is developed from endodermal cells
    D   The cardinal vein runs into the sinus venosus
    E   Cardiac pulsations are visible from the 34th day after conception

12. Which of the following is not a derivative of the vitelline vein?

    A   Lower inferior vena cava
    B   Inferior mesenteric vein
    C   Superior mesenteric vein
    D   Portal vein
    E   Hepatic vein

13. Which of the following statements best describes the development of the urogenital system?

    A   Sex cords are developed from coelomic epithelium
    B   Sex differentiation is present 35 days after fertilisation
    C   Myometrial walls are present in the fetal uterus by the 5th month
    D   Reproductive organs are developed from paraxial mesoderm
    E   In female sex organ development, the upper part of the gubernaculum becomes the round ligament

Answers

1. A False

    B True

    C True

    D False

    E False

    The trilaminar disc consists of the three germ cell layers: ectoderm, endoderm and mesoderm, and is formed at the region of the primitive streak. This forms during the 3rd week of development. There is a higher rate of growth of the ectoderm layer at each end of the disc, which changes the shape of the disc into a more oval nature.

    The process of neurulation refers to the development of the nervous system and involves the rounding of the neural plate with development of the cranial and caudal ends. The primitive streak is a depression in the caudal end of the disc and is usually evident by the end of the second week of development. The notochord provides the longitudinal axis for the embryo and becomes the vertebral column. The anterior neuropore (cranial) closes at day 24 and the posterior neuropore (caudal) closes at day 25.

2. A True

    B True

    C True

    D False

    E False

    Pharyngeal arches are responsible for forming the lower part of the face and the neck, and they develop from mesoderm. There are six pharyngeal arches, but the fifth arch regresses. (**Table 3.1**)

3. A True

    B False

    C True

    D False

    E False

    The urogenital system develops from mesoderm. The renal system develops from the nephrogenic cord. There are three parts to the embryonic urinary system that appear at different points in development. They all have a role in excretion and all develop at week 4.

    - **Pronephros**: limited function
    - **Mesonephros**: functions from week 6–10
    - **Metanephros**: functions at week 12

Pharyngeal arch	Muscle	Skeletal	Nerve	Artery
Table 3.1 Pharyngeal arches				
1st	Muscles mastication Anterior belly of digastric	Maxilla Mandible	Trigeminal nerve (CN V)	External carotid
2nd	Facial expression	Stapes Hyoid	Facial nerve (CN VII)	Stapedial artery
3rd	Stylopharyngeus	Inferior parathyroids Hyoid	Glossopharyngeal nerve (CN IX)	Common carotid
4th	Cricothyroid	Thyroid cartilage	Vagus nerve (CN X)	Subclavian artery Aortic arch
6th	Intrinsic muscle of larynx	Laryngeal cartilage	Vagus nerve (CN X)	Pulmonary artery

CN, cranial nerve

The mesonephric bud develops during the 5th week from the ureteric bud. It has an excretory role for approximately 4 weeks; however, it regresses by week 10. The permanent kidney develops from the metanephros and by the end of week 12, urine is produced.

4. A False

 B False

 C False

 D True

 E True

The embryonic alimentary system is broadly divided into the foregut, midgut and hindgut. Each part has a separate blood supply. **Table 3.2** shows the division of the alimentary system.

5. A True

 B True

 C False

 D False

 E True

Amniotic fluid volumes are approximately 50 mL at 12 weeks, and increases to about one litre towards the end of pregnancy. Fetal skin cells undergo keratinisation at about 25 weeks of pregnancy and prior to this, fluid arises by transfer across the skin. Amniotic fluid is produced by fetal excretion in urine, with contribution from lung secretions and amniotic membrane secretions. During the first trimester, the amniotic

Table 3.2 Embryological origins of the digestive system

	Section of alimentary system	Organs involved	Blood supply
Foregut	Oesophagus to D2	Oesophagus Stomach First two parts of duodenum	Coeliac trunk
Midgut	D3 to first 2/3 of transverse colon	Jejunum Ileum Caecum Appendix First 2/3 of transverse colon	Superior mesenteric
Hindgut	Last 1/3 of transverse colon to top of anal canal	Last 1/3 of transverse colon Rectum	Inferior mesenteric

fluid is mainly composed of water, with some electrolytes. From the second trimester composition of the fluid changes with addition of lipids, carbohydrates and proteins. Amniotic fluid is more acidic than the maternal blood.

6. **C**

Volume (mL)	Motility (% progressive)	Count (million/mL)	Morphology (% normal forms)
1.5–5.0	40	15	< 5

On average an ejaculate will have a volume of 2–5 mL seminal fluid. The average sperm count in this fluid is 60×10^6/mL and a low sperm count would be associated with a count of < 15 million/mL. Motility describes the action and movement of the sperm, and the proportion of which have forward motion. The progressive motility should be at least 40%. Another parameter that is used to classify sperm counts is the morphology. It is normal to have some abnormal spermatozoa; the minimum acceptable percentage of semen with normal morphology is 4%.

7. D It leads to the formation of the morula after the 16 cell stage

Compaction refers to the stage of cell division when the cells flatten out and it becomes impossible to determine cell outlines. This occurs between the 16 and 32 cell stage when the embryo becomes a morula. The reaction of the sperm with the ovum is known as capacitation.

8. A Endoderm: endocrine glands

The three embryonic germ cell layers are:

- Endoderm

- Mesoderm
- Ectoderm

Each of these layers give rise to different parts of the embryo as summarised in Table 3.3.

Table 3.3 Germ cell layers		
Ectoderm	Distal layer	Nervous system
		Skin epidermis
Mesoderm	Middle layer	Muscles (cardiac, skeletal)
		Connective tissue
		Blood vessels
		Bone
		Reproductive system
Endoderm	Proximal layer	Gastrointestinal tract
		Respiratory tract
		Endocrine glands

9. E Extraembryonic mesoderm

It is the cells of the extraembryonic mesoderm that develop into the chorionic villi.

The neural crest gives rise to the nervous system and melanocytes. Endoderm is one of the germ cell layers and produces the gastrointestinal tract, respiratory tract and endocrine organs. The primitive streak develops by the end of the second week in the bilaminar embryonic disc and functions to determine symmetry of the developing embryo. The hypoblast is a part of the inner cell mass and lies beneath the epiblast. It gives rise to extraembryonic endoderm.

10. E Metanephros – kidney

Gonadal development begins during the 4th week and begins at the mesonephros. The clitoris is formed from the genital tubercle. Initially the gonads are swellings and there is no differentiation until the 7th week. Sex differentiation is determined by the SRY gene which is located on the short arm of chromosome 11. In the female embryo the gonads develop from the paramesonephric ducts. The genital folds form the labia minora and the genital swellings form the labia majora. The bladder and urethra are derived from the primitive urogenital sinus and the ureters from the ureteric bud. Three excretory systems develop: pronephros, mesonephros and finally the metanephros, from which the definitive kidney is developed.

11. D The cardinal vein runs into the sinus venosus

There are two umbilical arteries and one vein. The ligamentum venosum is a remnant of the ductus venosus and is found on the inferior surface of the liver.

The ductus venosus is a variation of the fetal circulation which directs blood from the umbilical vein into the inferior vena cava. This allows oxygenated blood from the placenta to bypass the liver. The cardiac system is developed from angiogenic mesoderm cells. The anterior cardinal vein forms the internal jugular vein and combined with the common cardinal vein forms the superior vena cava. The cardinal vein does run into the sinus venosus.

12. B Inferior mesenteric vein

The vitelline veins take blood away from the yolk sac. The vitelline veins give rise to the hepatic veins, the inferior part of the inferior vena cava, the superior mesenteric vein and the portal vein. The inferior mesenteric vein is not a derivative of the vitelline vein.

13. A Sex cords are developed from coelomic epithelium

Sex differentiation occurs in the 9th week after fertilisation. Reproductive organs develop from intermediate mesoderm, rather than paraxial mesoderm. The gubernaculum assist in the descent of the gonads in both sex. In males only the lower part persists to become the scrotal ligament. In females, the upper part becomes the ovarian ligament and the lower part becomes the round ligament of the uterus.

Chapter 4

Endocrinology

Questions: MCQs

Answer each stem 'True' or 'False'.

1. Concerning thyroid function during pregnancy:
    A   Beta-human chorionic gonadotropin is partially thyrotrophic
    B   There can be a reduction in thyroid-stimulating hormone during the 1st trimester
    C   There is increased thyroxine-binding globulin
    D   Hyperemesis gravidarum is associated with abnormally reduced levels of T3 and T4
    E   There can be a 30–50% increase in T4 production during pregnancy

2. Parathyroid hormone (PTH):
    A   There are six parathyroid glands
    B   Parathyroid glands develop embryologically from the pharyngeal pouches
    C   Blood supply to the parathyroid glands is from the parathyroid arteries
    D   PTH is synthesised by the chief cells
    E   The gene for PTH is located on chromosome 11

3. With regard to prolactin:
    A   It controls the milk-ejection reflex
    B   It is released from the anterior pituitary gland in response to dopamine
    C   It is a peptide comprised of 198 amino acids
    D   Levels can be raised in primary hypothyroidism
    E   Levels can rise after an epileptic seizure

4. Concerning anatomy of the thyroid:
    A   It descends into the neck as the thyroglossal duct
    B   It is formed by the 3rd–4th week of development
    C   C cells are derived from the fifth arch
    D   The isthmus lies on tracheal rings 2–4
    E   The main blood supply is from the lateral thyroid artery

5. Regarding Graves's disease:
    A   It is caused by IgM antibody against the thyroid-stimulating hormone receptor
    B   It is a form of hypothyroidism
    C   Pretibial myxoedema can be present
    D   It does not affect the fetus
    E   Enophthalmos can be present

6. **With regard to cortisol:**
   A   It is produced by the zona fasciculata of the adrenal cortex
   B   The majority is transported in plasma bound to albumin
   C   Production has a circadian rhythm with highest production at night
   D   It is derived from cholesterol
   E   It is a mineralocorticoid

7. **Regarding the renin–angiotensin–aldosterone system (RAAS):**
   A   Renin is secreted from the juxtaglomerular cells of the kidney
   B   Renin stimulates production of angiotensinogen from angiotensin I
   C   Angiotensin II stimulates secretion of aldosterone from the adrenal medulla
   D   Angiotensin converting enzyme converts angiotensin I to angiotensin II
   E   Low blood pressure detected by carotid sinus chemoreceptors activate the RAAS

8. **Regarding Addison's disease:**
   A   It has an incidence of approximately 1/100,000
   B   It can be misdiagnosed as anorexia nervosa
   C   Patients may have hyperpigmentation
   D   Is associated with hypokalaemia and hyponatraemia
   E   It can be caused by Waterhouse–Friederichsen syndrome

9. **Phaeochromocytoma:**
   A   Is a cause of hypertension in < 1% of cases
   B   Has a triad of symptoms: sweating, palpitations and headaches
   C   Is linked with Carney complex
   D   Has an association with multiple endocrine neoplasia-1
   E   Treatment is with a cardioselective beta-blocker followed by an alpha-blocker, phenoxybenzamine

10. **Functions of insulin are:**
   A   Increases lipolysis
   B   Decreases gluconeogenesis
   C   Increases glycogen synthetase
   D   Suppresses ketogenesis
   E   Activates glycogen phosphorylase

11. **Regarding oestrogen:**
   A   The main oestrogen after menopause is oestrone
   B   The main oestrogen between puberty and menopause is oestriol
   C   Aromatase converts testosterone to oestradiol
   D   Oestradiol is weaker than oestrone
   E   Androstenedione is converted to oestrone

12. **Ovarian steroidogenesis:**
   A   Progesterone is produced by the ovarian theca cells only
   B   Testosterone is produced by the ovarian theca cells only

C   Oestradiol is produced by the ovarian granulosa cells
D   Theca cells have follicle-stimulating hormone (FSH) receptors
E   Granulosa cells are responsive to FSH and luteinising hormone

13. **Female reproductive system: the oocyte**

A   Primary oocytes are arrested at first mitotic division until ovulation
B   Completion of first meiotic division occurs in response to the luteinising hormone surge
C   First polar body is found in the sperm head
D   Completion of the first meiotic division leads to the secondary oocyte
E   Second meiotic division is not completed until after implantation

14. **Follicle-stimulating hormone:**

A   Is produced by the posterior pituitary gland
B   Has a molecular weight of 28,000 kDa
C   Has an α and a γ subunit
D   Is raised in postmenopausal women
E   Is a glycoprotein

15. **Luteinising hormone:**

A   Has an α subunit identical to that of thyroid-stimulating hormone
B   Maintains the corpus luteum
C   Reaches its peak at day 21 in the menstrual cycle
D   Is a steroid hormone
E   Is released in response to gonadotrophin-releasing hormone

16. **Regarding pubertal changes in the female:**

A   Thelarche precedes menarche
B   Adrenarche precedes thelarche
C   Tanner staging is a means to grading pubertal development
D   Menarche before the age of 12 years is considered precocious puberty
E   Changes occur in response to increasingly regular pulses of gonadotrophin-releasing hormone

17. **In regard to the menopause:**

A   The average age of the menopause in the UK is 51 years
B   Oestradiol levels can be used to aid diagnosis of the climacteric/menopause
C   Follicle-stimulating hormone and luteinising hormone rise
D   Progesterone levels rise
E   Urogenital atrophy is caused by falling levels of oestrogens

18. **In regard to hormone replacement therapy (HRT):**

A   HRT should contain both oestrogens and progestogens
B   Progestogens can prevent endometrial hyperplasia
C   Side effects include breast tenderness and bloating
D   Testosterone has no role in HRT
E   Tibolone is an artificial form of oestrodiol

19. **Prolactin:**

    A   Is a peptide hormone
    B   Has a molecular weight of 44,000
    C   Is produced by the anterior pituitary gland
    D   Production increases in response to dopamine release
    E   Has a similar structure to growth hormone

20. **Prolactin secretion is stimulated by:**

    A   Metoclopramide administration
    B   Thyrotrophin releasing factor
    C   Chlorpromazine administration
    D   Haloperidol
    E   Venepuncture

21. **Oxytocin:**

    A   Is stored in the hypothalamus
    B   Acts via a G-protein-coupled receptor
    C   Is a nonapeptide
    D   Is responsible for milk production
    E   Has an identical structure to vasopressin

22. **Human placental lactogen:**

    A   Is secreted by the syncytiotrophoblast
    B   Has a similar structure to prolactin
    C   Is secreted by the corpus luteum
    D   Is diabetogenic
    E   Consists of 190 amino acids

23. **Human chorionic gonadotropin:**

    A   Is a glycoprotein
    B   Can be used in fertility treatments to induce ovulation
    C   Is seen at suboptimal levels in gestational trophoblastic disease
    D   Rises throughout pregnancy to reach peak levels at term
    E   Is produced by the corpus luteum prior to blastocyst implantation

24. **Human chorionic gonadotropin:**

    A   May be secreted in males with testicular cancer
    B   Can be secreted by the pituitary gland
    C   Consists of α and γ subunits
    D   Helps to maintain the corpus luteum in early pregnancy
    E   Consists of 244 amino acids

25. **The hypothalamus synthesises:**

    A   Thyrotrophin-releasing hormone
    B   Prolactin
    C   Oxytocin
    D   Follicle-stimulating hormone
    E   Thyroid-stimulating hormone

26. **The anterior pituitary gland produces:**
    A   Vasopressin
    B   Thyroid-stimulating hormone
    C   Somatostatin
    D   Oxytocin
    E   Prolactin

27. **The posterior pituitary gland:**
    A   Stores oxytocin
    B   Releases nonapeptide hormones into the hypophyseal circulation
    C   Consists partially of axonal projections from the hypothalamus
    D   Is the site of vasopressin production
    E   Is also known as the adenohypophysis

28. **During pregnancy:**
    A   Prolactin levels increase
    B   Maternal iodine levels fall
    C   Relaxin levels peak in the second trimester
    D   Follicle-stimulating hormone levels rise
    E   Thyroid-stimulating hormone levels increase

29. **Regarding adrenal function during pregnancy:**
    A   Cortisol levels decrease throughout pregnancy
    B   Cortisol-binding globulin synthesis increases
    C   Aldosterone levels fall
    D   Angiotensin II levels fall
    E   Renin levels are unchanged

30. **Regarding calcium homeostasis in pregnancy:**
    A   Fetal plasma levels of calcium mirror those of the mother
    B   Plasma calcium concentrations are unchanged by pregnancy
    C   Albumin levels are decreased in pregnancy
    D   Parathyroid hormone secretion is increased
    E   1,25-dihydroxycholecalciferol production is unaltered

31. **In regard to thyroid function during pregnancy:**
    A   Synthesis of thyroid-binding globulin is increased
    B   Total T3 and T4 levels are decreased
    C   Levels of thyroid-stimulating hormone are unchanged during the first trimester
    D   Hyperemesis gravidarum may be caused by fluctuating levels of T4
    E   Free T4 levels start to fall in the first trimester

32. **Growth hormone:**
    A   Is secreted by the hypothalamus
    B   Is diabetogenic in action
    C   Has a molecular weight of 21,500 daltons

    D   Consists of 150 amino acids

    E   Is mainly catabolic in its actions

33. Growth hormone:

    A   Is secreted by the anterior pituitary gland

    B   Is released in a pulsatile manner every 90 minutes

    C   Stimulates protein synthesis

    D   Stimulates lipolysis

    E   Is released in lower quantities in patients with anorexia nervosa

Questions: SBAs

For each question, select the single best answer from the five options listed.

34. A 16-year-old girl is seen in the gynaecology outpatient department with primary amenorrhoea and excessive facial hair growth. Examination reveals normal genitalia, apart from an apparently large clitoris. Differential diagnosis includes congenital adrenal hyperplasia (CAH).

    CAH (21α-hydroxylase deficiency) is characterised by which of the following?

    A   Hypertension, hypokalaemia and hyponatraemia
    B   Hypertension, hyperkalaemia and hyponatraemia
    C   Hypotension, hyperkalaemia and hypernatraemia
    D   Hypotension, hyperkalaemia and hyponatraemia
    E   Hypotension, hypokalaemia and hyponatraemia

35. A 27-year-old woman is seen in the antenatal clinic. She suffered from hyperemesis gravidarum in the first trimester and routine thyroid function tests have revealed abnormalities.

    Which of the following is a recognised change in regulation of thyroid function in pregnancy?

    A   Decelerated rates of T4 and T3 degradation and production
    B   Decreased basal metabolic rate
    C   Increased total T4 and T3 in the first trimester
    D   Increased thyroid-stimulating hormone
    E   Reduced plasma iodine concentration in early pregnancy

36. During her pregnancy a 38-year-old woman is diagnosed with gestational diabetes requiring insulin treatment at 28 weeks of gestation.

    Which of the following statements bests describes the function of human placental lactogen?

    A   It enhances amino acid transfer across the placenta
    B   It has insulin-like properties
    C   It increases glucose utilisation
    D   It increases insulin sensitivity in pregnancy
    E   It is a growth hormone antagonist

37. A 34-year-old woman is admitted to labour ward at 31 weeks' gestation with threatened preterm labour. She is given two doses of steroids as a precaution.

    Which of the following describes the first step in the synthesis of steroids?

    A   Conversion of cholesterol to pregnenolone
    B   Conversion of corticosterone to deoxycorticosterone
    C   Conversion of dehydroepiandrosterone to androstenedione
    D   Conversion of dihydrotesterone to oestradiol
    E   Conversion of pregnenolone to progesterone

38. Which of the following is an action of cortisol?

A   Analgesia
B   Decrease glycogenesis
C   Decrease catabolism of proteins
D   Decrease gastric acid production
E   Increase gluconeogenesis

39. A 28-year-old woman is referred to the gynaecology clinic with primary infertility. On examination, she has a round face, prominent stretch marks on her abdomen and hirsutism.

Which of the following is not a feature of Cushing's syndrome?

A   Diabetes insipidus
B   Depression
C   Irregular menstrual cycles
D   Osteoporosis
E   Weight gain

40. A 26-year-old woman is referred to the gynaecology clinic with abdominal pain and amenorrhoea. You suspect she may have Cushing's syndrome and decide to send her for further tests.

Which of the following tests would be suitable for confirmation of the diagnosis?

A   Adrenocorticotrophic hormone levels
B   High dose dexamethasone suppression test
C   Low dose dexamethasone suppression test
D   Short synacthen test
E   Urinary free cortisol

41. A 52-year-old woman with Cushing's syndrome is referred to the preassessment clinic prior to a vaginal hysterectomy.

Which of the following is a feature of Cushing's syndrome?

A   Decreased plasma lactate dehydrogenase
B   Hypoglycaemia
C   Hypokalaemia
D   Hyponatraemia
E   Metabolic alkalosis

42. An 18-year-old woman is seen in the gynaecology clinic for investigation of amenorrhoea. You notice that she is overweight with hirsutism, a round face and acne. Although looking up recent blood tests, you notice that her plasma cortisol is high and her adrenocorticotrophic hormone (ACTH) is undetectable.

What is the most likely cause of these results?

A   Cushing's syndrome (adrenal origin)

B   Cushing's syndrome (ectopic ACTH production)
C   Cushing's syndrome (pituitary origin)
D   Polycystic ovarian syndrome
E   Primary adrenal failure

43. What is a site of action of antidiuretic hormone?

A   Bowman's capsule
B   Collecting duct
C   Glomerulus
D   Loop of Henle
E   Proximal convoluted tubule

44. A 72-year-old woman is seen in preassessment clinic prior to undergoing a routine vaginal hysterectomy for prolapse. Her blood pressure is found to be high and electrolytes deranged.

Which of the following is a secondary cause of hyperaldosteronism?

A   Conn's syndrome
B   Diabetes insipidus
C   Renal artery stenosis
D   Syndrome of inappropriate antidiuretic hormone secretion
E   Tuberculosis

45. A 60-year-old woman with a chronic disease is admitted to hospital acutely unwell. She has severe diarrhoea and vomiting. She is hypotensive with a blood pressure of 85/45 mmHg. You suspect, she has Addison's disease.

Which of the following is a recognised cause of Addison's disease?

A   Diabetes insipidus
B   HIV
C   Hyperparathyroidism
D   Pregnancy
E   Sarcoidosis

46. A 24-year-old woman is admitted with vomiting and diarrhoea at 26 weeks' gestation. Her electrolytes are deranged and fail to resolve after the acute event and she requires admission to the high-dependency unit. Addison's disease is suspected.

Which of the following is the most appropriate initial specific test for Addison's disease?

A   Dexamethasone suppression test
B   Short adrenocorticotrophic hormone (ACTH) inhibition test
C   Short ACTH stimulation test
D   Long ACTH inhibition test
E   Long ACTH stimulation test

47. Which is the first catecholamine to be produced in the synthesis of catecholamines?

    A Dopamine
    B Epinephrine
    C Norepinephrine
    D Phenylalanine
    E Tyrosine

48. A 48-year-old woman is found to have persistent hypertension during a work-up for gynaecology operation. Further investigation reveals a phaeochromocytoma.

Which of the following biochemical changes is associated with phaeochromocytoma?

    A Basophilia
    B Hyperglycaemia
    C Hyperkalaemia
    D Hypocalcaemia
    E Reduced urinary catecholamines

49. Which of the following actions is related to glucagon?

    A Decrease gluconeogenesis
    B Decrease ketone body production
    C Decrease plasma glucose
    D Increase glycogenolysis
    E Reduce lipolysis

50. A 32-year-old Asian woman is diagnosed at 28 weeks' gestation with gestational diabetes. Treatment with metformin is commenced.

Which of the following is an insulin antagonist?

    A Cortisol
    B Free fatty acids
    C Growth hormone
    D Prolactin
    E Somatostatin

51. A 51-year-old woman is started on hormonal replacement therapy (HRT). You consider the properties of oestrogen when discussing the contraindications to HRT treatment.

Which of the following is a property of oestrogen?

    A Decreases bone formation
    B Decreases circulating coagulation factors
    C Increases bowel motility
    D Reduce triglycerides in blood
    E Stimulates growth of endometrium

52. A 21-year-old woman is started on the mini pill. She asks you about the possible side effects of progesterone.

Which of the following is a property of progesterone?

A   Increases contractility of uterine smooth muscle
B   Increases respiratory drive
C   Inhibits lobular alveolar development of mammary glands
D   Promotes lactation during pregnancy
E   Reduces bone density

53. A 32-year-old woman is referred to the gynaecology clinic with secondary amenorrhoea. Day 21 progesterone levels indicate that she is not ovulating.

Which of the following statements best describes the events occurring at the midluteal phase of the menstrual cycle?

A   An increase in progesterone and selective rise in follicle-stimulating hormone (FSH)
B   High progesterone leads to low FSH and luteinising hormone (LH)
C   Oestradiol decreases and FSH increases
D   Oestradiol feedback becomes negative leading to LH surge
E   Peak of LH surge

54. A 34-year-old woman undergoes regular ultrasound scans for follicle tracking having been started on clomiphene treatment.

Which of the following statements most appropriately describes the mature ovarian follicle?

A   Its development is primarily controlled by luteinising hormone
B   It is surrounded by theca cells
C   It is usually the only primary follicle to develop during each cycle
D   It produces progesterone
E   It reaches a diameter of 20–30 mm prior to rupture

55. A 23-year-old woman is seen in the gynaecology clinic after an ultrasound scan reveals multiple cysts on both ovaries. She also complains of irregular menstrual cycles and has been trying to conceive for over 1 year.

Which of the following lead to clinical manifestations of polycystic ovarian syndrome?

A   Decrease in oestradiol levels
B   Decrease in prolactin
C   Decrease in testosterone and androstenedione
D   Increase in fasting insulin
E   Increase in sex hormone binding globulin

56. Which of the following increases sex hormone binding globulin?

A   Growth hormone
B   Hepatic cirrhosis
C   Hyperprolactinaemia
D   Hypogonadism
E   Hypothyroidism

Answers

1. A True

    B True

    C True

    D False

    E True

    Human chorionic gonadotrophin (hCG) is a glycoprotein which is thought to have thyrotrophic activity. This may cause some increased thyroid activity and therefore lead to a reduction in the levels of thyroid-stimulating hormone. Thyroxine-binding globulin is responsible for binding thyroxine in circulation, along with transthyretin and albumin. Hyperemesis gravidarum is a common condition of early pregnancy, associated with a rise in β-hCG. It is associated with an abnormally high level of free thyroid hormones and reduced thyroid stimulating hormone, and therefore thyroid function tests should be performed on women presenting with this condition.

2. A False

    B True

    C False

    D True

    E True

    Parathyroid hormone (PTH) is a polypeptide hormone secreted by the chief cells of the parathyroid glands. There are four parathyroid glands which develop from the pharyngeal pouches during embryological development. The superior glands develop from the third pouch and the inferior glands from the fourth pouch. They are located under the capsule at the posterior area of the thyroid gland and the blood supply is via the thyroid arteries. The gene for PTH is located on chromosome 11; with PTH being synthesised as a large preprohormone of 115 amino acids. It is cleaved to give a biologically active 84 amino acid peptide and then stored in the Golgi apparatus of the cytoplasm of the cell.

3. A False

    B False

    C True

    D True

    E True

    Prolactin is a long chain polypeptide hormone. It is produced by the anterior pituitary and is responsible for lactation. The milk ejection reflex is caused by oxytocin, produced by the posterior pituitary in response to suckling. Prolactin is released from the anterior pituitary gland in response to thyrotrophin-releasing hormone (TRH). Dopamine is an important inhibitor of prolactin release. Levels of prolactin may be found to be raised in primary hypothyroidism as a result of increased TRH. The levels of prolactin reach a peak in the bloodstream approximately 30 minutes after the onset of suckling. Prolactin shows diurnal variation and levels are higher during the evening and sleeping.

4. A True

B False

C True

D True

E False

Development of the thyroid gland begins at approximately 24th day after fertilisation. Thyroid hormones are secreted by the fetus by week 11 of development. The thyroid does descend into the neck as the thyroglossal duct and is formed by the 5–6th week of development. The inferior thyroid artery provides the main blood supply. The thyroglossal duct connects the thyroid gland to the tongue during embryological development and it is a remnant of this structure that may cause a thyroglossal duct in later life.

5. A False

B False

C True

D False

E False

Graves' disease is an autoimmune disease caused by an immunoglobulin G (IgG) autoantibody against the thyroid receptor which acts as a thyroid stimulator and leads to excess production of T4 and T3. This autoantibody has a binding site separate to thyroid-stimulating hormone, but changes the shape of the receptor. The signs and symptoms are those associated with hyperthyroidism; however, pretibial myxoedema and exophthalmus are common to Graves' disease. Pretibial myxoedema occurs in approximately 1–4% of patients with Graves' disease and appears as an indurated coloured region at the lower anterior leg. As the autoantibody is IgG, it is able to cross the placenta and may lead to fetal thyrotoxicosis and goitre. Ninety-five per cent of cases of hyperthyroidism in pregnancy are caused by Graves' disease. Other causes of hyperthyroidism in pregnancy include toxic thyroid adenoma or toxic multinodular goitre.

6. A True

B False

C False

D True

E False

Cortisol is a glucocorticoid steroid hormone produced by the zona fasciculata of the adrenal gland. It is transported bound to cortisol-binding globulin (80%) and albumin (15%). The remaining 5% of the hormone is free. It has circadian rhythm with highest production at 8 am. The functions of cortisol are important for the metabolism of carbohydrates, proteins and fats. Cortisol suppresses the immune system and this is important to remember in those patients that are on long-term steroid replacement therapy. The overall action of cortisol is to increase blood glucose level.

Actions of cortisol:

- Immunosuppressive and anti-inflammatory
- Increased lipolysis
- Increased gluconeogenesis, glycogenesis and glycogen storage in liver
- Breakdown of skeletal muscle and mobilisation of amino acids

7. A True

    B False

    C False

    D True

    E False

The renin–angiotensin–aldosterone system is activated when there is a reduction in blood pressure which is detected by baroreceptors located in the carotid sinus. A decrease in the filtered sodium concentration stimulates the macula densa of the kidney to release renin. A reduction in the perfusion of the juxtaglomerular apparatus of the kidney leads to a release of renin. Renin then acts on angiotensinogen to cleave an inactive peptide leading to the formation of angiotensin I. Angiotensin-converting enzyme, produced in the lungs, acts on angiotensin I converting it to angiotensin II. Angiotensin II is a vasoconstrictor of arterioles and causes release of aldosterone. The overall effect is to increase blood pressure.

8. A True

    B True

    C True

    D False

    E True

Addison's disease is also known as primary adrenocortical insufficiency. It has an incidence of approximately 0.8/100,000. Eighty per cent of cases are as a result of autoimmune disease and may be associated with other autoimmune conditions such as Graves' disease, pernicious anaemia and diabetes mellitus. Symptoms include fatigue, abdominal pain and other non-specific conditions such as nausea and vomiting. Adrenocorticotrophic hormone (ACTH) produced by the pituitary gland is responsible for the pigmentation seen in this condition, as levels are higher than normal. Classically there is hyponatraemia and hyperkalaemia, which may lead to associated ECG changes.

Diagnosis of Addison' disease is via the short Synacthen test. A cortisol level is taken 30 minutes after receiving a bolus of ACTH.

Waterhouse–Friderichsen syndrome is a haemorrhage into the adrenal cortex as a result of fulminant meningococcaemia. Other causes of adrenal haemorrhage include coagulopathic states, shock and pregnancy-associated causes.

9. A True

B True

C True

D False

E False

Phaeochromocytoma is a catecholamine producing tumour of the neuroendocrine cells of the adrenal medulla. It is a rare cause of hypertension, being responsible for approximately 1% of cases. It may be an autosomal dominant inherited condition. Most phaeochromocytoma are found unilaterally in the adrenal medulla. Symptoms may include headache and 'a sense of impending doom' associated with increased blood pressure. Multiple endocrine neoplasia (MEN) is a group of genetic tumour syndromes. Phaeochromocytoma is found in MEN-2a, along with medullary thyroid cancer and parathyroid hyperplasia. MEN-1 comprises parathyroid hyperplasia, pituitary adenoma and pancreatic tumours. Treatment can be surgical or medical; however, blood pressure control is usually necessary prior to operative management. Alpha-blockade is given by phenoxybenzamine and 24 hours later a cardioselective beta-blocker is given.

10. A False

B True

C True

D True

E False

The overall function of insulin is to decrease hepatic output of glucose. This occurs via the following mechanisms:

- Promote glycogen synthesis
  - Increase glycogen synthetase (muscle and liver)
  - Inhibit glycogen phosphorylase
- Decrease gluconeogenesis
- Suppress lipolysis
  - Inhibit triglyceride lipase
  - Increase fatty acid synthetase
- Suppress ketogenesis
  - Inhibit carnitine palmitoyltransferase
  - Increase acetyl coenzyme A carboxylase

11. A True

   B False

   C True

   D False

   E True

Three main oestrogens are:

- Oestrone (E1)
- Oestriol (E2)
- Oestradiol (E3)

Oestrone is the main oestrogen postmenopause and is weaker than oestradiol.

12. A False

   B True

   C True

   D False

   E True

The production of steroid hormones by the ovary depends on the menstrual cycle. Progesterone is produced by the ovarian theca and granulosa cells and is produced mainly during the luteal phase of the menstrual cycle. During the follicular phase of the cycle it is mainly oestrogen that is produced. Testosterone is produced by the theca only. Oestradiol, the end product of steroidogenesis, is produced only by the granulosa cells. In the ovarian follicles, theca cells have receptors for luteinising hormone (LH) and not follicle-stimulating hormone (FSH). Granulosa cells have receptors for FSH and for LH later on.

13. A False

   B True

   C False

   D True

   E False

Oogonia fill the ovaries during fetal life and these primordial germ cells divide by mitosis until shortly before birth. No further oocytes are produced after birth and at this time each female has approximately one million oocytes. Primary oocytes are contained in the ovary of the fetus and arrested after the first meiotic division until ovulation. Although the oogonia are arrested in the first prophase stage of meiosis, they are surrounded by a layer of granulosa cells. Oocytes surrounded by this protective layer are known as primordial follicles and are located in the cortex of the ovary. When the luteinising hormone surge occurs, the dominant follicle completes this first meiotic division to become a secondary oocyte. The first polar body is found in the ovum and contains half the chromosomes. Second meiotic division is not completed until fertilisation.

14. A False

   B True

   C False

   D True

   E True

Follicle-stimulating hormone (FSH) is a glycoprotein hormone produced by the anterior pituitary. FSH has a molecular weight of 30,000 and is comprised of 204 amino acids. FSH is similar in composition to other anterior pituitary gland hormones including thyroid-stimulating hormone and human chorionic gonadotrophin, and all of these hormones are made of an α subunit with a specific β subunit. FSH acts on the ovaries and the testes to promote gametogenesis, and it also has a role in hormone synthesis. FSH is raised in menopausal women because of the reduction in circulating oestradiol.

15. A True

   B True

   C False

   D False

   E True

Follicle-stimulating hormone (FSH) and luteinising hormone (LH) are both produced by the anterior pituitary gland and are glycoprotein hormones. Like thyroid-stimulating hormone (TSH), they consist of α- and β-subunits; the α subunit is identical in all three hormones. Both FSH and LH are released in response to pulses of gonadotrophin-releasing hormone (GnRH) from the hypothalamus.

FSH stimulates receptors on the granulosa cells of the female ovarian follicles to produce oestrogen; increased levels of oestrogen act via a negative feedback on the hypothalamus, thus leading to a decrease in the release in FSH.

Raised levels of oestrogen from the growing ovarian follicle lead to an increase in pulses of GnRH and a subsequent surge in LH, which in turns leads to ovulation at around day 14 of the menstrual cycle.

FSH levels are raised after the menopause, when decreasing levels of oestrogen, as a consequence of ovarian atresia, work via a positive feedback loop, thus increasing FSH levels in an attempt to stimulate oestrogen production.

16. A True

   B False

   C True

   D False

   E True

On average puberty in the UK occurs at around 12 years old; it describes a series of changes in endocrine function and physical appearance which accompany the change to adulthood. In females, thelarche, the process of breast development follows a growth spurt. It usually precedes adrenarche, the process of pubic hair development, which is then followed by menarche, the commencement of menstruation. Menarche prior to the age of 10 years is considered precocious. Failure to commence by the age of 16 years warrants further investigation.

Tanner staging is a means of grading pubertal breast and pubic hair development in female; it is also used in males to grade pubic hair and testicular development. Tanner staging is graded from I to IV, with the latter representing the adult form.

Puberty is associated with the commencement of gonadotrophin-releasing hormone pulses in late childhood, which become increasingly regular, gradually changing from nocturnal pulses to pulses occurring every 90 minutes. These pulses stimulate the production of follicle-stimulating and luteinising hormones with subsequent production of oestrogen and testosterone.

Growth hormone levels are increased during puberty and its actions, mediated by insulin-like growth factor-1 are thought to be responsible for the pubertal growth spurt.

17. A True

   B False

   C True

   D False

   E True

The menopause is a retrospective diagnosis, made when a woman has been amenorrhoeic for at least 1 year. The 'climacteric' encompasses the time from when a woman may experience classic menopausal symptoms, such as hot flushes, together with menstrual irregularity, up to the cessation of periods. With age there is an ovarian atresia, with fewer ovulatory cycles; this leads to lower levels of oestrogen production. Follicle-stimulating hormone (FSH) and luteinising hormone (LH) levels are subsequently raised in an attempt to increase oestrogen levels. Associated with the reduction in overall levels of oestradiol is the failure of endometrial proliferation and subsequent cessation of menstruation. Measuring FSH levels can be a useful investigation with levels above 30 IU/L aiding diagnosis of the menopause. The measurement of oestrodiol levels is not a useful tool in the diagnosis of the menopause as levels may fluctuate because of the continued peripheral conversion of androstenedione to oestrogens by ovarian tissue, adipose tissues, the liver and the adrenal glands. Oestrone is the predominant form of oestrogen postmenopausally. There is no role for the measurement of LH, oestrogen, testosterone or progesterone levels (**Table 4.1**).

Table 4.1 Hormones and the menopause	
Hormone	**Menopausal levels**
Follicle-stimulating hormone	Increased
Luteinising hormone	Increased
Oestrogens	Overall levels of oestradiol decrease
	Oestrogens still made peripheral conversion in tissues
	Oestrone predominant postmenopausal oestrogen
Testosterone	Unchanged
Progesterone	Decreased

18. A False

    B True

    C True

    D False

    E False

Hormone replacement therapy (HRT) aims to reduce symptoms of the menopause as well as reduce osteoporosis. HRT can be administered topically, orally, transdermally and via implants. The main constituent of all forms of HRT is oestrogen. In order to prevent endometrial hyperplasia because of unopposed oestrogen levels, all women with a uterus should also receive a form of HRT which contains a form of progestogen. Alternatively another source of progesterone can be administered, e.g. the levenorgestrel intrauterine system intrauterine system. In women who have had a hysterectomy an oestrogen only HRT is suitable. Synthetic progestogens are structurally different from progesterone but have similar activity.

Testosterone can improve the libido in postmenopausal women. Side effects of HRT include breast tenderness, bloating as well as headaches, nausea, depression and subjective reports of weight gain. Tibolone is a synthetic steroid drug that is classified as hormone replacement therapy. It is a chemically inert substance until it is absorbed when it then becomes active.

19. A True

    B False

    C True

    D False

    E True

Prolactin is a peptide hormone consisting of 198 amino acids, with a molecular weight of 24,000 daltons. It is a single peptide chain and is a somatotrophic hormone, being stored in somatotroph cells of the anterior pituitary gland. It has a similar structure to both growth hormone and placental lactogen. Secreted by the anterior pituitary gland, its secretion is responsible for lactogenesis and the development of breast tissue. Prolactin levels rise in pregnancy and during lactation.

20. A True

    B True

    C True

    D True

    E True

Prolactin secretion is stimulated by both serotonin and thyrotrophin-releasing factor. The main inhibitor of prolactin secretion is dopamine. Dopamine antagonists, including metoclopramide, domperidone, diazepam, haloperidol and phenothiazines such as chlorpromazine, therefore stimulate the production of prolactin. Prolactin inhibits the pulsatile release of gonadotrophin-releasing hormone and oestrogen. Stress can also cause the release of prolactin, and therefore a non-stressful venepuncture technique is required when measuring serum prolactin levels in the diagnosis of hyperprolactinaemia. Other stimulants of prolactin secretion include exercise and sleep.

21. A False

    B True

    C True

    D False

    E False

Oxytocin is produced by the supraoptic and paraventricular nuclei of the anterior hypothalamus and then transported to the posterior pituitary gland where it is stored for release. It is a nonapeptide, which consists of nine amino acids. It has a very similar structure to vasopressin (antidiuretic hormone), another nonapeptide also stored in the posterior pituitary gland. Oxytocin is involved in the release of breast milk, rather than its production. It is involved in the 'let down' reflex whereby stimulation of the nipples by the suckling infant leads to release of oxytocin, which then leads to milk ejection. Prolactin is responsible for milk production.

Oxytocin also plays an important role in the contraction of uterine muscle during labour.

22. A True

    B True

    C False

    D True

    E True

Human placental lactogen (HPL) is a polypeptide hormone produced by the syncytiotrophoblast of the placenta. It consists of 190 amino acids with two disulphide bonds. It has a similar structure to both prolactin and growth hormone. It is diabetogenic, i.e. it is anti-insulin, and is thought to modify the mother's metabolism in order to supply nutrients to the growing fetus. Levels of HPL increase throughout pregnancy, although interestingly human chorionic gonadotrophin is sometimes undetectable in normal pregnancy.

23. A False

B True

C False

D False

E False

Human chorionic gonadotrophin (hCG) is a peptide hormone consisting of 244 amino acids. It has an α subunit identical to follicle-stimulating hormone, luteinising hormone and thyroid-stimulating hormone and a β subunit. It has a peak in concentration level during the second trimester and usually reduces in the third trimester. In gestational trophoblastic disease, a fertilised ovum forms abnormal trophoblastic tissue which secretes large amounts of hCG. hCG is usually given during assisted conception regimens.

24. A True

B True

C False

D True

E True

Human chorionic gonadotrophin (hCG) is secreted by the syncytiotrophoblast and is thought to maintain the corpus luteum and stimulate it to produce progesterone. Levels of hCG increase throughout the first trimester, reaching a peak at around 12 weeks' gestation, although hCG is detectable throughout pregnancy. hCG may be given to stimulate ovulation in women with subfertility; its action due to its structural similarity to luteinising hormone. Serum hCG levels are massively elevated in gestational trophoblastic disease. In addition hCG levels are raised in germ cell tumours, e.g. of the testicles, as well as other forms of cancer such as pancreatic adenoma.

25. A True

B False

C True

D False

E False

Hormones synthesised by the hypothalamus include:

- Gonadotrophin-releasing hormone: stimulates luteinising hormone and follicle-stimulating hormone (FSH)
- Growth hormone (GH) releasing hormone: stimulates GH release
- Corticotrophin releasing hormone: stimulates adrenocorticotrophic hormone release
- Somatostatin
- Thyrotrophin-releasing hormone: thyroid-stimulating hormone (TSH) release

Prolactin, FSH and TSH are released from the pituitary gland.

26. A False

    B True

    C False

    D False

    E True

The anterior pituitary gland, also known as the adenohypophysis, sits in the sella turcica. The pea-sized pituitary gland sits immediately below the hypothalamus, to which is connected to via the pituitary stalk. The optic chiasm sits directly in front of the anterior pituitary gland. The anterior pituitary gland secretes the following: thyroid-stimulating hormone, adrenocorticotrophic hormone, prolactin, growth hormone, melanocyte-stimulating hormone and the gonadotrophins follicle-stimulating hormone and luteinising hormone.

27. A True

    B True

    C True

    D False

    E False

The pituitary gland sits in the depression at the base of the sphenoid bone called the sella turcica. It is comprised of two anatomical and functionally distinct parts: the anterior and posterior and each are responsible for storage and secretion of various hormones. The posterior pituitary, also known as the neurohypophysis, is not a true gland, but rather an extension of the axonal projections of the supraoptic and paraventricular nuclei of the hypothalamus. The anterior lobe of the pituitary gland is derived from the embryonic ectoderm. The posterior pituitary gland is not a site of hormone synthesis, but stores oxytocin and vasopressin, both synthesised by the hypothalamus. These nonapeptide hormones are stored in granules in the axon terminals ready for release into the hypophyseal circulation.

28. A True

    B True

    C False

D False

E True

Unsurprisingly prolactin levels rise during pregnancy. Maternal iodine levels fall due to the combined effects of increased urinary excretion and fetal demand. Relaxin has a variety of sources; in males it is produced by the prostate (present in semen). In females, relaxin is produced by the corpus luteum and the breast and in pregnancy by the placenta. It may have a role in ligament relaxation during pregnancy and cervical dilatation. Relaxin levels rise during the first trimester of pregnancy then fall at the end of the trimester only to peak again close to delivery. Follicle-stimulating hormone levels fall in pregnancy. Thyroid-stimulating hormone levels rise in pregnancy; this may be partly due to the thyrotrophic properties of human chorionic gonadotrophin.

29. A False

    B True

    C False

    D False

    E False

All levels of adrenal function are increased in pregnancy, and this includes corticotrophin releasing factor. Synthesis of both cortisol and cortisol-binding globulin is increased. Levels of aldosterone, angiotensin II and renin increase. The trophoblast increases the amount of ACTH produced with overall maternal levels remaining stable.

30. A False

    B False

    C True

    D True

    E False

Calcium homeostasis is markedly changed during pregnancy, because of changes in maternal physiology and the need to meet fetal demand. Serum albumin concentrations decrease in pregnancy because of the haemodilutional effects of volume expansion, leading to a reduction in levels of albumin-bound calcium. Unbound calcium levels remain the same. To meet fetal calcium demand there is increased production of parathyroid hormone and subsequent increases in 1,25-dihydroxycholecalciferol. Fetal plasma levels of calcium are higher than of the mother reflecting active transport across the placenta.

31. A True

    B False

    C False

D True

E True

Overall thyroid function is grossly unchanged during pregnancy, however, there are some notable changes. Synthesis of thyroid-binding globulin by the liver is increased; total levels of T3 and T4 increase as a result of this rise. Levels of free T4 do fall in the second and third trimester. Thyroid-stimulating hormone (TSH) levels show some fluctuation in the first trimester with increasing levels of human chorionic gonadotrophin (hCG) leading to a fall in overall TSH levels due to hCG's thyrotrophic activity. During pregnancy, the thyroid gland increases its uptake of iodine from the.

32. A False

B True

C True

D False

E False

Growth hormone (GH) is a peptide and consists of 191 amino acids. The locus for the growth hormone gene is on chromosome 17. It has a molecular weight of around 21,000 daltons and is structurally similar to both prolactin and human placental lactogen. It is secreted from the anterior pituitary gland somatotrophs in response to GH releasing hormone. Somatostatin is a direct inhibitor of GH. GH release stimulates the synthesis of insulin like growth factors and it stimulates lipolysis and gluconeogenesis.

Insulin growth factors stimulate bone growth and protein synthesis in muscles.

33. A True

B False

C True

D True

E False

Growth hormone (GH) is secreted by the somatotrophs of the anterior pituitary gland. Its release is stimulated and inhibited by hormones produced the hypothalamus, growth hormone releasing hormone and somatostatin respectively. The action of growth hormone is principally one of the anabolism and this is reflected in its role in lipolysis and its anti-insulinic properties.

GH is secreted in higher levels during puberty when more frequent pulsatile release occurs. The growth promoting actions of GH are mediated by insulin-like growth factor-1.

34. D Hypotension, hyperkalaemia and hyponatraemia

Ninety per cent of patients with congenital adrenal hyperplasia (CAH) have 21-hydroxylase deficiency. This enzyme has a function in both the production of glucocorticoids and mineralocorticoids, and therefore patients may have a 'salt wasting' form of the syndrome. A deficiency in mineralocorticoids leads to hypotension as a result of hypovolaemia, with hyponatraemia and hyperkalaemia. See **Figure 4.1** for steroidogenesis pathways.

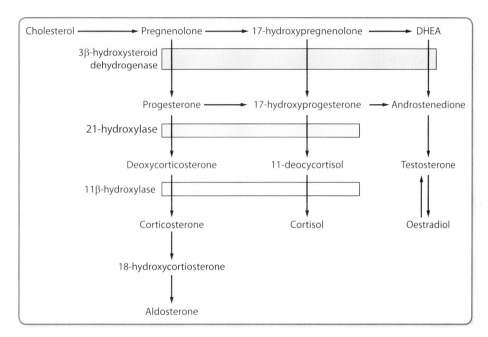

Figure 4.1 Steroidogenesis pathways.

Ten per cent of patients with CAH have a deficiency of 11β-hydroxylase. In this instance there remains a deficiency of glucocorticoids; however, there is an accumulation of deoxycortisol which may cause hypertension due to its glucocorticoid properties.

35. E Reduced plasma iodine concentration in early pregnancy

During the first trimester, the increased renal blood flow and glomerular filtration rate lead to increased level of iodine clearance from the plasma. Patients with already low levels of iodine are predisposed to developing goitre. In the first trimester rising levels of human chorionic gonadotrophin (hCG) to lead to a reduction in serum levels of thyroid-stimulating hormone (TSH) as it has thyrotropic properties, because of the structural similarity of hCG to TSH. Pregnancy is associated with increased thyroid binding globulin because of increased liver production, with subsequent elevation of total T4 and T3.

36. A It enhances amino acid transfer across the placenta

Human placental lactogen (HPL) is one of several peptides made by the placenta. Its structure and function is similar to growth hormone. It affects the maternal metabolism to provide increased nutrient supply to the fetus. HPL decreases maternal insulin sensitivity and therefore leads to greater amount of glucose in the blood. Lipolysis is induced which leads to fatty acids being released into the bloodstream. HPL decreases maternal glucose utilisation. HPL is only present in pregnancy and reaches its highest concentration by the 3rd trimester. It has previously been used as an indicator of fetal well being.

37. A Conversion of cholesterol to pregnenolone

All steroids are synthesised from cholesterol, with the first step of the pathway being the conversion of cholesterol to pregnenolone by cholesterol monooxygenase. Dihydrotesterone is produced from oestradiol by 5-alpha reductase (**Figure 4.1**).

38. B Decrease glycogenesis

The action of cortisol can be summarised as follows:

- Increasing plasma glucose
  - Increase gluconeogenesis
  - Increase glycogenesis
  - Increase glycogen storage
- Increase lipolysis
- Increase protein catabolism
- Sodium and water retention
- Anti-inflammatory
- Increased gastric acid production

39. A Diabetes insipidus

Cushing's syndrome is a state of excess of cortisol. Characteristic features include: truncal obesity, a red, puffy and rounded face, hypertension, depression, osteoporosis, diabetes mellitus, striae, hirsutism and amenorrhoea. Causes of excess cortisol production fall into four main categories:

1. Iatrogenic
2. Excess adrenocorticotrophic hormone (ACTH) production by pituitary tumour (Cushing's disease)
3. Adrenal cortical neoplasm producing steroid
4. Ectopic production of ACTH by non-pituitary tumour (e.g. lung tumour)

40. C Low dose dexamethasone suppression test

The best screening test is the overnight dexamethasone suppression test which is used to eliminate all those with no abnormality. False positives will be seen in alcoholics, those with anorexia nervosa and anyone taking enzyme inducer medication. If this test is positive, then further tests are done to localise the disease.

Low dose dexamethasone suppression test involves giving 0.5 mg/6 h orally for 48 hours and then measuring plasma cortisol at 0 hour and 48 hours. This test is used to confirm the diagnosis. Localisation of the disease is done via the high dose dexamethasone test (complete or partial suppression indicates Cushing's disease) and testing plasma adrenocorticotrophic hormone level.

41. C Hypokalaemia

Cushing's syndrome is a disorder of high serum cortisol, which has many causes and has been discussed previously. The most common cause is exogenous administration of steroid hormones. Cushing's disease refers to Cushing's syndrome caused specifically by a tumour of the pituitary gland, which secretes large amounts of adrenocorticotropic hormone, leading to high cortisol. Patients may have hyperglycaemia and insulin resistance, causing diabetes mellitus. All of the above are potential features of Cushing's syndrome, except for hyponatraemia. Findings of hyperglycaemia and hypokalaemia may be accompanied by hyponatraemia as a result of increased aldosterone levels.

42. A Cushing's syndrome (adrenal origin)

Cushing's syndrome as a result of an adrenal tumour leads to increased plasma cortisol and very low levels of ACTH , as shown in **Table 4.2**.

Table 4.2 Levels of cortisol and adrenocorticotrophic hormone (ACTH) in various pathologies		
	Cortisol	**ACTH**
Normal	Low – midnight High – 0800	Not raised
Primary adrenal failure	Low	High
Steroid therapy	Variable	Variable (may be normal or very low)
Cushing's (adrenal origin)	High	Low (undetectable)
Cushing's (pituitary origin)	High	High
Cushing's (ectopic ACTH production)	High	Very high

43. B Collecting duct

Antidiuretic hormone (ADH) or vasopressin is a peptide hormone that helps to regulate water homeostasis. It is released from the posterior pituitary in response to increased osmolality of plasma and acts on the distal tubule of the kidney to increase water absorption via insertion of aquaporins water channels into the membrane. By increasing the water reabsorption of the kidney, the osmolality of the urine is increased. Nephrogenic diabetes insipidus is caused when the kidney become unresponsive to ADH. Acquired forms a of nephrogenic diabetes insipidus may be triggered by hypokalaemia, pregnancy, hydronephrosis or drugs (e.g. lithium).

44. C Renal artery stenosis

Primary hyperaldosteronism is an excess production of aldosterone, independent of the renin–angiotensin–aldosterone system. Features suggestive of hyperaldosteronism include hypertension with hypokalaemia and alkalosis. Greater than 50% of cases are due to Conn's syndrome; a unilateral adrenocortical adenoma. The most appropriate form of treatment in this case is laparoscopic removal of the tumour. Other causes of primary hyperaldosteronism include bilateral adrenal hyperplasia; spironolactone therapy is often successful in treating these cases.

Secondary causes of hyperaldosteronism include renal artery stenosis which leads to a perceived hypoperfusion of the kidney and increased secretion of renin and aldosterone. The hypertension is often refractory to treatment, especially with angiotensin converting enzyme inhibitors.

Syndrome of inappropriate antidiuretic hormone (ADH) secretion has multiple causes including small cell carcinoma of the lung, stroke, encephalitis and postoperatively. Excessive secretion of ADH leads to hyponatraemia and fluid overload.

45. B HIV

Addison's disease is caused by primary adrenocortical insufficiency, most commonly with an autoimmune cause. It has an incidence of approximately 1/100,000 and is therefore relatively rare. Autoimmunity may lead to antibodies against the adrenal gland and may be associated with other autoimmune diseases, including thyroid disease, pernicious anaemia and diabetes. Other causes include tuberculosis and acute bleeding into the adrenal gland (Waterhouse–Friderichsen syndrome). HIV is now a common cause of Addison's disease in areas, where HIV is prevalent. Sarcoidosis is not classically known to cause Addison's disease.

46. C Short ACTH stimulation test

Addison's disease does not become apparent until 90% of the gland is destroyed. Hyperkalaemia and hyponatraemia are usual initial laboratory findings with symptoms of fatigue, abdominal pain, weakness, constipation, hyperpigmentation and weight loss. In severe cases of Addisonian crisis there may be postural hypotension, confusion. Diagnosis is usually confirmed with the short adrenocorticotrophic hormone (ACTH) stimulation test (also known as the Synacthen test), when plasma cortisol levels are tested before and after synthetic ACTH. The long ACTH stimulation test may be used once the results of the initial short test are noted to be abnormal.

In treating Addison's disease, it is essential to replace glucocorticoids (hydrocortisone) and mineralocorticoids (fludrocortisone). Hyperpigmentation is caused by an excess of ACTH which is released by the pituitary in order to trigger production of cortisol by the adrenal gland. In secondary adrenal failure there is low ACTH due to deficient corticotrophin-releasing hormone release by the hypothalamus.

47. A Dopamine

Catecholamines are derived from the amino acid tyrosine and have a half life in the circulation of a few minutes. The first step is the conversion of tyrosine to L-dopa by the enzyme tyrosine hydroxylase, and it is this reaction which forms the rate limiting step in the synthetic pathway. Dopamine is the first catecholamine to be produced, followed by norepinephrine and epinephrine. Catecholamines are degraded by catechol-O-methyltransferase (COMT) or monoamine oxidases (MAO).

48. B Hyperglycaemia

Phaeochromocytoma is a tumour that produces catecholamines and is a rare cause of resistant hypertension. It is usually found in the adrenal medulla, however 10% are found elsewhere. Other symptoms include palpitations and psychological symptoms. Investigation may reveal glycosuria in up to one-third of patients. Hyperglycaemia is caused primarily by the stimulation of lipolysis because of catecholamine production. Stimulation at β-adrenergic receptors leads to glycogenolysis and gluconeogenesis. Thirty per cent of patients have glycosuria during attacks. Investigations to establish a diagnosis of phaeochromocytoma include 24-hour urine collection for vanillylmandelic acid which is a catecholamine metabolite. Hyperkalaemia and basophilia are not typically associated with phaeochromocytoma.

49. D Increase glycogenolysis

Glucagon is a polypeptide composed of 21 amino acids. It is synthesised by the islet cells of the pancreas and is essential in the control of glucose homeostasis. Secretion is stimulated by low glucose states and is inhibited if blood sugars are raised. In states of low blood glucose, there is an increase in the activity of the sympathetic nervous system which causes an increase in circulating adrenaline. This in turn stimulates the β-adrenoreceptors and leads to an increase in glucagon. The main action of glucagon is to increase blood glucose and leads to a breakdown in stored fat and protein; it acts mainly on the liver.

50. E Somatostatin

Insulin is a peptide hormone synthesised and secreted by the β cells of the islet of Langerhans of the pancreas. It is secreted as a prohormone which gets converted to an active hormone by proteolytic cleavage of the C-peptide. Insulin is the main hormone controlling the blood glucose levels. Insulin is released in response to increased amino acids, free fatty acids and gastric hormone which are released in response to eating, including cholecystokinin, gastrin and secretin. Insulin release is inhibited by adrenaline and somatostatin.

51. E Stimulates growth of endometrium

Oestrogen causes the following effects on:

Coagulation

- Increase circulating coagulating factors, including plasminogen, factors II, VII, IX, X. Increase antithrombin III

Lipids
- Increase high-density lipoproteins
- Increase triglycerides
- Reduce low-density lipoproteins

Gastrointestinal
- Reduce bowel motility

Structural
- Stimulate endometrial growth
- Increase discharge and lubrication
- Increase bone formation
- Promote formation of secondary sexual characteristics

Fluid balance
- Increase salt and water retention

52. B Increases respiratory drive

Progesterone is a C-21 steroid hormone derived from cholesterol. As well as increasing respiratory drive it reduces bowel motility and increases basal body temperature. Levels increase during the luteal phase of the menstrual cycle in preparation for fertilisation of the ovum. If pregnancy does not occur, the corpus luteum degenerates and levels of progesterone fall. Progesterone protects the endometrium from cancer.

53. C Oestradiol decreases and FSH increases

During each menstrual cycle up to ten secondary follicles are recruited; of which one will become a dominant follicle and the rest regress. There is pulsatile production of gonadotrophin releasing hormones from the hypothalamus and subsequent release of follicle-stimulating hormone (FSH) and luteinising hormone (LH) from the pituitary. The developing follicle produces oestrogen under the influence of FSH. LH acts on the thecal cells of the ovary to produce androgens. There is feedback from the ovarian hormones to the pituitary and hypothalamus. The follicle stimulates the ovary to produce oestrogen which stimulates production of the glandular endometrium. As oestrogen levels increase, 14 days before the onset of menstruation it becomes high enough to trigger a surge of LH which in turn stimulates ovulation. Once the egg has been released, the corpus luteum causes increased production of progesterone and subsequent proliferation of endometrium. If fertilisation does not occur, hormones levels fall as a result of the failing corpus luteum and there is the onset of menstruation.

54. B It is surrounded by theca cells

A layer of thecal cells surrounds the mature follicle once it has reached the secondary stage with two layers of granulosa cells. Both of these layers of cells serve to protect the developing follicle. During development, an oocyte will grow up to 120 μm in diameter. Development is controlled primarily by follicle-stimulating hormone, rather than luteinising hormone and it does not produce progesterone.

55. D Increase in fasting insulin

Polycystic ovary syndrome (PCOS) is the most common endocrine disturbance affecting women. It can be familial. Signs and symptoms vary amongst women and even in an individual over time. Clinical symptoms range from obesity, to menstrual irregularities, to subfertility, hirsutism, and acne. Elevations in insulin are common in both thin and obese women with PCOS. It is thought that the insulin stimulates androgen secretion. There appears to be an insulin resistance in these women who then have an increase risk of developing diabetes.

56. C Hyperprolactinaemia

Sex hormone-binding globulin (SHBG) is synthesised in the liver. 80% of testosterone is bound to SHBG, 19% to albumin and 1% is unbound. Biological effects of circulating androgens depend primarily on the unbound fraction. Its production is decreased by androgens and insulin. On the other hand, oestrogen increases the production of SHBG and hence hirsutism is improved by taking the oral contraceptive pill and during pregnancy.

Chapter 5

Statistics and epidemiology

Questions: MCQs

Answer each stem 'True' or 'False'.

1. **Standard deviation:**
    A   Is the square root of the variance
    B   50% of the data set lies within one standard deviation from the mean
    C   95% of the data lies within two standard deviations from the mean
    D   Cannot be used for a data set with a skewed distribution
    E   One standard deviation is equal to the mode

2. **Concerning parametric data:**
    A   Analysis assumes a normal distribution
    B   Ordinal data is a form of parametric data
    C   The Mann–Whitney U test is a parametric test
    D   The *t*-test may be used to look at two sets of parametric data
    E   Parametric tests have more 'power' than non-parametric tests

3. **A valid screening test:**
    A   Is highly specific
    B   Is able to provide a diagnosis
    C   Is widely available
    D   Can identify rare conditions
    E   Is used only for treatable conditions

4. **In a sample of 10,000 women the age at the delivery of their first child showed a normal distribution. The mean age at delivery of their first child was 29 years old, with a standard deviation of 2 years.**
    A   Two standard deviations from the mean is 33 years old
    B   The variance is 3 years
    C   No primiparous woman would be older than 40 years of age
    D   The median age for a primiparous woman would be 29 years
    E   The standard error of the mean is 0.02

5. **Concerning a sample with a normal distribution:**
    A   It can also be described as having a Gaussian distribution
    B   50% of the data set lie within two standard deviations from the mean
    C   The median is higher than the mean
    D   It may be bimodal
    E   The mode lies at the centre of the distribution

6. **Regarding statistical tests:**
    A   Student's t-test can be used to compare the means of non-parametric data
    B   The χ^2 test can be used with categorical data
    C   The Mann–Whitney U test can be used for skewed data
    D   Fisher's exact test is a non-parametric test
    E   Non-parametric tests have greater power than parametric tests

7. **The standard error of the mean:**
    A   Is a measure of how close the sample mean is to the population mean
    B   Is also known as the standard deviation of the mean
    C   Is the square root of the sample size
    D   Is small when the sample mean is close to the population mean
    E   Is smaller with a larger sample size

8. **Concerning obtaining valid consent for a procedure:**
    A   Risks of side effects can be given as ratios
    B   All possible unexpected surgical interventions should be mentioned
    C   Verbal consent is acceptable in emergencies
    D   The patient can validly request the clinician gives consent on their behalf
    E   In the absence of prior counselling a woman can consent for sterilisation during a caesarean section

9. **The following are indirect causes of maternal mortality:**
    A   Pre-eclampsia
    B   Cardiac disease
    C   Suicide
    D   Thrombosis
    E   Epilepsy

Questions: SBAs

For each question, select the single best answer from the five options listed.

10. Which of the following is a quality of the median of a data set?

    A   It cannot be distorted by skewed data
    B   It is always higher than the mean
    C   It is obtained by dividing the sum of the data set by the number of values in the data set
    D   It is the middle value in a ranked set of data
    E   It is the most frequently occurring value in a data set

11. What is the World Health Organisation's definition of the perinatal mortality rate?

    A   The number of deaths in the 1st week of life per 1,000 live births
    B   The number of stillbirths and deaths in the first week of life per 1,000 live births
    C   The number of stillbirths and deaths in the first week of life per 10,000 live births
    D   The number of stillbirths and deaths in the first week of life per 100,000 live births
    E   The number of stillbirths and deaths in the first 28 days of life per 1,000 deliveries

12. The Eighth Confidential Enquiry into Maternal Deaths in the United Kingdom defines maternal mortality as:

    A   The number of deaths per 1000 pregnancies
    B   The number of deaths per 100,000 pregnancies
    C   The number of direct and indirect deaths per 100,000 mortalities
    D   The number of direct and indirect deaths per 10,000 mortalities
    E   The number of direct and indirect deaths per 100,000 pregnancies

13. Within what time frame does the Centre for Maternal and Child Enquiries (CMACE) consider maternal death to have occurred?

    A   During pregnancy
    B   During pregnancy or within 28 days of the end of the pregnancy
    C   During pregnancy or within 42 days of the end of the pregnancy
    D   Within 14 days of the end of the pregnancy
    E   Within 42 days of the end of the pregnancy

14. An early pregnancy unit undertakes a study to look at the average serum β-human chorionic gonadotrophin (β-hCG) level of women presenting to their unit with vaginal spotting over a 2-month period. The data collected has a normal distribution.

The following values are obtained:
- Mean = 500 IU/L
- N = 200
- Variance = 16

What is the data set's standard deviation?

A   2
B   3
C   4
D   9
E   12

15. An antenatal clinic undertakes a month long study looking at the diastolic blood pressure of women at their antenatal booking visit. The data collected has a normal Gaussian distribution.

The following values are obtained:
N = 93
Mean diastolic blood pressure = 82 mmHg
Variance = 9

What is the standard deviation of the data set?

A   2
B   3
C   5
D   12
E   18

16. One hundred women with postmenopausal bleeding have pelvic ultrasound scans to measure endometrial thickness and have a pipelle biopsy taken.

The findings of the scan – normal or thickened endometrial thickness – and the subsequent histology of the Pipelle biopsies – normal or showing endometrial cancer – are shown in the table below.

Pelvic scan result	Endometrial cancer on Pipelle (n)	Normal endometrium on Pipelle (n)	Total (n)
Abnormal	10	8	18
Normal	2	80	82
Total	12	88	100

What is the sensitivity (to the closest per cent) of the pelvic scan in detecting endometrial cancer?

A   25%
B   55%
C   83%
D   91%
E   98%

17. One hundred women with postmenopausal bleeding have pelvic ultrasound scans to measure endometrial thickness and have a pipelle biopsy taken.

The findings of the scan, normal or thickened endometrial thickness, and the subsequent histology of the Pipelle biopsies, normal or showing endometrial cancer, are shown in the table below.

Pelvic scan result	Endometrial cancer on Pipelle (n)	Normal endometrium on Pipelle (n)	Total (n)
Abnormal	10	8	18
Normal	2	80	82
Total	12	88	100

What is the specificity (to the closest per cent) of the pelvic scan in detecting endometrial cancer?

A 25%
B 55%
C 83%
D 91%
E 98%

18. Which of the following is an aim of clinical audit?

A To reject or accept a null hypothesis
B To assess the extent to which current practice meets a defined set of standards
C To assess differences between two different populations
D To establish what is best practice
E To extrapolate theory into practice

19. A study was designed to look at the relative risk of women with gestational diabetes mellitus (GDM) who delivered babies with a birth weight of over 4.5 kg. The study looked at all births in the Grace Maternity Unit over a period of 1 year and classified whether the woman had GDM or not, and whether their baby weighed more or less than 4.5 kg.

Birth weight	Diabetic (n)	Control (n)	Total
> 4.5 kg	80	50	130
< 4.5 kg	120	950	1070
Total	200	1000	1200

What is the relative risk of women with GDM delivering a baby weighing > 4.5 kg in this study?

A 0.05
B 0.1
C 0.4
D 8
E 150

Answers

1. A True

    B False

    C True

    D False

    E False

    Standard deviation is a measure of the scatter of the sample data around the mean. When data has a normal distribution, it is acceptable to consider the mean and the median to be equivalent. When there is a normal distribution, 68.1% of the data set will fall within one (+/–) standard deviation from the mean and 95.4% of the data set will sit within two (+/–) standard deviations from the mean (**Figure 5.1**). The standard deviation may be calculated by taking the square root of the variance. The standard deviation may used for a skewed data set; however, it is likely to be of limited use and interquartile ranges may be of more use. In order to obtain an accurate standard deviation for skewed data, it is advisable to apply logarithmic transformation.

    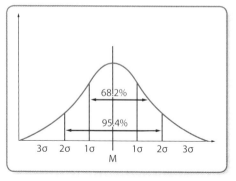

    Figure 5.1 A normal distribution. M, mean; σ, standard deviation.

2. A True

    B False

    C False

    D True

    E True

    Parametric data is essentially numerical data. It may be continuous, i.e. β-human chorionic gonadotrophin levels, or discrete, e.g. length of hospital stay. Non-parametric data may be ordinal data, e.g. first, second and third prizes in a competitive sport, or nominal data, e.g. Rhesus status being negative or positive. Parametric tests make a number of assumptions including that of a normal distribution. Parametric tests have more power than non-parametric tests, therefore we can have more confidence in their robustness and ability to find a statistically significance difference between data sets if the difference exists. Examples of parametric tests include Student's *t*-test and the one way analysis of variance (ANOVA) test.

Altman D, Bland JM. Parametric versus non-parametric methods for data analysis. BMJ 2009; 338:a3167.

3. A True

   B False

   C True

   D False

   E True

Screening tests are widely used as a means of identifying individuals who are at a high-risk of having or developing a disease or condition. Antenatal screening of pregnant women to assess the likelihood of their current pregnancy of being affected by a common trisomy, such as Trisomy 21, is an example of an effective screening programme. Screening tests should be widely available and should only used for either treatable conditions or in circumstances where the result allows affected individuals to make a decision on how to proceed, e.g. the termination of a pregnancy affected by a trisomy. Screening tests must be easily reproducible, cost-effective and acceptable to the population at risk. A screening test does not provide a final diagnosis; however, it must have a high sensitivity and specificity.

Programme Appraisal Criteria: Criteria for appraising the viability, effectiveness and appropriateness of a screening programme. UK National Screening Committee. www.screening.nhs.uk/criteria

4. A True

   B False

   C False

   D True

   E True

This data set shows a normal Gaussian distribution. On this basis, it is fair to assume that the median, mode and mean for the data set will be the same. Standard deviation (SD) is a measure of the scatter of the data set from the mean. In a data set with a normal distribution 68.2% of a data set will lie within one SD from the mean, whereas 95% of the sample will lie within approximately two (1.96) SDs from the mean. Variance is a measure of the extent to which each observation in the data set deviates from the data set mean. Variance may be calculated by squaring the standard deviation:

$$\text{Variance} = (\text{SD})^2$$

The standard error (SE) of the mean estimates how close the mean of the data set is to the mean of the population. The SE of the mean can be calculated by dividing the SD by the square root of the sample size:

$$\text{SE} = \text{SD}/\sqrt{\text{sample size}}$$

5. A True

    B False

    C False

    D False

    E True

    A data set with a normal distribution may also be described as having a Gaussian distribution. Pictorially a normal distribution may be represented using a bell-shaped curve, reflecting its unimodal properties. Within a normal distribution the majority of the sample set lie around the mean, giving the distribution a symmetrical shape. The mean and the median values are the same within a sample with a normal distribution. The population, from which the data set was taken, can be approximated by a normal distribution. The standard deviation (SD) is a measure of the spread of the data set around the mean. Approximately 68% of the data set in a normal distribution sits within one SD from the mean, whereas approximately 95% of the data set sits within two SDs from the mean.

6. A False

    B True

    C True

    D True

    E False

    The statistical test used to analyse a set of data must be carefully chosen and is dictated by the type of data, how it was obtained and the sample size. Parametric tests have greater power than non-parametric tests. Parametric tests make the assumption that the data has a normal distribution, whereas non-parametric tests do not. Parametric tests can only be used on parametric data, i.e. interval data. Ordinal and nominal data is classified as non-parametric data and can only be assessed using non-parametric statistical tests. Student's t-test is a simple and straightforward test that can be used to compare the means of two sample groups. The t-test can be performed on paired or unpaired parametric data. Two equivalent tests that can be used on non-parametric data are the Mann–Whitney U test and the Wilcoxon Rank Sum test. The Mann–Whitney U test may also be used on non-parametric skewed data. The Chi-square test is a non-parametric test and may be used with categorical data. Fisher's exact test is also a non-parametric test used for categorical data; however, it can be used for smaller sample sets.

    Greenhalgh T. How to read a paper: Statistics for the non-statistician. I: Different types of data need different statistical tests. BMJ 1997; 315:364.

7. A True

    B True

    C False

D True

E True

The standard error of the mean (SEM) is a measure of how close the sample mean of a data set is to the population mean (from which that sample has been taken from). The SEM is also known as the standard deviation of the mean. The SEM can be calculated by dividing the standard deviation by the square root of the sample size. The smaller the value obtained for the SEM, the closer the sample mean lies to the population mean. Further, the larger the sample size, the more representative the sample is of the population, and therefore the more accurate and, in theory smaller, the SEM.

$SEM = s \div \sqrt{n}$

Where; s = standard deviation, n = sample size.

8. A True

   B False

   C True

   D False

   E False

Risks of a procedure should be explained in a way that is most understandable by the patient. The use of numerical aids may be helpful. For some patients, the estimation of risk may be usefully explained using ratios, e.g. '1 in 1000' rather than as percentages, e.g. '0.1%'.

Valid consent for sterilisation cannot be obtained whilst the woman is having a caesarean section, unless counselling has previously taken place and provisional consent has already been given.

Royal College of Obstetricians and Gynaecologists. Obtaining Valid Consent. Clinical Governance Guide 6. London: RCOG, 2008.

9. A False

   B True

   C True

   D False

   E True

The 8th report of the Confidential Enquiries into Maternal Deaths in the United Kingdom classified causes as maternal death directly related, indirectly related or unrelated to pregnancy. Indirectly related causes are those that were not the direct result of obstetric complications but were made worse due to the physiological changes associated with pregnancy. Both conditions that were diagnosed prior to or during pregnancy can be classified as indirectly related causes. In the current report, as in recent previous reports, cardiac disease was the predominant indirectly related cause of maternal death. Suicide is classified as an indirectly related cause of maternal mortality because of the strong association with puerperal mental illness. Other indirect causes include epilepsy, diabetes and (within the UK) death from hormone-dependent malignancies. Causes such as pre-eclampsia and thrombosis are directly related causes of maternal mortality, i.e. death occurs as a direct consequence of an obstetric cause.

Centre for Maternal and Child Enquiries (CMACE). Saving Mothers' Lives: Reviewing Maternal Deaths to Make Motherhood Safer: 2006–2008. The Eighth Report on Confidential Enquiries into Maternal Deaths in the United Kingdom. BJOG 2011;118:1–203.

10. D It is the middle value in a ranked set of data

The median is one of the terms used to describe an 'average' of a set of data. The median is the middle value in a ranked data set. It should not be confused with the mode which refers to the most frequently occurring value in a data set. It also differs from the mean which is calculated by dividing the sum of data set by the number of values in the data set. An advantage of using the median is that it is not influenced by outliers or skewed data, which can affect the mean of a data set. The median figure in a data set may be higher or lower than the mean.

11. B The number of stillbirths and deaths in the first week of life per 1,000 live births

The World Health Organisation currently defines the perinatal mortality rate as the number of stillbirths and deaths in the first week of life per 1,000 live births (in a given period). It should not be confused with neonatal mortality, which is the number of deaths in the first completed 28 days of life per 1,000 live births. Perinatal mortality can be an important contributor to the overall neonatal mortality rate of a population.

World Health Organisation. Health Status Statistics: Mortality. Neonatal mortality rate (per 1000 live births). http://www.who.int

12. C The number of direct and indirect deaths per 100,000 mortalities

The Eighth Confidential Enquiries into Maternal Deaths in the United Kingdom defines maternal mortality as the number of direct and indirect deaths per 100, 000 mortalities. Direct causes of maternal mortality are those that result from obstetric complications and include sepsis, haemorrhage, pre-eclampsia/eclampsia and amniotic fluid embolism. Indirect causes are those that are not caused by obstetric complications but were made worse due to the physiological changes associated with pregnancy. These indirect causes may include conditions that were pre-existing or were diagnosed during pregnancy. Indirect causes of maternal mortality include conditions such as cardiac disease, diabetes, epilepsy and suicide.

Centre for Maternal and Child Enquiries (CMACE). Saving Mothers' Lives: Reviewing Maternal Deaths to Make Motherhood Safer: 2006–2008. The Eighth Report on Confidential Enquiries into Maternal Deaths in the United Kingdom. BJOG 2011;118:1–203.

13. C During pregnancy or within 42 days of the end of the pregnancy

According to the Centre for Maternal and Child Enquiries (CMACE) a maternal death is one that has occurred during pregnancy or within 42 days of the end of the pregnancy. The cause of the death should be related to pregnancy or, if due to a disease process, be of a nature that the condition had been made worse due to the physiological changes associated with pregnancy. Accidental deaths are not included. Deaths may be due to direct or indirect causes. Direct causes are those that are of a direct obstetric nature, i.e. eclampsia, as opposed to indirect causes which do not have a direct obstetric cause but relate to conditions which have become more severe in pregnancy.

Centre for Maternal and Child Enquiries (CMACE). Saving Mothers' Lives: Reviewing Maternal Deaths to Make Motherhood Safer: 2006–2008. The Eighth Report on Confidential Enquiries into Maternal Deaths in the United Kingdom. BJOG 2011;118:1–203.

14. C 4

The standard deviation of a sample is merely a measure of the scatter of the data set around the mean. The variance is a measure of how far each observation within the sample varies from the mean. Knowledge of the basic formula used to calculate standard deviation is key to answering this question. The variance can be calculated by taking the square root of the variance. There are other formulas that can be used to calculate the standard deviation but from the limited information given this simple formula should be used.

Worked answer:

Standard deviation = square root of the variance
Variance = 16
Square root of 16 = 4
Therefore, the standard deviation = 4

15. B 3

The standard deviation of the data set is a measure of how much the data is scattered from the data set mean. All the information required to calculate the standard deviation for the data set is given. The simple calculation of taking the square root of the variance is all that is required to obtain the standard deviation. Any other values given are distracters and can be ignored.

Worked answer:

Standard deviation = square root of the variance
Variance = 9
Square root of 9 = 3
Therefore the standard deviation = 3

16. C 83%

The sensitivity of a test, in this case the pelvic ultrasound, refers to the proportion of individuals with the disease in question who were correctly identified by the test. In this study, this can be considered as the proportion of women who were found on Pipelle biopsy to have endometrial cancer, who were correctly identified as having an abnormal pelvic ultrasound. In order for a test to be a useful investigation the specificity should be as close to 100% as possible. Sensitivity can be calculated by taking the number of subjects diagnosed with the condition using the initial/ screening test, divided by the total number of the all individuals diagnosed with the condition (whether detected by the screening test or not). To give a percentage the result is multiplied by 100.

Worked answer:

Sensitivity = endometrial cancer (with abnormal ultrasound) / endometrial cancer (with abnormal ultrasound) + endometrial cancer (with normal ultrasound) x 100

$10/(10 + 2) = 10/12 = 0.83$

$0.83 \times 100 = 83\%$

17. E 98%

The specificity of a test refers to the proportion of individuals who were confirmed not to have the disease who were correctly identified as normal by the test. In this scenario, it refers to the proportion of individuals without endometrial cancer who had a normal pelvic ultrasound scan. In similarity to sensitivity, ideally the specificity of a test should be as close to 100% as possible. Specificity can be calculated by dividing the number of individuals without the condition who had a normal result from the initial screening test by the total number of individuals without the condition (including those who initially had an abnormal initial test).

Worked answer:

Specificity = not diagnosed with endometrial cancer (with normal ultrasound) / not diagnosed with endometrial cancer (with normal ultrasound) + not diagnosed with endometrial cancer (with abnormal ultrasound) x 100

$80/(80 + 2) = 80/82 = 0.98$

$0.98 \times 100 = 98\%$

Loong T. Understanding sensitivity and specificity with the right side of the brain. BMJ 2003; 327:716.

18. B To assess the extent to which current practice meets a defined set of standards

It is important to be able to distinguish the difference between research and audit. Both are integral to the advancement of medical knowledge and clinical practice. Of the statements given for this question only the stem 'to assess the extent to which current practice meets a defined set of standards' is a valid aim of audit. All of the other stems actually refer to aims of research studies. Audit should occur regularly within a clinical setting to assess how practice standards are being met and the need to implement strategies for improvement. The process of audit is described as a continuous cycle, starting with defining the standards of the area of interest, collecting data, making an assessment of current practice and whether it meets the standards, followed by identifying and implementing any required changes in practice.

Wade D. Ethics, audit, and research: all shades of grey. BMJ 2005; 330:468

Hardman E, Joughin C. Clinical Audit: What it is and what it isn't. In: FOCUS on Clinical Audit in Child and Adolescent Mental Health Services. London: Royal College of Psychiatrists, 1998. http://www.rcpsych.ac.uk

19. D 8

Calculating relative risk is a means of quantifying the risk of an event, or a disease relative to exposure to a contributory factor. A calculated risk of an event/condition equal to one indicates that there is no difference between those exposed to the factor and those who were not. A relative risk of less than one suggests that the exposure group is less likely to develop the condition than the non-exposure, whereas a relative risk of greater than one indicates that the risk of condition is increased in the exposure group relative to the non-exposure group. For this study, the calculated relative risk of women with gestational diabetes mellitus (GDM), in this study, delivering a baby weighing > 4.5 kg was eight. This indicates that women with GDM had eight times the risk of having a baby weighing > 4.5 kg. **Table 5.1** sets out the groups for calculation of relative risk.

Table 5.1 Calculating relative risk			
Event/condition of interest	Exposed group	Non-exposed group	Total
Yes	A	B	A + B
No	C	D	C + D
Total	A + C	B + D	A + B + C + D

Relative risk can be calculated as below:

$$\text{Relative risk} = \frac{A/(A + C)}{B/(B + D)}$$

Using the data supplied in the question:

Proportion of diabetic mothers with babies > 4.5 kg = 80/200 = 0.4

Proportion of non-diabetic mothers with babies > 4.5 kg = 50/1000 = 0.05

Relative risk of diabetic women delivering a baby weighing 4.5 kg = 40/5 = 8

$$\text{Relative risk} = \frac{80/(80 + 120)}{50/(50 + 950)} = 8$$

Chapter 6

Genetics

Questions: MCQs

Answer each stem 'True' or 'False'.

1. **Concerning chromosomes:**
    - A Each consists of two identical chromatids
    - B They are best visualised during interphase
    - C The short arm of a chromosome is also known as the 'q' arm
    - D Humans have 23 pairs of autosomal chromosomes
    - E The centromere is the meeting point of two chromatids

2. **Cystic fibrosis is:**
    - A An X-linked recessive condition
    - B Associated with gene defect of chromosome 9
    - C Most commonly caused by deletion of F508
    - D Characterised by a defect in potassium ion transport
    - E Caused by a defect in the cystic fibrosis transmembrane conductance gene

3. **The following conditions show an X-linked form of inheritance:**
    - A Fragile X
    - B Duchenne's muscular dystrophy
    - C Turner's syndrome
    - D Christmas disease
    - E Prader–Willi syndrome

4. **The following conditions are caused by chromosome microdeletions:**
    - A Angelman syndrome
    - B Cri-du-chat
    - C Di-George syndrome
    - D Rett syndrome
    - E Tay–Sachs disease

5. **An increased nuchal translucency thickness may be seen in fetuses with:**
    - A Cardiac defects
    - B Down's syndrome
    - C Noonan's syndrome
    - D Patau's syndrome
    - E Turner's syndrome

6. **Regarding aneuploidies:**
   A   Trisomy 16 is the most common trisomy in miscarried fetuses
   B   Monosomy X is incompatible with life
   C   Individuals with triple X have multiorgan abnormalities
   D   Noonan's syndrome is caused by trisomy of chromosome 12
   E   The majority of trisomies follow a non-disjunction event at meiosis 1

Questions: SBAs

For each question, select the single best answer from the five options listed.

7. A woman presents at approximately 40 weeks' gestation in spontaneous labour;
    she is unbooked and has received no antenatal care. On abdominal palpation,
    she feels large of her reported gestational age. A small male infant is born by
    emergency caesarean section due to fetal distress. The baby is found to have
    microcephaly, a prominent occiput, a cleft lip and palate, clenched hands and
    polydactyl. Soon after birth, he has apnoeic episodes and has difficulty feeding.

    What chromosomal abnormality is the most likely cause of this baby's presentation?

    A   Microdeletion of chromosome 15
    B   Microdeletion of chromosome 22
    C   Trisomy 13
    D   Trisomy 18
    E   Trisomy 21

8. A 32-year-old woman is 15 weeks pregnant with her second pregnancy. She opts
    to have antenatal screening and has blood taken as part of the quadruple test.
    The result shows reduced levels of α-fetoprotein and unconjugated oestriol with
    elevated β-human chorionic gonadotrophin.

    Which of the following is the most likely explanation for the screening results:

    A   Down's syndrome
    B   Edwards' syndrome
    C   Multiple pregnancy
    D   Neural tube defect
    E   Normal pregnancy

9. A 39-year-old multiparous woman is 13 weeks pregnant. She has serum screening
    as part of the combined test. Analysis shows an elevated level of α-fetoprotein and
    a normal level of pregnancy-associated plasma protein A.

    What diagnosis are the screening results suggestive of?

    A   Down's syndrome
    B   Edwards' syndrome
    C   Multiple pregnancy
    D   Neural tube defect
    E   Normal pregnancy

10. A 37-year-old primiparous woman is 14 weeks pregnant. Following serum
    screening, the pregnancy is found to have an increased risk of trisomy 21. She
    wishes to have further testing to confirm whether the fetus is affected.

    In view of her current gestation what is the most appropriate diagnostic test?

    A   Amniocentesis
    B   Cell-free fetal DNA sampling

C   Chorionic villus sampling
D   Cordocentesis
E   Nuchal translucency imaging

11. A 29-year-old woman seeks genetic counselling as she has a number of her female relatives who have had either breast or ovarian cancer. Both her mother and her sister have been diagnosed with breast cancer. DNA sequencing subsequently shows that she carries a mutated form of the *BRCA1* gene.

Via which mode of inheritance is the *BRCA1* gene mutation transmitted?

A   Autosomal dominant inheritance
B   Autosomal recessive inheritance
C   Mitochondrial inheritance
D   X-linked dominant inheritance
E   X-linked recessive inheritance

12. A 34-year-old woman delivers a male baby with Down's syndrome. Chromosomal analysis following his birth is suggestive of familial Down's syndrome.

What chromosomal event best describes the aetiology of Familial Down's syndrome?

A   Microdeletion
B   Nonsense mutation
C   Reciprocal translocation
D   Robertsonian translocation
E   Triplet repeat expansion

13. A couple are both known to carry the trait for a haemoglobinopathy. They decline any invasive testing when they conceive their first pregnancy. At an anomaly scan at 20 weeks' gestation the fetus is found to have severe hydrops. In utero death occurs at 22 weeks' gestation.

What is the most likely cause of the fetal demise?

A   Alpha-thalassaemia with deletion of 4α-globin genes
B   Beta-thalassaemia major
C   Glucose-6-dehydrogenase deficiency
D   Haemoglobin H disease
E   Sickle cell disease

Answers

1. A True

    B False

    C False

    D False

    E True

    Chromosomes consist of long strands of DNA which have been elaborately folded and coiled. Within the strands of DNA are sequences which are genes. In eukaryotic cells, they are found in the cell nuclei, where the DNA material is packaged as chromatin. Each chromosome consists of two identical chromatids which are held together in the midline at the centromere. The shape of chromosomes may be described according to the position of the centromere. The short arm of a chromosome is known as the 'P' arm, whereas the long arm is known as the 'Q' arm. Humans have 22 autosomal chromosome pairs and one pair of sex chromosomes in each cell. Chromosomes are best visualised in the metaphase of mitosis. Giemsa staining may be used to aid visualisation of gene rich areas, which aids chromosome identification in a process called G-banding. See **Figure 6.1** for the basic structure of a chromosome.

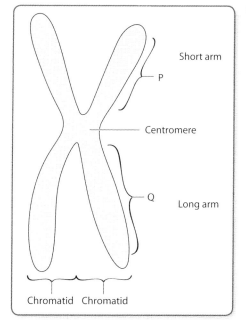

Figure 6.1 Basic structure of a chromosome.

2. A False

    B False

C True

D False

E True

Cystic fibrosis (CF) is an autosomal recessive condition affecting exocrine function. CF is typically found in Caucasian populations and is considered a life-limiting condition. It is often associated with manifestations such as severe lung disease, pancreatic insufficiency and infertility.

CF is caused by a defect in the cystic fibrosis transmembrane conductance regulator (CFTR) gene found on chromosome 7. This leads to a defect in the CTFR protein which normally acts as a chloride channel. There is defective transport of chloride ions across epithelial cell membranes and an accumulation of intracellular sodium leading to an excess of thick secretions on mucosal surfaces. CF is caused by a large number of mutations in the CFTR gene; however, the most commonly identified defect is a deletion of the 508th codon of the gene, leading to the absence of a phenylalanine residue. This mutation is usually denoted as ΔF508.

3. A True

   B True

   C False

   D True

   E False

Fragile X is inherited by X-linked dominant inheritance, caused by defect in the *FMR1* gene. X-linked dominant conditions can affect both males and females; as males (XY) contribute the Y chromosome to their male offspring they cannot pass on their defective X chromosome to their sons, however all of their daughters inherit their X chromosome.

Duchenne's muscular dystrophy shows an X-linked recessive inheritance; the defective gene is carried on the X chromosome, leading to males inheriting the one defective X chromosome from their mother expressing the condition. Female offspring who inherit one defective X chromosome act as carriers only due to the presence of two X chromosomes. Other X-linked recessive conditions include haemophilia A, Christmas disease (haemophilia B) and glucose-6-phosphate dehydrogenase deficiency. Prader–Willi syndrome is not an X-linked condition and is associated with a deletion of the paternally derived chromosome 15. Turner's syndrome affects females and is an abnormality of the sex chromosomes, typically due a loss of a Barr body leading to monosomy X.

4. A True

   B True

   C True

   D False

   E False

A series of syndromes have been identified that arise due to chromosomal microdeletions. A microdeletion refers to the loss of a small subset of genes which are found adjacent to each other on a chromosome. Syndromes caused by microdeletions tend to have common characteristics including learning difficulties, dysmorphic facial features and organ abnormalities such as cardiac anomalies often occurring. Many cases of Angelman syndrome are caused by a microdeletion associated with the loss the maternally inherited chromosome 15; its equivalent is Prader–Willi syndrome which can be caused by loss of the paternally inherited chromosome 15. Di-George and Shprintzen syndromes are both associated with deletion of the proximal long arm of chromosome 22. Cri-du-chat syndrome is caused by a loss of part of the short arm of chromosome 5 (**Table 6.1**).

Table 6.1 Examples of syndromes caused by chromosome microdeletions

Microdeletion syndrome	Chromosome affected
Cri-du-chat	5
Williams	7
Angelman	15
Prader–Willi	15
Smith–Magenis	17
Di-George	22

5. **A** True

   B True

   C True

   D True

   E True

Nuchal translucency refers to the measurement of the subcutaneous fluid at the back of the fetal neck using ultrasound. Increased nuchal translucency thickness, when measured between 11 and 14 weeks' gestation, has been associated with a number of chromosomal abnormalities and structural defects. Down's syndrome is the most commonly referred cause of increased nuchal thickness. Used alongside the serum markers used in the combined test, data obtained from nuchal translucency measurement is capable of identifying 90% of fetuses affected by Down's syndrome. Fetuses with Patau's syndrome and Edwards' syndrome may also have an increased nuchal thickness, as do female fetuses affected by the monosomy Turner's syndrome. Noonan's syndrome is an autosomal dominant condition which may be first detected by ultrasound in fetuses with a normal karyotype alongside nuchal oedema and pleural effusions. In addition to the syndromes described above there is a strong association between increased nuchal thickness and major cardiac abnormalities.

6. A True

    B False

    C False

    D False

    E True

    Aneuploidy refers to an abnormal number of chromosomes and can occur both to autosomes and the sex chromosomes. The majority of trisomies occur following a non-disjunction event which occurs in the meiotic division. The most common trisomy found in miscarried fetuses is trisomy 16 which is incompatible with life. Trisomy 21 is the most common trisomy compatible with life. Babies with trisomies 13 and 18 have a considerably shortened life expectancy, with the majority not surviving infancy. Individuals with a trisomy of the X chromosome typically have normal lives and their aneuploidy is often not diagnosed. The loss of an autosome, i.e. a monosomy of a chromosome, is not compatible with life; however, fetuses affected by the monosomy of the X sex chromosome, i.e. Turner's syndrome, can survive (albeit with a high incidence of miscarriage). Noonan's syndrome is an autosomal recessive condition associated with mutations of four genes leading to multiple organ defects.

    Connor JM. Medical Genetics for the MRCOG and Beyond. London: RCOG Press, 2005.

7. D Trisomy 18

This baby has Edwards' syndrome, also known as trisomy 18. The syndrome is caused by an extra copy of chromosome 18 due an error in meiotic dysjunction. In addition to a true trisomy 18, individuals may be mosaic for trisomy 18, i.e. they have some cells with an extra copy of chromosome 18 because of a translocation defect. Trisomy 18 can be detected as part of antenatal screening such as the quadruple test, however in the absence of antenatal care it may not be detected until delivery. Both polyhydramnios and oligohydramnios may be observed in these pregnancies, the former as a possible indicator of defective fetal swallowing, and the latter reflecting abnormalities in the renal tract. There may intrauterine growth restriction. Fetuses affected by trisomy 18 typically have cardiac abnormalities of varying degrees of severity. The appearance of the baby typifies many of the features of a baby with trisomy 18. Other associated features include rocker-bottom feet, micro penis, radial aplasia and low-set ears. There is gross delay in psychomotor development and the rare individuals who survive infancy typically have severe intellectual disability.

8. A Down's syndrome

Down's syndrome, trisomy 21, is one of a number of conditions that may be screened for using serum markers, as part of the quadruple test. Reduced serum α-fetoprotein (AFP) is associated with pregnancies affected by Down's syndrome. AFP is produced by the fetal liver and yolk sac. Reduced levels of AFP are thought to be secondary to the smaller size of fetuses affected by Down's syndrome. Beta-human chorionic gonadotrophin levels are often elevated in Down's syndrome pregnancies. The quadruple test does not aim to provide a definitive diagnosis, but is a screening test with both false positive and false negative results.

Connor JM. Medical Genetics for the MRCOG and Beyond. London: RCOG Press, 2005.

9. D Neural tube defect

The combined test uses serum markers together with fetal nuchal translucency measurement in order to obtain an estimate as to how likely it is that a particular fetus is affected by a chromosomal or genetic disorder. Alpha-fetoprotein (AFP) is produced by the fetal liver and yolk sac. High levels of AFP are suggestive of neural tube defects, such as spina bifida, or more rarely anencephaly. This raised level is a consequence of flow of AFP from the open neural tube of the fetus, into the amniotic fluid (and secondarily maternal serum). Pregnancy-associated plasma protein A (PAPP-A) is produced by the fetus and also by the placenta. Reduced levels of PAPP-A in maternal serum can be suggestive of a fetus with an aneuploidy, such as Down's syndrome. Intrauterine growth restriction has also been associated with reduced levels of PAPP-A.

Connor JM. Medical Genetics for the MRCOG and Beyond. London: RCOG Press, 2005.

10. C Chorionic villus sampling

Chorionic villus sampling can be performed from 11 weeks' gestation and provides a means of culturing fetal placental tissue in order to determine fetal karyotyping. Amniocentesis involves the aspiration of fetal cells found in amniotic fluid in order to perform chromosomal analysis and should ideally be performed from 15 weeks' gestation. Cordocentesis involves the sampling of fetal blood from the umbilical vein in order to perform chromosomal analysis; it may also be used to detect fetal infection and anaemia. Although currently not widely used, cell-free fetal DNA sampling detects naturally occurring fetal DNA and RNA in maternal blood. This technique can be used in the determination of fetal sex and rhesus status and in paternally inherited dominant single gene disorders. In the future, this technique may be used to detect other genetic diseases as well as fetal aneuploidies. Nuchal translucency imaging using ultrasound is a screening test for fetal abnormalities as a thickened nuchal fold is associated with aneuploidies such as Turner's and Down's syndromes.

Royal College of Obstetricians and Gynaecologists. Amniocentesis and Chorionic Villus Sampling. Green-top Guideline 8. London: RCOG, 2010.
Wright C, Chitty L. Cell-free fetal DNA and RNA in maternal blood: implications for safer antenatal testing. BMJ 2009; 339:b2451.

11. A Autosomal dominant inheritance

BRCA stands for breast cancer susceptibility gene. The *BRCA1* gene is found on chromosome 17, whereas the *BRCA2* gene is found on chromosome 13. Both the *BRCA1* and *BRCA2* genes are in fact tumour suppressor genes which code for the DNA repair proteins *BRCA1* protein and *BRCA2* protein. Mutations in each gene lead to a defective form of the DNA repair protein, with the consequence of increased tumorigenesis. Both *BRCA* genes are passed on via autosomal dominant inheritance. This means that only one defective copy of the gene is required for the gene to be expressed. An individual with a parent carrying the mutated *BRCA1* gene has a one in two chance of inheriting the gene themselves. See **Figure 6.2** for diagrammatic representation of autosomal inheritance.

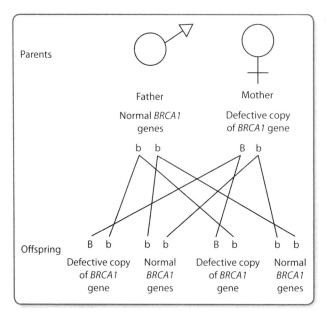

Figure 6.2 Autosomal dominant inheritance.

Families that carry either *BRCA1* or *BRCA2* mutations have a high incidence of breast and ovarian cancers (particularly of early onset), with individuals with the defective genes having an estimated 80% lifetime risk of breast cancer and up to a 40% lifetime risk of ovarian cancer.

Connor JM. Medical Genetics for the MRCOG and Beyond. London: RCOG Press, 2005.
National Cancer Institute at the National Institutes of Health. Fact Sheet: BRCA1 and BRCA2: Cancer Risk and Genetic Testing. Bethesda: National Cancer Institute, 2009. http://www.cancer.gov

12. D Robertsonian translocation

Familial Down's syndrome refers to trisomy 21 that occurs following a Robertsonian translocation. These translocations only occur in humans at chromosomes 13, 14, 15, 21 and 22. These chromosomes are acrocentric, i.e. they have very short arms. This form of translocation occurs when there is fusion of one acrocentric chromosome onto another acrocentric chromosome, so that their long arms become fused, with the loss of the insignificant genetic material found in the short arms. This may result in either a balanced Robertsonian translocation, whereby there is the no overall loss or excess of chromosomal material, or an unbalanced translocation. In the latter there may be an extra copy of one of the chromosomes, i.e. a trisomy or a monosomy. Down's syndrome caused by a Robertsonian translocation is usually caused by the inheritance of two normal copies of chromosome 21 (one from each parent) and the inheritance of a balanced translocation chromosome from one parent. This translocation chromosome, typically chromosome 14, has a copy of chromosome 21 fused to its long arm, leading to trisomy 21. Couples where one partner carries such a translocation chromosome have around a 10% chance of each of their pregnancies being affected by Down's syndrome.

13. A Alpha-thalassaemia with deletion of 4α-globin genes

Alpha-thalassaemia is an autosomal recessive condition associated with deletions in genes responsible for the production of α-globin chains. This couple both have α-thalassaemia trait, which means they each have either 2α-globin gene deletions on the same chromosomes or two chromosomes each with an α-globin gene deletion. Severity of α-thalassaemia is largely dependent on the number of α-globin genes affected. Individuals with the α-thalassaemia trait are usually minimally affected other than a mild anaemia. However in fetuses with deletions in all of the 4α-globin chains there is a complete absence of α-globin production. In early fetal life embryonic globin and gamma chains form functional units. At later gestations there is formation of haemoglobin Bart's (excess gamma chains which form tetramers) which has a high affinity for oxygen and therefore little oxygen delivery capacity. Hydrops fetalis is seen in fetuses with this profound absence of α-globin. Previously thought to be incompatible with life some fetuses may now survive with intrauterine transfusion.

Chapter 7

Physiology

Questions: MCQs

Answer each stem 'True' or 'False'.

1. **Methods of contraception:**
   A The levonorgestrel intrauterine system works by preventing sperm fertilising an egg
   B Male sterilisation involves cutting the vas deferens
   C The contraceptive implant works by preventing ovulation
   D The contraceptive patch is suitable for those with a body mass index >40
   E The combined oral contraceptive pill is contraindicated in migraine with aura

2. **Regarding spermatogenesis:**
   A Each spermatid contains 23 chromosomes
   B Spermatogenesis is completed in 40 days
   C Each spermatogonium develops into a single spermatid
   D Spermatids mature in the Leydig cells
   E Spermatogenesis occurs through mitotic division

3. **Regarding angiotensin-converting enzyme:**
   A Is produced by the liver
   B Potentiates the action of bradykinin
   C Is inhibited by the drug ramipril
   D Converts angiotensin II to angiotensin III
   E Levels can be raised in primary biliary cirrhosis

4. **Concerning the renal system during normal pregnancy:**
   A Serum creatinine is raised
   B The kidneys increase in length
   C Renal blood flow peaks during the second trimester
   D Plasma osmolality decreases
   E Glomerular filtration rate increases

5. **Concerning liver function tests in normal pregnancy:**
   A Bilirubin is increased
   B Total protein is increased
   C Bile acids increase
   D Alkaline phosphatase is decreased
   E Albumin decreases

6. **During the third stage of labour:**

   A   Oxytocin levels rise
   B   Raised prostaglandins levels cause myometrial contraction
   C   Beta-agonists can be used to manage this stage
   D   Use of synthetic prostaglandins is contraindicated
   E   Ergometrine is contraindicated if there is a fibroid uterus

7. **Concerning the luteoplacental shift:**

   A   It occurs at around 12 weeks' gestation
   B   It coincides with a decrease in 17α-hydroxyprogesterone production
   C   Human chorionic gonadotrophin production decreases after the shift
   D   Refers to the transition of human placental lactogen production from the corpus luteum to the placenta
   E   Failure of the corpus luteum prior to the shift is linked with miscarriage

8. **Concerning oxytocin:**

   A   It is a nonapeptide
   B   Oxytocin agonists are used to manage threatened preterm labour
   C   It can be given to increase uterine tone post delivery
   D   Administration can cause hyponatraemia
   E   It is made in the anterior pituitary gland

9. **Ergometrine:**

   A   Administration can cause hypertension
   B   Can be used to augment labour
   C   Can be used in the third stage of labour
   D   Is a serotonin agonist
   E   Is a constituent of the drug oxytocin

10. **The electrocardiogram of a pregnant woman can show:**

   A   Left axis deviation
   B   T-wave inversion in lead II
   C   Prolongation of the PR interval
   D   Q waves in aVF
   E   Increased heart rate

11. **Lactation is suppressed by:**

   A   Cabergoline
   B   Progesterone-only contraceptive pill
   C   Bromocriptine
   D   Metoclopramide
   E   Levothyroxine

12. **Pulmonary surfactant:**

   A   Is made by type II pneumocytes
   B   Is predominantly formed from proteins
   C   Production is promoted by maternal diabetes

    D   Contains dipalmitoylphosphatidylcholine
    E   Reduces pulmonary surface tension

13. **Control of respiration and mechanics of ventilation:**
    A   Intrathoracic muscles are innervated from T4–T11
    B   The diaphragm is innervated by the phrenic nerve
    C   Aortic arch chemoreceptors are innervated by the glossopharyngeal nerve
    D   Aortic arch chemoreceptors are sensitive to changes in pO_2
    E   Carotid body chemoreceptors are innervated by the vagus nerve

14. **With regards to the liver:**
    A   Kupffer cells are phagocytic
    B   Fibrinogen is synthesised in the liver
    C   Bilirubin is a breakdown product of haemoglobin
    D   Physiological jaundice of the neonate occurs as a result of failure of excretion of bilirubin
    E   High-density lipoprotein is the most abundant lipoprotein found in the liver

15. **Urine:**
    A   pH is relatively acidic compared to plasma
    B   Composition changes with diet
    C   Usually contains a trace of glucose
    D   Creatinine levels are lower than in plasma
    E   In normal circumstances it is protein free

Questions: SBAs

16. A 32-year-old primiparous woman suffers a massive antepartum haemorrhage and undergoes an emergency caesarean section. During the caesarean section she suffers a massive obstetric haemorrhage requiring transfusion of blood and clotting factors. As a result of these events, she develops disseminated intravascular coagulopathy.

    Which of the following laboratory results would be expected in this condition?

    A   Decreased activated partial thromboplastin time
    B   Increased factor VII levels
    C   Increased fibrinogen
    D   Increased soluble fibrin
    E   Thrombocytopenia

17. A 23-year-old woman develops a fever and has offensive vaginal discharge and abdominal pain. You are concerned that she is septic and wish to administer intravenous antibiotics. Prior to administration you wish to calculate her estimated glomerular filtration rate (eGFR) in order to dose her antibiotic therapy appropriately.

    Which of the following factors is included when calculating eGFR?

    A   Creatinine
    B   Diabetic status
    C   Height
    D   Medication
    E   Weight

18. A 25-year-old primiparous woman attends antenatal clinic for a routine check at 28 weeks' gestation. Her urine dipstick shows glucose 2+. On questioning, she has just eaten a doughnut.

    Which of the following describes the sequential handling of glucose by the kidney?

    A   Filtered, reabsorbed and secreted
    B   Filtered, reabsorbed and not secreted
    C   Filtered, secreted, but not reabsorbed
    D   Filtered and neither secreted or reabsorbed
    E   Unfiltered, secreted

19. A 37-year-old woman attends her general practitioner for contraceptive advice. She is a smoker of 10 cigarettes a day and has had two children. She is keen to try the progesterone-only pill and asks you how it works.

    Which is the most appropriate answer?

    A   Creates a hostile environment for fertilisation to occur

 B Creates an inflammatory reaction
 C Inhibits ovulation
 D Prevents implantation
 E Thickens cervical mucus

20. A 72-year-old woman undergoes a total abdominal hysterectomy. She has chronic obstructive pulmonary disease. Postoperatively, she is difficult to extubate and has a prolonged stay on the intensive care unit.

Which of the following is the most important direct stimulus to respiration?

 A Decreased arterial pH
 B Decreased arterial pO_2
 C Decreased arterial pCO_2
 D Increased H^+ concentration of the cerebrospinal fluid (CSF)
 E Increased pCO_2 of the CSF

21. A 27-year-old woman attends antenatal clinic at 32 weeks' gestation complaining of gradual increasing shortness of breath through pregnancy. Although you feel it is important to exclude serious pathology, you are aware that this could be a normal symptom of advancing pregnancy.

Which of the following contributors to lung volume and capacity occurs in normal pregnancy?

 A Chest compliance increases
 B Expiratory reserve volume increases
 C Residual volume decreases
 D Tidal volume decreases by up to 40%
 E Vital capacity decreases

22. A 32-year-old woman is readmitted to the postnatal ward 10 days after an emergency caesarean section with a swollen painful calf. Her observations are stable. Her body mass index is 37. You want to rule out a deep vein thrombosis.

Which of the following clotting factors are increased in normal pregnancy?

 A Factor VII
 B Factors VII and VII
 C Factors VII, VIII and X
 D Factors VII, VIII, X and XI
 E Factors VII, VIII, X, XI and XIII

23. With regard to the cardiac cycle what is the definition of stroke volume?

 A Stroke volume = cardiac output / body surface area
 B Stroke volume = end diastolic volume – end systolic volume
 C Stroke volume = end systolic volume – end diastolic volume
 D Stroke volume = end systolic volume + end diastolic volume
 E Stroke volume = end diastolic volume + end systolic volume

24. A 2-week-old neonate is admitted to hospital with failure to thrive, tachypnoea and difficulty feeding. He is thought to have a circulatory defect.

    Administration of prostaglandin antagonists soon after birth can be used to therapeutically close which patent structure of fetal origin?

    A   Ductus arteriosus
    B   Ductus venosus
    C   Foramen ovale
    D   Fossa ovalis
    E   Ligamentum venosum

25. A 67-year-old woman is admitted to hospital with frequency of urination and extreme thirst. Her blood tests reveal deranged urea and electrolytes. Provisional diagnosis is diabetes insipidus.

    Which hormone acts in the nephron, to increase the permeability of the collecting ducts to water?

    A   Aldosterone
    B   Angiotensin
    C   Atrial natriuretic peptide
    D   Parathyroid hormone
    E   Vasopressin

26. A 22-year-old woman is breastfeeding an hour after delivery. During lactation the 'let-down' reflex is stimulated by the action of which hormone?

    A   Human placental lactogen
    B   Oestrogen
    C   Oxytocin
    D   Prolactin
    E   Progesterone

27. A 27-year-old woman is being treated for primary infertility. A pelvic ultrasound shows multiple small ovarian follicles present in both ovaries. She is having ultrasound tracking of her ovaries as she has an irregular cycle.

    What is the approximate size of the dominant ovarian follicle at the time of ovulation?

    A   1–2 mm
    B   5 mm
    C   20 mm
    D   30–40 mm
    E   50 mm

28. A 33-year-old woman attends antenatal clinic at 33 weeks' gestation complaining of shortness of breath.

    Which of the following causes a shift of oxygen dissociation to the left?

A   Decreased haemoglobin
B   Decreased 2,3-diphosphoglycerate
C   Increased acidity
D   Increased carbon dioxide
E   Increased temperature

29. Which of the following substances is unable to bind with fetal haemoglobin?

A   2,3-diphosphoglycerate
B   Carbon dioxide
C   Carbon monoxide
D   Nitrous oxide
E   Oxygen

30. A 72-year-old woman is undergoing lung function tests prior to abdominal surgery.

Which of the following gives the correct lung volume equation?

A   Functional residual capacity = residual volume + tidal volume
B   Inspiratory capacity = tidal volume + expiratory reserve volume
C   Inspiratory capacity = inspiratory reserve volume – tidal volume
D   Total lung capacity = inspiratory capacity + residual volume
E   Vital capacity = inspiratory capacity + expiratory reserve volume

Answers

1. A False

    B True

    C True

    D False

    E True

    The levonorgestrel intrauterine system is a plastic device containing progesterone, which works by releasing hormone slowly into the system. The progesterone works to thin the endometrium and so preventing implantation. It also thickens the cervical mucus. Male sterilisation is a permanent form of contraception caused by cutting, sealing or tying the vas deferens, which carries the sperm from testicles to the penis. It is very effective, with less than a 1% failure rate.

    The contraceptive implant is placed into the non-dominant upper arm. It releases progesterone and causes the usual progesterone effects as well as preventing ovulation. It can be left in situ for 3 years, but can be taken out sooner with a potential return to fertility immediately. The contraceptive patch is not suitable for those women with a large body mass index or smokers. The combined oral contraceptive pill is contraindicated for use as a contraceptive in patients with migraine with aura.

    National Institute for Health and Clinical Excellence. Long-acting reversible contraception. Clinical Guideline CG30. London: NICE, 2005. http://guidance.nice.org.uk/CG30

2. A True

    B False

    C False

    D False

    E True

    Spermatogenesis (**Figure 7.1**) refers to the process that produces mature sperm (spermatozoa) from primitive germ cells (spermatogonia). Starting in adolescence and continuing throughout male adulthood spermatogenesis takes around 70 days to complete. During this time the spermatogonia found at the basal lamina of the seminiferous tubules begin to mature, eventually becoming primary spermatocytes. Both spermatogonia and primary spermatocytes contain a diploid number of chromosomes, which is reduced to haploid number (23 chromosomes) as a result of meiotic division. The primary spermatocyte divides by meiosis into two secondary spermatocytes (first meiotic division), each of which then divide again (second meiotic division) to form two spermatids each. These haploid spermatids then undergo a process of maturation attached to the Sertoli cells, eventually becoming mature spermatozoa.

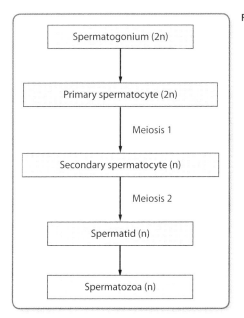

Figure 7.1 Spermatogenesis.

3. A False

    B False

    C True

    D False

    E True

Angiotensin-converting enzyme (ACE) is produced predominantly by the endothelial cells of the lungs, but also in the kidneys. ACE catalyses the conversion of angiotensin I to angiotensin II which is a vasoconstrictor and key regulator of extracellular volume as part of the renin–angiotensin system. ACE is also known to cause breakdown of the peptide bradykinin, a potent vasodilator. ACE may be raised in a number of pathologies including primary biliary cirrhosis, sarcoidosis and Gaucher's disease.

ACE inhibitors such as ramipril and enalapril prevent angiotensin II formation and induce a state of relative vasodilation.

4. A False

    B True

    C True

    D True

    E True

Pregnancy is associated with both a large increase in circulating volume, as well as dilatation of the urinary collecting systems. The kidneys normally increase in length. Renal blood flow dramatically increases by around 50% reaching a peak in the second trimester and then falls slightly in the third trimester. The glomerular filtration rate increases considerably, with resulting reduction in serum levels of creatinine, urea and plasma osmolality.

5. A False

    B False

    C False

    D False

    E True

Bilirubin levels are largely unaltered in pregnancy, however the other liver function tests show considerable change.

Albumin, total protein and the transaminases (alanine transaminase and aspartate transaminase) fall throughout pregnancy. These changes may largely be explained by pregnancy-related volume expansion.

Alkaline phosphatase (ALP) however, increases throughout pregnancy and reaches its peak during the third trimester reflecting placental production of ALP. Having taken these normal changes into account, interpretation of liver function tests in pregnancy can aid the diagnosis of conditions such as hyperemesis gravidarum, obstetric cholestasis, pre-eclampsia, haemolysis, elevated liver enzymes, and low platelet (HELLP) syndrome and acute fatty liver (**Table 7.1**).

Table 7.1 Tests of liver function: pregnant and non-pregnant values

Liver function test	Non-pregnant state	Pregnant state
Alkaline phosphatase (IU/L)	30–130	32–418
Aspartate aminotransferase (IU/L)	7–40	10–30
Alanine aminotransferase (IU/L)	0–40	6–32
Albumin (g/L)	35–46	28–37
Total protein (g/L)	64–86	48–64
Bilirubin (μmol/L)	0–17	3–16

Adapted from: Appendix 2: Normal laboratory values in pregnancy/non-pregnancy. In: Handbook of Obstetric Medicine, 4th edn. London: Informa Healthcare, 2010: 273–274.

6. A False

    B True

    C False

    D False

    E False

The third stage of labour is defined as the time from delivery of the baby to the delivery of the placenta and membranes. It may be managed physiologically or more commonly, actively. Physiological management involves delivery of the placenta by maternal effort. No oxytocin or ergometrine is used.

Active management of the third stage, however involves clamping of the cord, the use of uterotonics such as oxytocin and ergometrine, and delivery of the placenta by controlled cord traction.

Side effects of oxytocin include nausea and vomiting. Rarer side effects include arrhythmias, disseminated intravascular coagulation and water intoxication and hyponatraemia. Ergometrine may also be associated with side effects such as nausea and vomiting, arrhythmias, chest pain and palpitations. Active management of the third stage is recommended to avoid postpartum haemorrhage in women at risk of postpartum haemorrhage, such as grand multiparous women.

7. **A** False

   B True

   C False

   D False

   E True

The term 'luteoplacental' shift refers to the transition that occurs in early pregnancy when the placenta takes over progesterone production from the ageing corpus luteum. This shift occurs at around 7–8 weeks' gestation. The corpus luteum secretes 17α-hydroxyprogesterone throughout the luteal phase of the menstrual cycle; should fertilisation not occur the corpus luteum fails 14 days after ovulation, progesterone levels significantly reduce and menstruation occurs. When fertilisation has occurred human chorionic gonadotrophin produced by the syncytiotrophoblast stimulates the corpus luteum to continue producing progesterone. At around 7–8 weeks' gestation the placenta becomes the main source of progesterone synthesis. The corpus luteum begins to fail and eventually will become a corpus albicans. Failure of the corpus luteum to maintain progesterone levels prior to the 'shift' is associated with first trimester miscarriage. Progesterone support is required in assisted conception pregnancies until the shift has occurred.

Csapo A. The luteo-placental shift, the guardian of pre-natal life. Postgrad Med J 1969;45(519):57–64.

8. **A** True

   B False

   C True

   D True

   E False

Oxytocin is a nonapeptide hormone which is made in the hypothalamus and released from the posterior pituitary gland. Numbers of oxytocin receptors in uterine muscle increase close to term, and increased release of oxytocin in labour is thought to aid uterine muscle contraction.

Oxytocin is also involved in the 'let-down' reflex of milk ejection as part of lactation. Synthetic forms of oxytocin, such as 'syntocinon', can be given to augment labour or to prevent/manage postpartum haemorrhage by stimulating uterine contraction.

Oxytocin has a similar structure to that of vasopressin (antidiuretic hormone), and therefore administration can be associated with hyponatraemia.

'Atosiban' is a tocolytic agent and is an oxytocin antagonist. It is used in cases of threatened preterm labour.

9. A True

    B False

    C True

    D True

    E False

Ergometrine is an ergot alkaloid that is known to act as a serotonin, dopaminergic and α-adrenergic agonist. Although its true mechanism of action is not fully understood, ergometrine is known to aid both vasoconstriction and uterine contraction thus making it a useful drug for the management of the third stage of labour and the prevention postpartum haemorrhage.

Use of ergometrine is contraindicated in the first and second stage of labour. Ergometrine is often given in combination with a synthetic oxytocin in the form of 'syntometrine'. Known to cause vasoconstriction, ergometrine should be given with caution to women with raised or borderline blood pressure and significant renal disease. Administration in such cases may be associated with further increases in blood pressure, and hence its use is contraindicated in women with pre-eclampsia.

10. A True

    B False

    C False

    D True

    E True

In pregnancy, the normal electrocardiogram (ECG) is slightly different from that of the non-pregnant state, with changes reflecting the altered physiology of pregnancy. As pregnancy is associated with increased blood volume, increased stroke volume and increased cardiac output there is associated hypertrophy of the heart and enlargement of the left side of the heart. The gravid uterus also pushes the diaphragm up, and therefore the heart is displaced forward and to the left.

The combination of these changes lead to left-axis deviation on the ECG. There may also be T-wave inversion or flattening in Lead III and the presence of Q waves in both leads aVF and III.

Ciliberto CF, Marx GF. Physiological changes associated with pregnancy. Update Anaesthesia 1998; 9:1-3.

11. A True

B False

C True

D False

E False

Lactation suppression may be instigated by interruption of the normal balance of lactation promoters and inhibitors. Prolactin is the main promoter of lactation and is produced by the pituitary gland. It is inhibited by dopamine agonists such as cabergoline and bromocriptine. These drugs can be given to suppress lactation in HIV positive women or those who are not breastfeeding because they have had a stillbirth.

Dopamine antagonists unsurprisingly have the opposite effect and drugs such as metoclopramide and domperidone are sometimes used to increase milk production.

With regards to postnatal contraception the progesterone-only contraceptive pill is often the contraceptive of choice in breastfeeding women in the postpartum period. It does not interfere with lactation. The combined oral contraceptive pill, however, is relatively contraindicated due to its oestrogen content and concerns with regards to it reducing the volume and quality of breast milk.

12. A True

B False

C False

D True

E True

Pulmonary surfactant is a naturally occurring substance produced by type II pneumocytes. It predominantly consists of lipids [such as dipalmitoylphosphatidylcholine (DPPC)] which are linked with a series of surfactant proteins (A, B, C and D) and organised into hydrophobic and hydrophilic complexes. Pulmonary surfactant increases lung compliance and reduces pulmonary surface tension which helps prevent atelectasis.

Surfactant production begins in the fetus relatively late in pregnancy and is therefore suboptimal in infants born prematurely. Respiratory distress syndrome is a major cause of mortality and morbidity in premature infants due to lack of surfactant and lung immaturity. The administration of intramuscular glucocorticoids such as dexamethasone and betamethasone is associated with increased fetal surfactant production and enhanced lung maturity and therefore has benefit when there is risk of delivery before 34 weeks' gestation.

13. A False

   B True

   C False

   D True

   E False

Expansion of the chest cavity occurs as a result of contraction of the intrathoracic muscles which are innervated from the T1–T11 nerves. There is also influence from the diaphragm which is innervated by the phrenic nerve, C3–C5. There are two important controls to respiration, the central chemoreceptors (medulla) and peripheral chemoreceptors (aortic arch and carotid body). The aortic arch receptors are innervated by the vagus nerve and the carotid body receptors by the glossopharyngeal nerve. The carotid body chemoreceptors are the only ones sensitive to changes in the partial pressure of oxygen. Both peripheral and central chemoreceptors are sensitive to changes in both pCO_2 and pH. If there is an increase in the level of pCO_2 detected, then there is an associated increase in ventilation to reduce the pH.

14. A True

   B True

   C True

   D False

   E False

An adult liver weighs approximately 1 kg and is composed of lobules. Each lobule surrounds a central vein which then drains into a hepatic vein. Kupffer cells are phagocytic and line the sinusoids. Bilirubin is a breakdown product of haemoglobin and is then secreted by the liver.

The synthesis of lipoproteins occurs in the liver, but the main lipoprotein to be manufactured is VLDL. Plasma proteins are derived from the liver and nearly all albumin and fibrinogen are synthesised here. The neonatal liver weighs approximately 150 g and is immature at birth. Physiological jaundice occurs as a result of the neonatal liver's failure to conjugate the bilirubin. High levels of unconjugated bilirubin mean that it cannot be completely bound to albumin and may cross the blood-brain barrier, causing kernicterus.

15. A True

   B True

   C False

   D False

   E True

Table 7.2 summarises the properties of urine.

Table 7.2 Properties of urine

	Urine	Plasma
pH	5.0–7.0	7.35–7.45
Protein	0	65–80
Glucose	0	4.0–6.0
Na	50–120	135–145
K	20–70	3.5–5.0
Osmolality	100–1000	280–295
Creatinine	5–20	0.06–0.12

16. E Thrombocytopaenia

Disseminated intravascular coagulopathy (DIC) is a condition, where there is generalised and widespread pathological activation of the clotting system. There is clotting within the microvasculature which causes consumption of coagulation products. Pathological changes include inflammatory activation, suppression of anticoagulation and inhibition of fibrinolysis. The obstruction of the microvascular vessels can cause disruption of blood flow to major organs, potentially leading to multiorgan failure.

DIC usually occurs as a result of activation of the intrinsic coagulation pathway. There are usually increased levels of soluble fibrin. Diagnosis is by blood tests which usually reveal:

- Thrombocytopaenia
- Prolonged activated partial thromboplastin time
- Low fibrinogen
- Increased fibrinogen degradation products

Treatment is via reversal of the underlying cause. Fresh frozen plasma may be given as well as platelets depending on the degree of thrombocytopaenia.

17. A Creatinine

Estimated glomerular filtration rate is used as a marker of renal function and used in clinical practice, e.g. for calculations of renal function in the use of nephrotoxic drugs. It is often calculated using the modification of diet in renal disease (MDRD) equation which takes into account the age, creatinine levels, gender and ethnic group. Weight, height, comorbidities and medication are not used in this formula. It must be remembered that estimated glomerular filtration rate (eGFR) is still an estimate and may be inaccurate in certain circumstances, e.g. malnourished patients and amputees. It should not be used in children or pregnant women. For Afro-Caribbean patients, the eGFR may be 21% higher than estimated. Normal GFR is > 90 mL/min/1.73 m^2.

18. B Filtered, reabsorbed and not secreted

In the normally-functioning kidneys glucose is filtered, reabsorbed via secondary active transport and is on the whole not secreted in the urine. Virtually all glucose is reabsorbed in the apical region of proximal convoluted tubule of the kidney via Na/glucose transporters and also by glucose transporters (GLUTs). When the level of plasma glucose exceeds the filtering capacity of the kidneys, then the amount of glucose excreted in the urine increases. The renal threshold for glucose, that is the amount of plasma glucose that the kidneys are able to filter without it being excreted in large amounts in the urine, is around 200 mg/dL. Glycosuria may be suggestive of diabetes mellitus and requires further investigation.

19. E Thickens cervical mucus

If taken appropriately, the progesterone-only pill (POP) is approximately 99% effective. Its main mechanism of action is by thickening the cervical secretions. It also thins the endometrium and makes the embryo less likely to implant. The POP is only effective if taken at the same time every day or within a 3-hour window. This is due to the mechanism of action of the POP which loses efficacy if there is a delay in taking it. The combined oral contraceptive pill works by inhibiting ovulation. The intrauterine contraceptive device provides a hostile environment and prevents implantation. It may also cause an inflammatory reaction. The copper of the copper coil also prevents the sperm from entering the uterus.

20. D Increased H$^+$ concentration of the cerebrospinal fluid

The main stimulus to the respiratory centre comes from the chemoreceptors. These are central and peripheral. The central chemoreceptors are found on the surface of the upper medulla. Peripheral chemoreceptors are around the aortic arch, innervated by the vagus nerve, and in the carotid body, innervated by the glossopharyngeal nerve. The central chemoreceptors are only sensitive to changes in the pH. The carotid body receptors are sensitive to changes in pO_2. Both the carod body and aortic arch receptors are sensitive to changes in pCO_2 and pH. Variations in CO_2 are altered via a change in ventilation. A rise in CO_2 leads to an increase in ventilation and hypoxia increases the respiratory centre sensitivity to CO_2. The response to hypoxia is less marked than the response to CO_2. The response to respiration as a result of acidosis is reduced because of the production of deoxygenated haemoglobin which acts as a buffer.

21. C Residual volume decreases

Table 7.3 summarises the change in lung function tests that occur as a result of pregnancy.

Table 7.3 Changes in respiratory system during pregnancy		
Increase	**Decrease**	**No change**
Tidal volume – up to 40%	Total lung capacity	Vital capacity
	Residual volume	Respiratory rate
	Expiratory reserve volume – approximately 200 mL	Lung compliance
	Inspiratory reserve volume	FEV1/PEFR
	Chest compliance	
	Airway resistance	

FEV1, forced expiratory volume in 1 second; PEFR, peak expiratory flow rate.

22. C Factors VII, VIII and X

In order to prepare the body to achieve rapid haemostasis after delivery, pregnancy is essentially a hypercoagulant state. As a consequence there is an increase in the majority of clotting factors during pregnancy, in particular factors VII, VIII and X. Factors XI and XIII do not change significantly during pregnancy.

Fibrinogen and erythrocyte sedimentation ratio may be doubled by term. There is an increase in antithrombin III and fibrinogen degradation products. The inhibition of fibrinolysis is partly mediated through placental plasminogen activator inhibitor (PAI2). PAI2 is a coagulation factor that is produced by the placenta and is only detectable in the blood during pregnancy. It activates tissue plasminogen activator and urokinase and is found in monocytes and macrophages.

The procoagulant state of pregnancy is one of the processes in place to prevent excess bleeding after delivery. Other mechanisms include uterine contraction and the development of a fibrin mesh which covers the placental site.

23. B Stroke volume = end diastolic volume – end systolic volume

The cardiac cycle is the repeated action of contraction and relaxation that leads to the pumping of blood from the heart and maintenance of circulation. Myocardial cells contract during electrical excitation and relax during repolarisation. During diastole the heart chambers relax and fill with blood. During systole, there is contraction of the ventricles and ejection of blood into the circulation. The atria contract together, with contraction of the ventricles occurring 0.1–0.2 seconds later.

Concerning the left side of the heart: at the beginning of ventricular systole, the mitral valve is open and the pressure in the left atrium is greater than that in the ventricle. As the pressure in the left atrium builds up, the mitral valve closes. Stroke volume is the calculated by subtracting the end systolic volume from the end diastolic volume. This is actually around 60–70% of blood left in the ventricles at the end of diastole. Stroke volume usually refers to the left ventricle, although it can be applied to both. Both ventricles have an equivalent stroke volume, which in the average sized adult is approximately 70 mL.

24. A Ductus arteriosus

The ductus arteriosus is one of the three circulatory shunts that exist in the fetal circulation. It is the fetal connection between the pulmonary artery and the aorta, allowing oxygenated fetal blood to be carried from the right ventricle and around the body, largely bypassing the lungs. It remains open throughout the fetal period due to high levels of vasodilating prostaglandins and also due to the low oxygen tension associated with the non-functioning pulmonary circulatory system. The ductus arteriosus usually closes permanently in the first few days of life as prostaglandin levels fall and as oxygen tensions dramatically rise after the first breath, leading to a rise in systemic circulatory pressure and fall in pressure of the previously high-resistance pulmonary circulation. A patent ductus arteriosus (PDA) is associated with prematurity and with other causes including maternal rubella infection during pregnancy. Children with a PDA may be asymptomatic, however young babies may present in the few weeks of life with tachypnoea, failure to thrive and difficulties with feeding. Prostaglandin antagonists such as non-steroidal anti-inflammatory drugs (NSAIDs) may be used to therapeutically close a PDA. Usage of NSAIDs can cause constriction of the fetal ductus arteriosus and hence all NSAIDs should be avoided in the third trimester of pregnancy.

25. E Vasopressin

Nephrons are the functional unit of the kidney and are responsible for the filtration of blood, excretion of waste products and the regulation of water balance. The collecting duct is the terminal part of the nephron and receives filtrate that has already passed through the glomerulus (the main functional filtration unit), the loop of Henle and the proximal and distal convoluted tubules. By the time the filtrate reaches the collecting duct it has already undergone a process of reabsorption of substances such as sodium chloride, water, bicarbonate, potassium and calcium. At the collecting duct vasopressin, also known as antidiuretic hormone, increases permeability to water allowing for water molecules to be reabsorbed. Vasopressin enables the production of concentrated urine by acting on the aquaporins (water channels) of the collecting duct, allowing them to facilitate the passive reabsorption of water (**Figure 7.2**).

Chapter 38: Renal Function and Micturition. In: Barrett KE, Barman SM, Boitano S, Brooks H. Ganong's Review of Medical Physiology, 23rd edn. New York: McGraw-Hill, 2010.

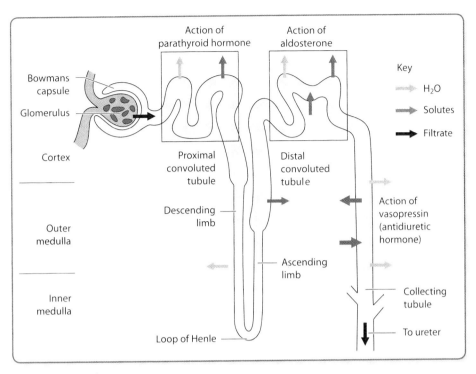

Figure 7.2 The nephron.

26. C Oxytocin

The 'let-down reflex', also known as the milk ejection reflex, describes the release of breast milk following the stimulus of suckling. The reflex is controlled by the action of the hormone oxytocin which is released from the hypothalamus in response to suckling, and causes contraction of the myoepithelial cells of the milk ducts subsequently leading to milk ejection. Conditioning of this reflex naturally occurs to the extent that milk ejection may occur in lactating women in response to stimuli such as the sound of crying babies. Actual production of milk is largely under the control of prolactin which is released from the anterior pituitary gland in increasing amounts from early pregnancy.

27. C 20 mm

The dominant ovarian follicle grows considerably throughout folliculogenesis and by the time of ovulation has reached approximately 20 mm in size. It reaches the surface of the ovary and its release is due to necrobiosis of the overlying tissue. The rise in basal body temperature is thought to be due to the thermogenic effect of progesterone on the brain. The actual process of follicular rupture takes a few minutes. Mittelschmerz is the midcycle lower abdominal pain experienced by almost 1 in 4 women. This is thought to be caused by the release of follicular fluid leading to peritoneal irritation.

28. B Decreased 2,3-diphosphoglycerate

The oxygen dissociation curve is a graph which demonstrates the percentage saturation of haemoglobin at different partial pressures of oxygen. At higher partial pressures of oxygen, the haemoglobin binds with oxygen to form oxyhaemoglobin.

Each molecule of haemoglobin can bind with four molecules of oxygen. The sigmoid shape of the curve is a result of 'cooperation' between the oxygen binding site, i.e. occupancy of one of the binding sites makes it easier for the second to bind and the same with the third and fourth.

A right shift in the oxygen dissociation curve indicates a reduced oxygen affinity (**Figure 7.3**). This occurs when there is an increase in:

- Temperature
- Acidity
- 2,3-diphosphoglycerate
- Carbon dioxide

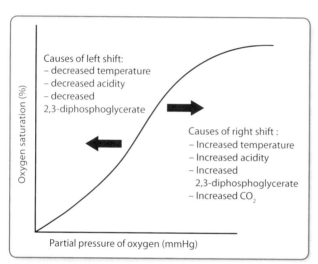

Figure 7.3 Oxygen dissociation curve with factors causing left and right shift.

29. A 2,3-diphosphoglycerate

The oxygen dissociation curve for fetal haemoglobin (HbF) is a sigmoid shape. HbF consists of two α chains and two γ chains. HbF has a higher affinity for oxygen and there is therefore a left shift in the fetal oxygen dissociation curve. The reason for this shift is the reduced binding of 2,3-diphosphoglyceric acid (2,3-DPG). 2,3-DPG has a higher affinity for the β chains in the adult haemoglobin (HbA). This difference in binding capacity between HbA and HbF ensures that HbF has a greater affinity for oxygen than HbA. The P_{50} is defined as the partial pressure of oxygen at which the oxygen-carrying protein is 50% saturated and this is lower in HbF due to the reduced sensitivity of 2,3-DPG (**Figure 7.4**).

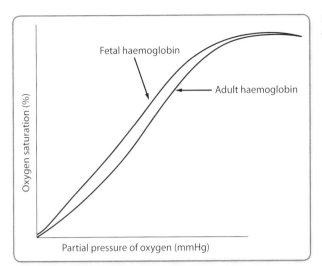

Figure 7.4 Fetal-maternal oxygen dissociation curves.

30. E Vital capacity = inspiratory capacity + expiratory reserve volume

Vital capacity describes the maximum volume of air that a person can exhale after maximum inspiration. It is therefore the combination of inspiratory capacity and the expiratory reserve volume. The inspiratory capacity is the combination of inspiratory reserve volume plus the tidal volume and is approximately 2.4 L in a female adult. The expiratory reserve volume is determined by the functional residual volume minus the residual volume. Vital capacity may be measured by spirometry and forms one element of a basic lung function test.

Chapter 8

Biophysics

Questions: MCQs

Answer each stem 'True' or 'False'.

1. **Ultrasound causes:**
   - A Cavitation
   - B Heating
   - C Microstreaming
   - D Decreased velocity of blood flow
   - E Ionisation

2. **Soft markers for chromosomal abnormalities seen on ultrasound scan include:**
   - A Choroid plexus cyst
   - B Echogenic bowel
   - C Exomphalos
   - D Fetal hydrops
   - E Mild renal pelvic dilatation

3. **Concerning electrosurgery:**
   - A Bipolar diathermy can be used to cut tissue
   - B Monopolar diathermy necessitates the use of a return electrode
   - C Diathermy uses low-frequency electrical currents
   - D Desiccation of tissue can be achieved using both mono- and bipolar diathermy
   - E Direct coupling is achieved by adhering to strict safety protocols

4. **Concerning the normal electrocardiogram:**
   - A The PR interval is 0.2–0.4 seconds
   - B The duration of the QRS complex should be >0.12 seconds
   - C Each QRS complex is preceded by a P-wave
   - D The QT interval is 0.35–0.42 seconds
   - E The paper speed is set at 25 mm/s

5. **Concerning the hysterosalpingogram:**
   - A It is performed in the luteal phase of the menstrual cycle
   - B It uses ultrasound
   - C It may used to investigate secondary subfertility
   - D A pregnancy test must be performed before the procedure
   - E It is contraindicated in individuals with a history of *Chlamydia*

6. **Ultrasound:**

   A   Has no known adverse effects on tissue
   B   Can have thermal effects on tissue
   C   Can cause streaming
   D   Can cause fulguration
   E   Safety protocols necessitate the use of thermal indices

Questions: SBAs

For each question, select the single best answer from the five options listed.

7. Which of the following describes the mode used in creating standard grey scale ultrasound images?

    A   A-mode
    B   B-mode
    C   Doppler mode
    D   M-mode
    E   None of above

8. Which of the following is a recognised parameter used in fetal biophysical profiling?

    A   Abdominal circumference
    B   Amniotic fluid index
    C   Biparietal diameter
    D   Head circumference
    E   Femur length

9. Which of the following is an acute side-effect of radiotherapy?

    A   Epithelial surface damage
    B   Hair loss
    C   Infertility
    D   Lymphoedema
    E   Tissue fibrosis

10. Which of the following modalities uses an ionising form of radiation?

    A   Electrocautery
    B   Laser
    C   Magnetic resonance imaging
    D   Ultrasound
    E   X-ray

11. The standard chest X-ray is equivalent to what duration of natural background radiation:

    A   2–3 days
    B   10 days
    C   2 months
    D   18 months
    E   5 years

12. At what crown–rump length would you first expect to see a fetal heart beat using transvaginal ultrasonography?

A   >2 mm
B   >3 mm
C   >4 mm
D   >5 mm
E   >6 mm

13. A 68-year-old woman developed left-sided chest pain a day after she has had total abdominal hysterectomy and bilateral-salpingo-oophorectomy. A 12-lead electrocardiogram is performed and is suggestive of an anterior ST elevation myocardial infarction.

Which of the following leads would be most likely to show ST elevation in this patient?

A   I, aVL, V_5-V_6
B   I, II and III
C   II, III and aVF
D V_1-V_4
E   All of the above

14. Which of the following is a late side-effect of radiotherapy?

A   Fatigue
B   Lymphoedema
C   Mouth ulcers
D   Nausea
E   Oedema

15. Which of the following best describes acoustic impedance?

A   It is an estimate of mean velocity of flow within a vessel
B   It is the apparent bending of waves
C   It is the opposition to the passage of sound waves and is a function of density and elasticity
D   It is when reflected waves from a moving interface undergo a frequency shift
E   It is the angle at which the wave is incident on the surface equals the angle of reflection

Answers

1. A True

    B True

    C True

    D False

    E False

    Ultrasonography uses high frequency sound waves to create images that are widely used in many area of medical practice. Although generally considered a safe modality of imaging it can cause a number of tissue effects. Ultrasound causes heating of the surrounding tissues, the extent of which is dependant on the tissue type, the distance between the transducer and the tissue and the intensity of the ultrasound used. Cavitation describes the formation of gas cavities within tissue secondary to ultrasound. Although cavitation is not thought to occur in diagnostic ultrasonography, it can be practically applied in lithotripsy. Microstreaming is the generation of fluid circulation within tissue, which can be either intra- or extracellular. Ionisation does not occur as a result of the usage of ultrasound.

2. A True

    B True

    C False

    D False

    E True

    Soft markers are more common in a fetus with chromosomal abnormalities. However, the presence of these markers alone is not sufficient to provide a definitive diagnosis as they often spontaneously resolve. Choroid plexus cysts may be seen in a fetus with trisomy 18; however, when seen in an otherwise normal fetus they are of questionable significance. Echogenic bowel describes bowel that appears bright on ultrasound and can indicate chromosomal abnormalities, bowel obstruction and cystic fibrosis. It always requires further investigation. Exomphalos is persistent protrusion of the bowel through the abdominal wall at the base of the umbilicus. This may be normal before 10 weeks of gestation. The ongoing presence of exomphalos may be indicative of chromosomal abnormalities or other organ malformation. Fetal hydrops refers to the accumulation of serous fluid in fetal tissue and may be associated with diagnoses such as parvovirus infection and anaemia. Mild renal pelvic dilatation is associated with only a small risk of chromosomal abnormalities.

3. A False

    B True

    C False

    D True

    E False

Electrosurgery uses high-frequency AC electrical currents to achieve cutting, coagulation, desiccation and fulguration (destruction) of tissue. Modern surgical techniques use monopolar, bipolar and tripolar diathermy. Monopolar diathermy uses high-frequency currents applied to tissue by a hand-held electrode. The current passes through the surgeon's electrode through the patient and leaves the patient via a return electrode which is attached to the patient. In bipolar diathermy each blade of the forceps held by the surgeon is actually an electrode and the current passes from one electrode, through any held tissue, and back into the return electrode blade of the forceps. Monopolar diathermy can be used to achieve cutting and coagulation, whereas cutting is not possible using bipolar diathermy. Both techniques can be used for tissue desiccation. Strict adherence to safety protocols is essential. Direct coupling is one of the hazards associated with monopolar diathermy and refers to tissue damage caused by the electrode touching another conducting instrument close by. Overall bipolar diathermy is considered safer than its monopolar equivalent.

4. A False

    B False

    C True

    D True

    E True

The electrocardiogram (ECG) records the electrical activity of the heart. The standard 12-lead ECG makes use of electrode placement in order to build a picture of electrical activity in various planes of the heart. By convention the standard paper speed is set as 25 mm/s. The normal PR interval is 0.12–0.20 s and represents sequential sinoatrial node and atrial depolarisation. Longer intervals may indicate heart block, whereas a reduced interval may indicate an accessory conduction pathway such as Wolff–Parkinson–White syndrome, or the presence of an AV junctional rhythm. The QRS complex, which represents ventricular contraction, should have a duration of less than or equal to 0.12 s. A longer QRS duration may indicate conduction anomalies such as a bundle branch block. The QT interval is measured from the beginning of the QRS complex to the end of the T wave. The normal QT interval is 0.35–0.42 s. A shorter interval may indicate abnormalities such as hypercalcaemia, whereas causes of a prolonged interval include myocarditis and hypocalcaemia.

5. A False

    B False

    C True

    D False

    E False

The hysterosalpingogram (HSG) is a radiological means of assessing tubal patency. Typically one of the basic investigations used to investigate both primary and secondary subfertility the HSG may also be used to confirm successful bilateral tubal ligation surgery, i.e. sterilisation. The technique requires the use of a cervical catheter which is used to inject a radio-opaque contrast agent into the uterus and through the fallopian tubes. X-ray images are obtained to show the passage of the contrast agent into the uterus and, when there is tubal patency, to visualise the bilateral spill out of each fallopian tube. The procedure must be performed during the follicular phase of the menstrual cycle and within 10 days of menstruation to prevent radiation exposure to an early embryo. An HSG should not be performed when there is co-existing, untreated pelvic infection.

StratOG.net. Epidemiology, ethical and legal issues of subfertility. London: StratOG, 2012. www.rcog.org.uk/stratog

6. A False

   B True

   C True

   D False

   E True

Overall, ultrasound is considered a safe imaging modality. Nevertheless its usage does require monitoring to ensure that there are no adverse effects related to its use. The main concerns regarding the usage of ultrasound relate to thermal effects related to the heating of local tissue. In order to reduce the potential impact of exposing an embryo or fetus to the thermal effects to ultrasound, exposure should be kept to a minimum. Particular caution should be applied when using a transvaginal probe in early pregnancy. Thermal indices are used, as a measure of tissue heating effects and safety protocols necessitate the use of minimising the thermal index (to < 1) and keeping scanning time as short as possible to prevent tissue heating. Fulguration is the destruction of tissue using electrosurgery.

Ambramowicz JS, Kossoff G, Marsal K, Ter Haar G. Safety Statement, 2000 (reconfirmed 2003). Ultrasound Obstet Gynecol 2003; 21:100.
Salvesen K, Lees C, Ambramowicz J, et al. ISUOG statement on the safe use of Doppler in the 11 to 13+6-week fetal ultrasound examination. Ultrasound Obstet Gynecol, 2011; 37:628.

7. B B-mode

A-mode is the simplest form of ultrasound and is now rarely used. It creates wave spikes as the ultrasound comes into contact with various tissues. The distance between the spikes can be measured. The A in A-mode refers to the amplitude of the ultrasound used. B-mode, or brightness mode, is widely used in ultrasound to create two-dimensional greyscale images obtained from a linear array of transducers, which simultaneously scan a tissue plane. M-mode incorporates movement with successive A- or B-mode images. Doppler mode is used to assess movement and therefore is the mode used for looking at blood flow. There are various different types of Doppler used including pulsed wave, continuous and colour.

8. B Amniotic fluid index

Biophysical profiling provides a means of formally assessing fetal well-being.

This may be indicated in the context of reduced fetal movements or growth restriction. There are five biophysical variables which are assessed in biophysical profiling. Fetal tone, breathing, movement and heart rate are recorded, alongside an assessment of the amniotic fluid index. The assessment of the fetal heart rate is described as a non-stress test. A score is given for each variable and the total can then guide further management. The fetal head circumference, abdominal circumference, femur length and biparietal diameter are parameters used to assess fetal growth and are not part of biophysical profiling.

9. A Epithelial surface damage

Although radiotherapy is used in the treatment of a wide range of malignancies, patients exposed to it may experience a number of side-effects, both acute and late. Epithelial surface damage is an example of an acute side-effect of radiotherapy and may manifest in the form of mouth ulcers. Radiotherapy for vulval cancer is particularly associated with severe skin reactions, due to the high dosages of radiation required. Other acute side-effects of radiotherapy include gastrointestinal symptoms, cystitis, fatigue and oedema. **Table 8.3** lists acute and late side-effects of radiotherapy.

StratOG.net, Principles of Radiotherapy. London: stratOG, 2010. www.rcog.org.uk/stratog

10. E X-ray

High energy forms of radiation capable of separating an electron from an atom are described as 'ionising'. Forms of ionising radiation can have therapeutic properties, but require close regulation to prevent excessive exposure. **Table 8.1** lists sources of ionising and non-ionising radiation.

Table 8.1 Examples of ionising and non-ionising radiation	
Ionising radiation	**Non-ionising radiation**
X-ray	Electrocautery
Radiotherapy	Laser
Positron emission tomography	MRI
Radionucleotides, e.g. barium swallow	Ultrasound
	Microwaves
	Diathermy

11. A 2–3 days

Radiation dosage is measured in millisieverts (mSv) and is often referred to as the effective dose. Exposure to radiation can also be described in terms of the equivalent duration of natural background radiation associated with the exposure. For different imaging modalities, **Table 8.2** gives the time it would take to receive an equivalent radiation does from natural background radiation dose.

Table 8.2 Imaging modalities with equivalent natural background radiation	
Modality	**Time period for effective dose from natural background radiation**
Chest X-ray	7–10 days
CT of abdomen	3 years
Lumbar spine X-ray	6 months
Intravenous urogram	1 year

12. A >2 mm

Fetal heart action should be evident when the crown–rump length (CRL) is >2 mm. However, in 5–10% of embryos there will be no fetal heart action visible until >4 mm. When using ultrasound to diagnose the viability of a pregnancy, a CRL of ≥7 mm and absence of fetal heart action suggests a non-viable pregnancy. In these cases a further scan may be indicated after an interval of at least 1 week.

Royal College of Obstetricians and Gynaecologists. The Management of Early Pregnancy Loss. Green-top Guideline 25. London: RCOG, 2006.
Royal College of Obstetricians and Gynaecologists. Addendum to GTG No 25. The Management of Early Pregnancy Loss, 2011. www.rcog.org.uk

13. D V_1–V_4

Bearing in mind that varying electrode placement allows the electrocardiogram to create a pictorial representation of electrical activity in the heart it is possible to localise pathological changes in the heart's conduction pathways. Leads V_1–V_4 detect electrical activity in the anterior part of the heart along the horizontal plane. Therefore, when there is a considerable change in the heart conduction pathways as a consequence of an anterior myocardial infarction we may expect to see ST wave elevation in these leads. An inferior ST elevation myocardial infarction (STEMI) would be represented as ST wave elevation in leads II, III and aVF. Electrical activity in the lateral aspect of the heart is monitored by V_5 and V_6, as well by as leads I and aVL. Thus, a lateral STEMI is likely to be seen as ST elevation in leads I, aVL and V_5 to V_6.

14. B Lymphoedema

Radiotherapy is a form of ionising radiation that is widely used in the treatment of cancers, but may also be used to for a variety of non-malignant conditions. Radiotherapy is effective in damaging the cellular DNA and thus causing cellular death. The ionising radiation is targeted at localised areas to avoid generalised exposure to its effects. Like any intervention, radiotherapy has side effects which can be classified to acute or late (**Table 8.3**). Lymphoedema is one such late side effect and typically occurs following pelvic and breast radiotherapy.

StratOG.net, Principles of Radiotherapy. London: stratOG, 2010. www.rcog.org.uk/stratog

Table 8.3 Side-effects of radiotherapy	
Acute side-effects of radiotherapy	**Late side-effects of radiotherapy**
–	Lymphoedema
Oedema	Hair loss
Gastrointestinal symptoms: nausea, vomiting, diarrhoea, abdominal pain	Development of further cancers
Fatigue	Tissue fibrosis
Epithelial surface damage, e.g. mouth ulcers	Infertility

15. C It is the opposition to the passage of sound waves and is a function of density and elasticity

Acoustic impedance is a term used in the description of ultrasound behaviour within a tissue. It represents the opposition to the passage of sound waves and is a function of density and elasticity. Refraction is the change in direction of the wave as a result in change of speed. Diffraction describes the bending of waves during its passage as a result of interaction with obstacles. Reflected waves from a moving object undergoing a frequency shift is the Doppler effect. Colour Doppler provides an estimate of mean velocity of flow within a vessel.

Chapter 9

Clinical management

Questions: MCQs

Answer each stem 'True' or 'False'.

1. Acute pelvic inflammatory disease can present with:
   A Superficial dyspareunia
   B Cervical tenderness
   C Heavy menstrual bleeding
   D Lower abdominal pain radiating to the loins
   E Postcoital bleeding

2. Concerning pelvic inflammatory disease due to *Neisseria gonorrhoeae*:
   A Normally presents with associated cough
   B Is sensitive to quinolones
   C Testing is from a high vaginal swab
   D A urethral swab increases diagnostic yield
   E Does not increase risk of subfertility

3. In regard to pelvic inflammatory disease:
   A It is rare in cases of intrauterine pregnancies
   B It cannot be treated in early pregnancy as there are no safe drugs
   C It is most prevalent in women aged between 25 and 35 years
   D It does not increase the risk of subfertility if treated with intravenously antibiotics
   E Treatment for the index partner is necessary only with proven *Chlamydia* infection

4. With regards to semen analysis:
   A Men should abstain from ejaculation for 7 days prior to providing a sample
   B It should reach the laboratory within 24 hours of being produced
   C If abnormal it should be repeated after 3 months
   D Sperm can be collected in a normal condom
   E The result should be available prior to any form of ovulation induction

5. The following are appropriate initial investigations for menorrhagia:
   A Pelvic ultrasound scan
   B Full blood count
   C Hormone profile
   D Hysteroscopy
   E MRI pelvis

6. **The following laboratory tests should be carried out on all women who present with heavy menstrual bleeding:**

   A Hormone profile
   B Serum ferritin
   C Thyroid function test
   D Coagulation function
   E Full blood count

7. **With regards to the diagnosis of malaria in pregnancy:**

   A Severe malaria is defined as parasitaemia of $> 50\,\%$
   B Her full blood count will show normal haemoglobin but low platelets
   C She is not likely to have the disease if she has been compliant with prophylaxis
   D A rapid detection test should be performed to exclude malaria
   E Three negative malaria smears 12–24 hours apart will rule out malaria if the patient is febrile

8. **With regard to the management of HIV positive women presenting in active labour and wishing to have a vaginal delivery:**

   A A recent viral load result should be confirmed as < 50 copies/mL
   B Highly active antiretroviral treatment should be administered throughout the labour
   C Fetal blood sampling can be performed to assess fetal wellbeing
   D The membranes should be ruptured as early as possible to expedite delivery
   E An induction of labour is contraindicated

9. **Regarding caesarean section:**

   A Approximately 1 in 6 women will have a caesarean section in the United Kingdom
   B Body mass an index of >50 is a clear indication for elective caesarean section
   C Women with an uncomplicated singleton breech at 34 weeks' gestation should be recommended to have an elective caesarean section
   D All preterm and small for gestational age babies need an elective caesarean section delivery
   E Risk of a hysterectomy at a caesarean section is roughly 5%

10. **Regarding preconception management of women with pre-existing diabetes:**

    A She should be taking 800 µg of folic acid
    B She should be commenced on a statin to lower her cholesterol
    C She should have monthly haemoglobin A1C (HbA1C) measurement
    D She should be discouraged from pregnancy if her HbA1C is 8%
    E Metformin should be stopped prior to conception

11. **Recognised risk factors for postpartum haemorrhage are:**

    A Multiple pregnancy
    B Previous caesarean section with a low lying placenta
    C Antepartum haemorrhage
    D Polyhydramnios
    E Young age

Questions: SBAs

For each question, select the single best answer from the five options listed.

12. A 26-year-old woman attends the emergency department feeling unwell and complaining of lower abdominal pain. On examination she has a temperature of 39 °C and a pulse rate of 110 beats per minute. She has lower abdominal tenderness with guarding and cervical excitation. A speculum examination reveals profuse discharge.

    What is the most appropriate management?

    A   Admit for intravenous antibiotics and supportive care
    B   Book for a diagnostic laparoscopy
    C   Organise a pelvic ultrasound scan
    D   Refer for a surgical review
    E   Refer to a sexual health clinic for screening and partner contact tracing

13. A 27-year-old female teacher, who is 14 weeks pregnant, presents to her general practitioner as she is concerned because one of her students was sent home today with chickenpox. Her varicella zoster virus IgG antibody is positive.

    What is the correct advice to give her?

    A   Chickenpox is not contagious once the rash appears so she need not worry
    B   She is immune to chickenpox and no further action needs to be taken
    C   She should have be referred to fetal medicine unit for a scan to exclude abnormality
    D   She should not attend the hospital as she may infect other pregnant women
    E   She should receive varicella zoster immune globulin within the next 24 hours for it to be effective

14. A 28-year-old patient attends out patient clinic with primary subfertility. Her partner's semen analysis and her hysterosalpingogram are normal. Her follicle-stimulating hormone is 2.3 IU/mL, luteinising hormone is 6.8 IU/mL, and her day 21 progesterone is 19 ng/mL.

    What is the most likely cause for her subfertility?

    A   Asherman's syndrome
    B   Endometriosis
    C   Hypogonadotrophic hypogonadism
    D   Premature menopause
    E   Polycystic ovaries

15. A 22-year-old patient, who is 35 weeks pregnant, presents to the hospital complaining of heavy painless bleeding. She is pale, has a pulse rate of 140 beats per minute, and a blood pressure of 70/40 mmHg. Her abdomen is soft and non-tender.

    What is the most likely diagnosis?

    A   Concealed abruption
    B   Placenta praevia
    C   Premature labour
    D   Revealed abruption
    E   Vasa praevia

16. A 40-year-old woman complains of heavy regular periods for 5 years. Ultrasound scan has revealed no abnormality. Her family is complete.

    What is the most appropriate first line treatment for this patient?

    A   Combined contraceptive pill
    B   Laparoscopic assisted vaginal hysterectomy
    C   Levonorgestrel-releasing intrauterine system (IUS)
    D   Norethisterone tablet 5 mg three times daily from day 5 to 26
    E   Tranexamic acid

17. A 35-year-old woman attends gynaecology outpatient department with an incidental ultrasound finding of a-4 cm simple ovarian cyst.

    What is the most appropriate plan of management?

    A   Consider further imaging (i.e. MRI)
    B   Laparoscopic cystectomy
    C   Reassure and discharge
    D   Serum CA-125 test
    E   Yearly ultrasound follow-up

18. A 22-year-old woman with a past history of *Chlamydia* attends the emergency department complaining of severe abdominal pain. She has mild vaginal bleeding. Her pulse rate is 120 beats per minute, with a blood pressure of 60/40 mmHg and she has a distended tender abdomen.

    What is the most likely diagnosis?

    A   Acute appendicitis
    B   Complete miscarriage
    C   Ruptured ectopic pregnancy
    D   Threatened miscarriage
    E   Urinary tract infection

19. You are asked to review a 20-year-old woman in the emergency department. She has a positive pregnancy test, and is unsure of her last menstrual period. On examination, her pulse is 70 beats per minute and her blood pressure is 110/70 mmHg. Her abdomen is soft and non-tender. Speculum examination reveals a closed cervix and mild bleeding.

    What is the most appropriate plan of management?

    A   Admit the patient and arrange an evacuation of retained products of conception
    B   Admit the patient for a laparoscopy as an ectopic pregnancy cannot be excluded

C   Admit the patient for hourly observations
D   Arrange the next available ultrasound scan as an outpatient
E   Discharge the patient with the diagnosis of complete miscarriage

20. A 30-year-old patient, who is hypertensive and obese with a body mass index of 38, requests contraception. She has had two previous caesarean sections.

What is the most effective and safest form of contraception for her?

A   Laparoscopic sterilisation
B   Combined oral contraceptive pill
C   Subdermal implant
D   Barrier contraception
E   Intrauterine device

21. A 44-year-old is 28 weeks pregnant with ovum donation. She presents with headache and reports seeing 'flashing lights'. Her blood pressure is 172/112 mmHg and her pulse rate is 78 beats per minute. Urine dipstick shows protein +++, leucocytes trace, nitrites negative, blood trace.

Which is the most appropriate immediate management for this patient?

A   Request an urgent scan for fetal growth
B   Administer antihypertensives to lower her blood pressure
C   Administer ramipril
D   Avoid steroid injections as it will worsen her blood pressure
E   Immediate delivery of the baby by category one caesarean section

22. The risk of malignancy index (RMI) is used to score the risk of ovarian cancer in women.

Which of the following is correct with regards to the basis of its calculation?

A   Classification of post menopausal is a woman who has had no periods for 2 years or over age of 51 years
B   Premenopausal status is scored as 3
C   Serum CA-125 levels are measured on a scale of 1 to 10
D   Ultrasound scan must show a cyst of at least 10 cm in size
E   Ultrasound score × menopausal status × CA-125

23. A 27-year-old woman attends the antenatal clinic at 14 weeks' gestation in her third pregnancy. She had a deep vein thrombosis, when she broke her leg during a skiing trip at age 20 years. Her thrombophilia screen outside of pregnancy was negative. She has no family history of venous thromboembolism.

Which of the following is the most appropriate action?

A   Aspirin 150 mg from conception to 36 weeks' gestation
B   Low-molecular weight heparin therapy immediately
C   Low-molecular weight heparin therapy from 24 weeks' gestation until onset of labour

    D   Low-molecular weight heparin therapy for 6 weeks postnatally

    E   Referral to haematology for repeat thrombophilia screen now she is pregnant

24. A 47-year-old premenopausal woman undergoes a hysteroscopy for investigation of severe menorrhagia. Histology of endometrial biopsy shows simple hyperplasia.

What would be the most appropriate recommendation?

    A   Commence hormone replacement therapy

    B   Hysterectomy

    C   Insertion of a levonorgestrel-releasing intrauterine system (IUS)

    D   Ultrasound scan in 6 months

    E   No treatment is required

25. A 32-year-old primiparous woman is in labour. Labour was induced at 40+12 weeks for post- dates and oxytocin augmentation has been used. Following delivery of the fetal head the midwife is unable to deliver the body using gentle traction. She suspects there is 'shoulder dystocia' and the emergency buzzer is pulled.

Which of the following is the most appropriate first line measure to be taken in order to deliver the baby?

    A   Episiotomy

    B   Fundal pressure

    C   McRoberts' manoeuvre

    D   Symphysiotomy

    E   Zavanelli manoeuvre

26. A 28-year-old primiparous woman is 24 weeks pregnant. She presents to the Maternity Day Unit with a history of reduced fetal movements over the last 18 hours. She is well and has no medical or obstetric history of note.

What is the most appropriate means of assessing fetal well-being in this pregnancy?

    A   Auscultation of the fetal heart using a handheld Doppler device

    B   Biophysical profiling

    C   Cardiotocograph

    D   Completion of 24-hour kick chart

    E   Ultrasound scan

Answers

1. A False

    B True

    C False

    D False

    E True

    Acute pelvic inflammatory disease (PID) lacks definitive clinical diagnostic criteria but certain clinical features are highly suggestive of PID and treatment should start without delay. Women with PID may present with:

    - Lower abdominal pain
    - Abnormal discharge
    - Pain during intercourse
    - Pyrexia
    - Cervical motion and adnexal tenderness on bimanual examination.

    Differential diagnosis must always include ectopic pregnancy, appendicitis, an ovarian cyst accident, urinary tract infection, and gastrointestinal disorders.

    Royal College of Obstetricians and Gynaecologists. Management of Acute Pelvic Inflammatory Disease. Green-top Guideline 32. London: RCOG, 2008.

2. A False

    B False

    C False

    D True

    E False

    Gonorrhoea is the second most common sexually transmitted bacterial infection in the United Kingdom. It may sometimes be asymptomatic, but if left untreated it can cause subfertility. Women with Gonorrhoea may present with abnormal discharge, lower abdominal pain or dysuria. Testing should be with an endocervical specimen; however, an additional sample from the urethra increases diagnostic yield when testing by nucleic acid amplification test is not available. A pregnancy test should be performed in all women who attend with lower abdominal pain or are suspected to have pelvic inflammatory disease.

    Royal College of Obstetricians and Gynaecologists. Management of Acute Pelvic Inflammatory Disease. Green-top Guideline 32. London: RCOG, 2008.

3. A True

    B False

    C False

D False

E False

Pelvic inflammatory disease (PID) is rarely seen with intrauterine pregnancy and hence diagnosis of PID should be made with caution when looking for differential diagnosis in pregnancy. All drugs used in pregnancy for any reason should be looked at from risk benefit ratio and if benefits outweigh risks, they can be used. Treated or untreated, PID does increase the risk of subfertility. Therefore, it is essential that even if there is no robust evidence of PID on tests performed, if symptomatic, treatment should be offered.

Royal College of Obstetricians and Gynaecologists. Management of Acute Pelvic Inflammatory Disease. Green-top Guideline 32. London: RCOG, 2008.

4. A False

B False

C True

D False

E True

Abstinence of 2–3 days prior to performing a semen analysis is considered to be ideal, as shorter abstinence may result in production difficulties. Longer abstinence usually results in collection of dead sperm and debris in larger proportions. The sample once produced should reach the laboratory, ideally, within 45–60 minutes to assess the motility accurately. Normal condoms contain spermicides, so sperm should only be collected either directly in the aseptic pot or into non-spermicidal condoms.

National Institute for Health and Clinical Excellence. Fertility Assessment and Management for People with Fertility Problems. Clinical Guideline CG11. London: NICE, 2004.

5. A False

B True

C False

D False

E False

Menorrhagia refers to heavy menstrual bleeding. Blood loss may be such that it affects many aspects of a woman's life, including her physical health and overall quality of life.

A full blood count should be performed at presentation. If uterine structural abnormalities such as fibroids are suspected, then ultrasound is a first line diagnostic tool. A biopsy of the lining of the womb may be indicated in women above 45 years old or those who present with persistent intermenstrual bleeding. Pharmaceutical management, if appropriate, should be considered. Initial management includes the insertion of a levonorgestrel-releasing intrauterine system (IUS) as a first choice, with other options including tranexamic acid or the combined oral contraceptive. Norethisterone or long-acting injected progestogens may also be considered.

Other treatments for heavy menstrual bleeding, other than hysterectomy, include endometrial ablation, and in the presence of fibroids include myomectomy and uterine artery embolisation.

National Institute for Health and Clinical Excellence. Heavy Menstrual Bleeding. Clinical Guideline CG44. London: NICE, 2007.

6. A False

    B False

    C False

    D False

    E True

Women with heavy menstrual bleeding require a full blood count at their first presentation. Thyroid function tests should only be performed if the signs and symptoms of thyroid disease are present. A coagulation screen function should not be performed, unless the history is suggestive of a coagulation abnormality. A hormonal profile is not indicated. An assessment of serum ferritin is not usually required.

National Institute for Health and Clinical Excellence. Heavy Menstrual Bleeding. Clinical Guideline CG44. London: NICE, 2007.

7. A False

    B False

    C False

    D False

    E True

Malaria can be difficult to diagnose and may present as a flu-like illness. Pregnant women with parasitaemia of 2% or more are at risk of developing severe malaria which can manifest with respiratory distress, impaired consciousness or pulmonary oedema. Laboratory investigation may reveal severe anaemia, thrombocytopaenia, hypoglycaemia and impaired renal function.

Malaria in pregnancy requires microscopic diagnosis. The current gold standard for the detection of malaria is the preparation of thick and thin blood films. Although less sensitive, rapid detection techniques can be used, but they can miss the low levels of parasitaemia that may be present in pregnant women, and they are less able to detect the presence of *Plasmodium vivax*. In a febrile patient, three negative malaria smears 12–24 hours apart are needed to exclude diagnosis of malaria. Pregnant women with malaria should be admitted to hospital for treatment. Choloroquine is used for treatment of *P. vivax*, *P. ovale* or *P. malariae*. All newborns of mothers who have had malaria in pregnancy should be screened as there is a risk of vertical transmission.

Royal College of Obstetricians and Gynaecologists. The Diagnosis and Treatment of Malaria in Pregnancy. Green-top Guideline 54B. London: RCOG, 2010.

8. A True

    B True

    C False

    D False

    E False

Women with HIV in pregnancy should be advised to take antiretroviral therapy and this should be continued throughout labour. They should also be tested for hepatitis C, varicella zoster, measles and toxoplasma.

Women with a viral load of <50 copies/mL can opt for a vaginal delivery. In case of prolonged pregnancy in these women, a membrane sweep may be performed and prostaglandins may be used.

In order to reduce the chance of vertical transmission, membranes should be kept intact for as long as possible and invasive procedures, such as fetal blood sampling and fetal heart monitoring via a scalp electrode, should be avoided. If instrumental delivery is required, forceps should be used in preference over performing a ventouse delivery.

Royal College of Obstetricians and Gynaecologists. Management of HIV in Pregnancy. Green-top Guideline 29. London: RCOG, 2010.

9. A False

    B False

    C False

    D False

    E False

At the time of writing, the caesarean section rate in the United Kingdom was around 25%. A raised body mass index alone should not be an indicator for elective caesarean section. An external cephalic version should be offered to women with an uncomplicated singleton breech pregnancy at 36 weeks' gestation, rather than automatically recommending an elective caesarean section. Small for gestational age babies do not require delivery by elective caesarean. The risk of hysterectomy, due to a postpartum haemorrage, at a caesarean section is very low, at around 0.03%.

National Institute for Health and Clinical Excellence. Caesarean Section. Clinical Guidance CG132. London: NICE, 2011.

10. A False

    B False

    C True

D True

E False

Women with diabetes should have preconception counseling and advised of the importance of achieving good glycaemic control prior to conception. They should be advised to take 5 mg of folic acid daily prior to conception and continue this until 12 weeks' gestation. They should be referred for retinal screening. If they are being prescribed cholesterol-lowering drugs, these should be stopped.

Monthly haemoglobin A1C (HbA1C) measurement is recommended to ensure good control prior to conception. If possible, women should aim for an HbA1C of 6.1% or as close to it as possible to reduce the chance of congenital malformations. Women whose HbA1C is above 10% should be strongly advised not to become pregnant.

National Institute for Health and Clinical Excellence. Diabetes in Pregnancy: Management of Diabetes and its Complications from Preconception to the Postnatal Period. Clinical Guidelines CG63. London: NICE, 2008.

11. A True

B True

C True

D True

E False

Postpartum haemorrhage (PPH) can be considered as either primary or secondary. A primary PPH is the loss of more than 500 mL of blood within 24 hours of delivery. A secondary PPH is the loss of large volumes of blood which occurs between 24 hours and 6 weeks after delivery.

The majority of PPHs are caused ultimately by uterine atony, which is more likely in multiple pregnancy, polyhydramnios and prolonged labour. Abnormal placentation is associated with increased risk of antepartum and postpartum haemorrhage. Other risk factors for PPH include a previous history of PPH, previous antepartum haemorrhage, multiparity and advancing maternal age.

Royal College of Obstetricians and Gynaecologists. Prevention and Management of Postpartum Haemorrhage. Green-top Guideline 52. London: RCOG, 2009.

12. A Admit for intravenous antibiotics and supportive care

Pelvic inflammatory disease (PID) is a common problem in young women. Untreated PID can lead to long-term subfertility, be associated with chronic pelvic pain and increase the risk of ectopic pregnancy. Hence, a low threshold for treatment is required. Admission to hospital may be necessary in clinically severe cases, and when other surgical emergencies need to be excluded. Intravenous antibiotics for at least 24 hours are recommended. Women should be given a detailed explanation of the diagnosis and its possible long term implications, and the importance of contact tracing reinforced.

Royal College of Obstetricians and Gynaecologists. Management of Acute Pelvic Inflammatory Disease. Green-top Guideline 32. London: RCOG, 2008.

13. B She is immune to chickenpox and no further action needs to be taken

The incubation period of chickenpox is 1–3 weeks. Chickenpox is infectious from 48 hours before the rash appears and remains so until the vesicles crust over. If a woman is not immune, varicella vaccination can be offered pre-pregnancy or postpartum.

Women who are varicella zoster virus IgG-negative should avoid contact with chickenpox and shingles in pregnancy. Varicella zoster immunoglobulin (VZIG) should be given to non-immune pregnant women who have been exposed. VZIG should not be given once chickenpox has developed.

Chickenpox in the first trimester does not increase risk of miscarriage.

Royal College of Obstetricians and Gynaecologists. Chickenpox in Pregnancy. Green-top Guideline 13. London: RCOG, 2007.

14. E Polycystic ovaries

Polycystic ovaries are one of the most common endocrinological conditions associated with subfertility and anovulation. The hormone picture is usually 1:3 ratio of early follicular phase follicle-stimulating hormone (FSH):luteinising hormone (LH) along with an ovulatory day 21 progesterone (< 30 ng/mL) levels. Women going through premature menopause will have raised FSH and LH levels in early follicular phase. Endometriosis and Asherman's syndrome do not alter the FSH/LH ratio. Hypogonadotrophic hypogonadism results into very low FSH and LH levels without any alterations in the ratio.

National Institute for Health and Clinical Excellence. Fertility Assessment and Management for People with Fertility Problems. Clinical Guideline CG11. London: NICE, 2004.

15. B Placenta praevia

Placenta praevia is the partial or complete insertion of the placenta into the lower segment of the uterus. It is graded from I to IV, where grades I and II are classified as minor placenta praevia and grades III and IV as major placenta praevia. Minor placenta praevia is present when the placenta has inserted into the lower segment and is close to the cervical os. Major placenta praevia is present when the placenta lies over the cervical os. Women with placenta praevia may present with painless bleeding.

Vasa praevia is present when fetal vessels are found across the membranes over the internal os, below the presenting part. Bleeding from a placenta praevia carries risk to maternal life, whereas vasa praevia is associated with high levels of fetal morbidity and mortality due to fetal haemorrhage if immediate delivery is not undertaken.

Royal College of Obstetricians and Gynaecologists. Placenta Praevia, Placenta Praevia Accreta and Vasa Praevia: Diagnosis and Management. Green-top Guideline 27. London: RCOG, 2011.

16. C Levonorgestrel-releasing intrauterine system

Heavy menstrual bleeding is a common problem. Once preliminary investigations, such as an ultrasound of the pelvis, have been completed there are a number of interventions that can be tried in sequential order. The use of a levonorgestrel-releasing intrauterine system (IUS) is currently the first-line recommended management option. Using this form of IUS the majority of women will have a reduction in their menstrual flow and in some women it may cause amenorrhoea. A second-line option is the use of the tranexamic acid. The use of northisterone or injectable progestogens are reserved as third-line treatments.

National Institute for Health and Clinical Excellence. Heavy Menstrual Bleeding. Clinical Guideline CG44. London: NICE, 2007.

17. C Reassure and discharge

The majority of ovarian cysts in premenopausal women are benign, with the risk of malignancy being 1–3 per 1000. Simple thin-walled cysts which are <s50mm in diameter can be managed conservatively, and most of these are resolve w thin 3 months. A pelvic ultrasound is the most appropriate way of assessing an ovarian cyst, with the transvaginal route being more sensitive. See **Figure 9.1** for an ultrasound image of an ovarian cyst.

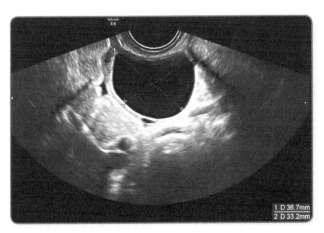

Figure 9.1 Ultrasound of ovarian cyst.

It is important to remember that CA-125 has an increased rate of false positives in premenopausal women. Its value may be raised in other conditions such as endometriosis, pelvic infection, endometriosis, and when a woman has fibroids. Therefore in the presence of a simple ovarian cyst taking a serum CA-125 level is not essential.

However, in women under 40 years old with the ultrasound finding of a complex ovarian mass, tumour markers such as hCG, α-fetoprotein, and lactate should be measured to exclude germ cell tumours.

Royal College of Obstetricians and Gynaecologists. Management of Suspected Ovarian Masses in Premenopausal Women. Green-top Guideline 62. London: RCOG, 2011.

18. C Ruptured ectopic pregnancy

An ectopic pregnancy is one that is implanted outside the womb. It must be excluded in any woman who presents with abdominal or bowel symptoms with a positive pregnancy test. Previous pelvic inflammatory disease (PID) is a known risk factor. Other risk factors for ectopic pregnancy include previous pelvis or tubal surgery, endometriosis, assisted conception or a history of subfertility, smoking and the presence of an in situ intrauterine device.

The fallopian tube is the most common site of an ectopic pregnancy; however, they may also be abdominal, ovarian or cervical. The majority of ectopic pregnancies are in the ampullary segment of the fallopian tube.

The isthmic segment of the tube is narrower than the ampullary portion. As a consequence rupture occurs at earlier gestations with isthmic ectopic pregnancies. In contrast, rupture of the interstitial segment of the fallopian tube can occur at the relatively late gestation of 12 to 14 weeks.

Potdar N, Konje JC. Chapter 25: Ectopic Pregnancy. In: Shaw RW, Luesley D, Monga A (eds). Gynaecology, 4th edn. Edinburgh: Churchill Livingstone, 2011: 363–381.

19. D Arrange the next available ultrasound scan as an outpatient

Miscarriage is the most common complication of pregnancy. Threatened miscarriage is defined as uterine bleeding with a closed cervix. It can affect up to 25% of pregnancies. Clinical examination will reveal a soft, non-tender uterus.

An inevitable miscarriage is either complete or incomplete depending on whether all the pregnancy tissue has been expelled from the uterus or not. An incomplete miscarriage will present with ongoing bleeding, abdominal pain and an open cervix.

An early pregnancy assessment unit is an appropriate setting for referral of a haemodynamically stable patient in early pregnancy. Women need to know that until then an ectopic pregnancy cannot be excluded, and they must return earlier if they experience severe pain or become unwell.

Royal College of Obstetricians and Gynaecologists. The Management of Early Pregnancy Loss. Green-top Guideline 25. London: RCOG, 2006.

20. C Subdermal implant

The subdermal implant is a progestogen-based contraception and is a form of long-acting reversible contraception. Once inserted, it is licensed for contraceptive use for 3 years. The main mode of action is inhibition of ovulation, but as it contains progestogen it also has progestogerone contraception effects, including changes to cervical mucus and inhibition of normal endometrial development. Benefits include efficacy (pregnancy <1 in 1000 over 3 years), length of efficacy and no user reliability. It obviously does not protect against sexually transmitted infections and the major side effect of its use is irregular bleeding, which patients should be counselled about prior to insertion. Up to 20% of women will have no bleeding and up to half of women will experience irregular or infrequent bleeding. UK medical eligibility criteria IV (absolute contraindication) is current breast cancer. Previous ectopic pregnancy is not a contraindication for use.

Fleming CF. Long-acting reversible contraceptives. The Obstetrician & Gynaecologist 2009;11:83–88. Faculty of Sexual and Reproductive Healthcare. Progestogen-only Implant. London: RCOG, 2008.

21. B Administer antihypertensives to lower her blood pressure

This patient has pre-eclampsia, as indicated by her hypertension, proteinuria and symptoms.

When a patient has severe pre-eclampsia it is important to keep her blood pressure <150/80–100mmHg. Suitable antihypertensives include oral or intravenous labetalol, intravenous hydralazine or oral nifedipine. These are the first line treatments as uncontrolled hypertension leads to both maternal and neonatal morbidity and mortality.

If this patient's pre-eclampsia cannot be controlled she may require delivery. If delivery is thought to be likely in the next 7 days a course of steroids should be considered if the gestation is <37 weeks.

National Institute for Health and Clinical Excellence. Hypertension in Pregnancy. Clinical Guideline CG107. London: NICE, 2010.

22. E Ultrasound score × menopausal status × CA-125

The risk of malignancy index (RMI) uses three presurgical features in order to stratify an overall risk of having a malignant ovarian tumour. It is calculated as RMI = U x M x CA-125, where:

- U is the ultrasound result and gives a point for specific characteristics of the ovarian mass
- M is the menopausal status; being postmenopausal confers higher risk
- CA-125 is the serum level of the tumour marker, Cancer Antigen 125

National Institute for Health and Clinical Excellence. Ovarian Cancer: the Recognition and Initial Management of Ovarian Cancer. Clinical Guideline CG122. London: NICE, 2011.

23. D Low-molecular weight heparin therapy for 6 weeks postnatally

Any woman who has had only one thromboembolic event in the past, with no other known risk factors, still needs to be monitored closely during her pregnancy. A prophylactic dose of low molecular weight heparin is needed for 6 weeks after delivery.

Factor V Leiden is the most common inherited thrombophilic disorder. The risk of thromboembolic events can be increased by approximately 30 times in individuals who are homozygous for the disease.

This patient is most at risk of developing a thromboembolic event postnatally and the most appropriate course of action is to give low molecular weight heparin for 6 weeks postnatally.

Royal College of Obstetricians and Gynaecologists. Reducing the Risk of Thrombosis and Embolism during Pregnancy and the Puerperium. Green-top Guideline 37. London: RCOG, 2009.

24. C Insertion of a levonorgestrel-releasing intrauterine system (IUS)

Endometrial hyperplasia is a premalignant condition and these patients are more likely to develop endometrial carcinoma. One important cause is unopposed oestrogens, therefore oestrogen-only hormone replacement therapy would be contraindicated in this case. An ultrasound in 6 months time would not be the most appropriate management as it is not a diagnostic tool, and would only be of benefit to determine endometrial thickness. Use of progestogens helps to maintain a thin endometrium and prevent development of endometrial cancer.

25. C McRoberts' manoeuvre

Failure to deliver the fetal body, following delivery of the head, which requires the use of manoeuvres to release the impacted fetal shoulder is known as shoulder dystocia. This event is considered an obstetric emergency as the fetus can quickly become compromised and help should be called for immediately. The McRoberts' position requires flexion and abduction of both of the maternal hips. This manoeuvre is often sufficient to deliver the baby. Fundal pressure should not be applied at any point. Episiotomy may be performed to provide additional room for further internal manoeuvres but in itself does not aid delivery. The Zavanelli manoeuvre, which involves replacement of the baby's head prior to emergency caesarean section, is one of the last manoeuvres to resort to if all else has failed.

Royal College of Obstetricians and Gynaecologists. Shoulder Dystocia. Green-top Guideline 42. London: RCOG 2012.

26. A Auscultation of the fetal heart using a handheld Doppler device

The perception of reduced fetal movement (RFM) is a common obstetric presentation. In the majority of presentations of RFM, fetal well-being is confirmed and the pregnancy goes on to have a successful outcome. Nevertheless, the sudden reduction in fetal movements or cessation of any movement perception must be taken seriously and is often reported by women who have had a stillbirth. Between 24 and 28 weeks' gestation the most appropriate investigation is auscultation of fetal heart using a handheld Doppler device. At this gestation there is neither role for cardiotocography (CTG) nor ultrasound assessment (unless there are other concerns regarding fetal growth). After 28 weeks a CTG is an appropriate method of assessing well-being. Prior to 24 weeks' gestation fetal well-being should be assessed using a handheld Doppler device (as for pregnancies of 24–28 weeks' gestation). The completion of a 24-hour kick chart following normal investigation of fetal well-being is not indicated at any gestation. Biophysical profiling is not indicated in low-risk pregnancies with RFM. Any woman who has further episodes of RFM should be advised to re-present to her care providers as soon as possible.

Royal College of Obstetricians and Gynaecologists. Reduced Fetal Movements. Green-top Guideline 57. London: RCOG, 2011.

Chapter 10

Data interpretation

Questions: MCQs

Answer each stem 'True' or 'False'.

1. Concerning cardiotocograph (CTG) monitoring:
   A The paper speed is 1 cm per minute in the UK
   B The CTG is a legal document
   C Variability <5 beats for <90 minutes is a non-reassuring feature
   D As per National Institute for Health and Clinical Excellence guidance, two abnormal features are needed to classify the CTG as pathological
   E Fetal blood sampling may be considered in fetuses over 32 weeks' gestation

2. Regarding the diagnosis of diabetes in pregnancy:
   A An oral glucose tolerance test is most appropriately performed at 20 weeks' gestation
   B Diabetes is diagnosed if a fasting glucose level is > 7.0 mmol/L
   C Diabetes is diagnosed if a 2-hour glucose level is > 10.1 mmol/L
   D Impaired glucose tolerance is diagnosed if 2-hour glucose level is ≥8.2 and <10.1 mmol/L
   E Polyhydramnios can indicate gestational diabetes

3. A positive result for protein on urine dipstick can indicate:
   A Pre-eclampsia
   B Urinary tract infection
   C Renal colic
   D Normal pregnancy
   E Hydronephrosis

4. Regarding serum β-human chorionic gonadotrophin (β-hCG):
   A High levels of β-hCG can indicate gestational trophoblastic disease
   B An increase in β-hCG of 50% in 48 hours is considered normal
   C An intrauterine pregnancy should be visible on transvaginal scan when the β-hCG is ≥500 IU/L
   D Serum β-hCG monitoring has no role when there is a known intrauterine pregnancy confirmed on ultrasound
   E Serial β-hCG monitoring typically involves checking levels every 24 hours

5. **Regarding normal semen analysis:**
   A   Total motility should be $>80\%$
   B   The count should be at least 15 million sperm/mL
   C   A volume of 1 mL is acceptable
   D   The average ejaculate should have a minimum of 39 million sperm
   E   Analysis should be performed within 90 minutes of production

Questions: SBAs

For each question, select the single best answer from the five options listed.

6. A fetal blood sample is performed on a primiparous 24-year-old woman at 7 cm dilatation due to a pathological cardiotocograph (CTG). The result shows a pH of 7.24.

    Which is the most appropriate action based on this result?

    A   A repeat sample should be performed in 30 minutes
    B   It is a normal result and the patient should be reassured
    C   No further sample should be performed unless there is a terminal CTG
    D   Proceed straight to caesarean section
    E   The patient should be placed into left lateral position

7. An 18-year-old pregnant woman attends antenatal clinic at 32 weeks' gestation. Her urine sample reveals protein + and leucocytes +. She is asymptomatic of a urinary tract infection and is otherwise well.

    What is the most appropriate action?

    A   Antibiotics and send urine for culture
    B   Blood tests including a full blood count and renal function
    C   Renal ultrasound scan and antibiotics
    D   Routine urine dipstick at next appointment
    E   Send urine for culture and treat if positive

8. A 22-year-old primiparous woman books her pregnancy at 11 weeks' gestation. Her booking blood tests reveal a haemoglobin level of 10.1 g/dL. Electrophoresis reveals haemoglobin karyotype HbAS.

    What is the diagnosis?

    A   Beta-thalassaemia major
    B   Beta-thalassaemia trait
    C   Hereditary spherocytosis
    D   Sickle cell anaemia
    E   Sickle cell trait

9. A 32-year-old woman is being continuously monitored during labour using a cardiotocograph (CTG). She has had one previous caesarean section for breech presentation at term. She is currently 40 weeks' gestation and in spontaneous labour. The baseline of the CTG is 115 beats per minute.

    Regarding CTG analysis, what is the accepted range for the baseline rate?

    A   80–100 beats per minute
    B   90–120 beats per minute
    C   100–150 beats per minute
    D   110–160 beats per minute
    E   120–180 beats per minute

10. A 32-year-old multiparous pregnant woman attends the antenatal clinic for review at 28 weeks' gestation. She mentions that her 4-year-old daughter has chickenpox. She is unsure whether she has had chickenpox before. Serology results are as follows:

Varicella zoster virus IgM: negative
Varicella zoster virus IgG: positive

What do the serology results suggest regarding her immune status with respect to chickenpox?

A   Acute episode of shingles
B   Varicella zoster – chronic carrier
C   Varicella zoster – current acute infection
D   Varicella zoster – no acute infection, no previous exposure
E   Varicella zoster – previous exposure

11. A 40-year-old primiparous woman is admitted and investigated for raised blood pressure. Protein shows +++ on urine dipstick. A 24-hour urine collection is sent for protein calculation.

What level of urinary protein excretion in 24 hours indicates significant proteinuria?

A   >0.1 g
B   >0.2 g
C   >0.3 g
D   >0.4 g
E   >0.5 g

12. A 27-year-old primiparous woman presents with mild abdominal pain and some vaginal spotting. Her last menstrual period was 5 weeks ago. Her serum β-human chorionic gonadotrophin (β-hCG) on presentation is 258 IU/L. As she is clinically stable, with no risk factors for ectopic pregnancy, she goes home and returns to the early pregnancy unit 2 days later for a repeat serum β-hCG.

The results of her serial serum β-hCG as follows:
Day 1: β-hCG 258 IU/L
Day 3: β-hCG 460 IU/L

Which of the statements below best describes this patient's serum β-hCG trend?

A   Normal rise, cannot exclude ectopic pregnancy
B   Normal rise, confirmatory of a viable intrauterine pregnancy
C   Suboptimal rise, suggestive of early miscarriage
D   Suboptimal rise, suggestive of ectopic pregnancy
E   None of the above

13. A couple with primary subfertility, who have been trying to conceive for over 12 months, attend a reproductive medicine clinic. The male partner has already given a semen sample for analysis. The results of semen analysis are as follows:

Normal morphology: 15%
Volume: 4.5 mL
Sperm count: 12 million sperm/mL
Total motility: 61%

What does this analysis indicate?

A   Normal semen analysis
B   Reduced normal morphology, with all other parameters normal
C   Reduced sperm count, with all other parameters normal
D   Reduced total motility, with all other parameters normal
E   Reduced volume, with all other parameters normal

14. A 34-year-old primiparous woman is induced at 40 weeks' gestation and 12 days
    for post-dates. The fetus is being continuously monitored via a cardiotocograph
    (CTG). At 6 cm dilatation the CTG becomes pathological and fetal blood samples
    (FBS) are taken.

    The results of the FBS are as follows:
    Sample 1: pH 7.19
    Sample 2: pH7.20

    What are the most appropriate interpretation and action based on the FBS results?

    A   Abnormal result, consider immediate delivery of baby
    B   Abnormal result, repeat sample within 30 minutes if CTG remains
        pathological
    C   Borderline result, repeat within 30 minutes if CTG remains pathological
    D   Normal result, no further action required
    E   Normal result, repeat sample within one hour if CTG remains pathological

15. A 37-year-old multiparous woman with gestational diabetes is in labour. The
    labour is being continuously monitored using a cardiotocograph (CTG). She is
    reviewed by the obstetric team and the parameters of the CTG are noted.

    Baseline: 130 beats per minute
    Accelerations: present
    Variability: < 5 beats per minute for 50 minutes
    Decelerations: typical variable decelerations with more than 50% of contractions
                   for 30 minutes
    Contractions: three to four contractions in 10 minutes

    On the basis of this report how is the CTG best classified?

    A   Normal CTG
    B   Normal CTG with one non-reassuring feature
    C   Suspicious CTG with one non-reassuring feature
    D   Pathological CTG with one abnormal feature
    E   Pathological CTG with two non-reassuring features

16. A 23-year-old woman is admitted at 6 weeks' gestation with severe hyperemesis
    gravidarum. Her serum potassium is 2.7 mmol/L.

What is the normal range of serum potassium?

A   2.5–3.0 mmol/L
B   2.7–3.5 mmol/L
C   3.0–4.0 mmol/L
D   3.5–5.0 mmol/L
E   4.0–5.5 mmol/L

17. A 64-year-old woman undergoes a total abdominal hysterectomy and bilateral salpingo-oophorectomy for endometrial carcinoma. The staging of the specimen is described as stage Ib.

What is the definition of stage Ib endometrial cancer?

A   Endocervical invasion only
B   Extension to adjacent organs
C   Extension to vagina
D   Less than half the myometrial depth invaded
E   Limited to endometrium

18. An 82-year-old woman is undergoing investigation for postmenopausal bleeding. Her serum lactate dehydrogenase (LDH) is found to be raised.

Which of the following conditions is associated with a normal level of LDH?

A   Haemolysis
B   Myocardial infarction
C   Paget's disease
D   Pulmonary embolism
E   Tumour necrosis

19. A 54-year-old woman is investigated for abdominal bloating and weight loss. A range of blood tests are sent as part of her investigations.

Which of the following serum levels would be increased if the she had hepatocellular cancer?

A   Alpha-fetoprotein
B   CA 15-3
C   Carcinoembryonic antigen
D   Creatinine kinase
E   Neurone specific enolase

20. A 67-year-old woman is undergoing investigation for postmenopausal bleeding. An ultrasound scan shows her endometrial thickness to be 6 mm.

What is considered a normal endometrial thickness for a postmenopausal woman?

A   <2 mm
B   <3 mm
C   <4 mm
D   <6 mm
E   <8 mm

21. A 32-year-old primiparous woman attends the maternity day unit at 34 weeks' gestation complaining of itching of the palms of her hands. Her blood tests show raised bile acids of 17 μmol/L. Her alanine aminotransferase is raised to 180 IU/L.

What is the most likely diagnosis?

A   Alcoholic liver disease
B   Dermat itis
C   Gallstones
D   Hepatitis B
E   Obstetric cholestasis

22. A 38-year-old woman attends a colposcopy clinic following an abnormal result of moderate dyskaryosis at cervical screening. The results of the biopsy taken at colposcopy indicate cervical intraepithelial neoplasia (CIN) II.

What is the extent of cervical involvement in CIN II?

A   1/4 thickness of squamous epithelium affected
B   1/3 thickness of squamous epithelium affected
C   2/3 thickness of squamous epithelium affected
D   Full thickness of squamous epithelium affected
E   None of the above

23. A 25-year-old nulliparous woman attends cervical screening for the first time. The results of her smear test show borderline nuclear changes.

What is the appropriate follow-up for this woman?

A   Immediate referral to colposcopy
B   Repeat smear in 1 year
C   Repeat smear in 3 years
D   Repeat smear in 3 months
E   Repeat smear in 6 months

24. A 25-year-old primiparous woman has a forceps delivery. She sustains trauma to the perineum. You perform a per rectal examination. You note that <50% of the thickness of the external sphincter has been torn.

What grade of perineal tear has the patient sustained?

A   Fourth degree tear
B   Second degree tear
C   Third degree tear – class A
D   Third degree tear – class B
E   Third degree tear – class C

25. A 38-year-old multiparous woman is admitted with a heavy antepartum haemorrhage (APH) at 26 weeks' gestation. She has had three previous caesarean sections. On examination, her abdomen is soft and non-tender.

What is the most likely cause of this woman's APH?

A Abruption
B Placenta praevia
C Trauma
D Vasa praevia
E Uterine rupture

26. A 32-year-old primiparous woman with gestational diabetes is 32 weeks pregnant. At her antenatal clinic review her symphysis fundal height is measured as 38 cm. She is referred for an urgent scan to assess fetal growth and amniotic fluid index.

Which amniotic fluid index would indicate polyhydramnios?

A ≥5 cm
B ≥10 cm
C ≥15 cm
D ≥18 cm
E ≥22 cm

Answers

1. A **True**

    B **True**

    C **True**

    D **False**

    E **False**

    A cardiotocograph (CTG) is a legal document and should therefore be appropriately stored for 25 years. It should always be dated and timed, and labelled with the woman's details. See **Table 10.1** for CTG classification.

    Fetal blood sampling (FBS) should be considered if there is a pathological trace and there are no contraindications. FBS may be performed in a fetus from 34 weeks' gestation.

    National Institute for Health and Clinical Excellence. Intrapartum Care. Clinical Guideline CG55. London: NICE, 2007.

Table 10.1 Interpretation and classification of the cardiotocograph (CTG)

Feature on CTG	Reassuring	Non-reassuring	Abnormal
Baseline rate (bpm)	110–160	100–109	<100
		161–180	>180
			Sinusoidal trace ≥10 minutes
Variability (bpm)	≥5	≤5 for 40–90 minutes	<5 for ≥90 minutes
Accelerations	Present	The absence of accelerations in an otherwise normal trace is of unknown significance	The absence of accelerations in an otherwise normal trace is of unknown significance
Decelerations	None	Typical variable decelerations with > 50% of contractions for > 90 minutes	Atypical variable decelerations with >50% of contractions or late decelerations, for >30 minutes
		Single prolonged deceleration lasting up to 3 minutes	Single prolonged deceleration for > 3 minutes

Adapted from: National Institute for Health and Clinical Excellence. Intrapartum Care. Clinical Guideline CG55. London: NICE, 2007.

2. A **False**

    B **True**

    C **False**

    D **False**

    E **True**

Gestational diabetes mellitus (GDM) is defined as the onset of diabetes during pregnancy. If indicated, an oral glucose tolerance test is performed at 27–28 weeks' gestation. Universal screening is currently not advocated in the UK. Risk factors for gestational diabetes include previous GDM, previous large baby (>4.5 kg), polycystic ovarian syndrome, obesity and polyhydramnios. An oral glucose tolerance test involves taking a fasting glucose level followed by giving a 75 g glucose load. Glucose levels are then taken 2 hours later. Diabetes is diagnosed if a fasting glucose level is >7.0 mmol/L or a 2-hour level of >11.1 mmol/L. Impaired glucose tolerance is diagnosed if the 2-hour glucose level is >7.8–<11.0 mmol/L.

National Institute for Health and Clinical Excellence Diabetes in Pregnancy. Clinical Guideline CG63. London: NICE, 2008.

3. A True

    B True

    C False

    D True

    E True

The differential diagnosis for proteinuria includes:

1. **Pre-eclampsia:** only significant once it reaches ≥0.3 g in 24 hours. May be associated with other features including headache, visual disturbance and raised blood pressure.
2. **Normal pregnancy:** proteinuria may be a normal finding in pregnancy due to changes in the renal system including increased glomerular filtration rate and increased protein excretion.
3. **Urinary tract infection:** including lower urinary tract infection and pyelonephritis. There may also be leucocytes and nitrites on urine dipstick to support evidence of infection.
4. **Renal tract disease:** may be associated with microscopic haematuria. Renal damage may be as a result of diabetes or autoimmune conditions.

4. A True

    B False

    C False

    D True

    E False

Serum β-human chorionic gonadotrophin (β-hCG) monitoring is typically used to aid the diagnosis and management of pregnancies of unknown location. An intrauterine pregnancy, if present, should be visible on transvaginal ultrasound scan when the serum β-hCG level is ≥1500 IU/L, although an early pregnancy may be visible at from levels of around 1000 IU/L. Serum β-hCG is typically repeated 48 hours after the first sample, and may be repeated at several 48 hourly intervals. A rise in β-hCG of at least 66% every 48 hours is considered normal. A diagnosis of miscarriage or ectopic pregnancy cannot be based on serum β-hCG levels alone. Once an intrauterine pregnancy has been confirmed on ultrasound a serum β-hCG is not useful. Elevated levels of β-hCG may indicate gestational trophoblastic disease or a multiple pregnancy.

5. A False

   B True

   C False

   D True

   E False

Semen analysis is a routine investigation when assessing a couple's subfertility problems. Based on the World Health Organisation's (WHO) redefined reference ranges for semen analysis the minimum acceptable semen count is now considered to be 15 million sperm/mL. The average ejaculate sample should have a minimum of 39 million sperm. Total motility is calculated by adding the percentages of progressive and non-progressive motile forms. The WHO states that the normal total motility percentage is 40%. The minimum normal volume of ejaculate is 1.5 mL. The minimum acceptable percentage of semen with normal morphology is 4%. Analysis should be performed within 60 minutes to ensure the accuracy of the results.

Cooper TG, Noonan E, von Eckardstein S, et al. World Health Organization reference values for human semen characteristics. Human Reproduction Update 2009: 1–15.

6. A A repeat sample should be performed in 30 minutes

This fetal blood sample (FBS) shows a pH of 7.24, which is classified as suspicious. The sample should be repeated in no more than 30 minutes, or sooner if clinically indicated. See **Table 10.2** for a FBS action plan.

Table 10.2 Interpretation of fetal blood sampling (FBS) results		
Result (pH)	**Interpretation**	**Action**
≥ 7.25	Normal	Repeat FBS if cardiotocograph remains pathological or suspicious
7.21–7.24	Suspicious	Repeat FBS in 30 minutes or sooner if indicated
≤ 7.20	Abnormal	Delivery

7. E Send urine for culture and treat if positive

Urine tract infection (UTI) is defined as the presence of 100,000/mL organisms in an asymptomatic patient or 100/mL organisms with increased white cell count in a symptomatic patient. In an asymptomatic patient, the diagnosis of a urinary tract infection should be made once the presence of a pathogen has been confirmed on culture. Asymptomatic bacteriuria is the presence of 100,000/mL of organisms in the absence of symptoms on at least two occasions. These are treated as there is a risk of cystitis and ascending infection which may increase maternal or fetal morbidity. Urinalysis should be performed on pregnant women routinely at all antenatal clinic visits. The presence of protein, leucocytes and nitrites all suggest the presence of a UTI. A renal ultrasound scan would only be indicated in the presence of recurrent pyelonephritis or if renal abnormality or disease is suspected.

8. E Sickle cell trait

Sickle cell conditions are due to the production of abnormal β peptide chains leading to abnormal haemoglobin. The gene which codes for the β chain of haemoglobin has an amino acid substitution which results in the production of HbS rather than HbA. Individuals with sickle cell anaemia are homozygous with HbSS. Heterozygotes have HbAS and have sickle cell trait. Sickle cell trait is thought to be protective against falciparum malaria. Sickle cell anaemia results in the production of fragile erythrocytes which leads to their early destruction and subsequent haemolysis. In sickle cell trait there may be mild anaemia, however there is usually no evidence of haemolysis, i.e. normal lactate dehydrogenase, bilirubin and a normal reticulocyte count. Ideally these patients should have pre-pregnancy counselling and screening of their partner. If this has not been undertaken prior to conception, then it should be arranged as soon as it is identified to determine the risk of HbSS in the fetus.

9. D 110–160 beats per minute

Cardiotocography (CTG) or electronic fetal monitoring is commonly used during pregnancy and labour to determine fetal well-being. A range of parameters are studied including baseline fetal heart rate which is considered normal if between 110–160 beats per minute. Fetal cardiac activity is controlled via the sympathetic and parasympathetic autonomic nervous systems, with other influences coming from oxygenation and baroreceptors. Fetal baseline heart rate generally falls as the pregnancy increases and this is a result of the parasympathetic system becoming more developed. Intrapartum fetal tachycardia, when associated with maternal tachycardia, may be as a result of infection and chorioamnionitis should be considered.

10. E Varicella zoster – previous exposure

Varicella zoster virus is a member of the herpes virus family and causes chickenpox. The majority of adults in the UK are immune to chickenpox. It is transmitted via droplet infection and has a relatively long incubation period of approximately 2 weeks. Chickenpox infection is more severe in pregnancy and there is a higher rate of complications, such as varicella pneumonitis. Once there has been exposure to the virus there will be initial production of varicella IgM antibodies, followed by the production of long-term immunity through IgG antibodies. In the case illustrated, the patient has IgG positive result and is therefore immune to varicella zoster through previous exposure. There is therefore no risk to the fetus and no indication for immunoglobulin. If IgM was positive and IgG negative, this would suggest recent infection with no prior immunity and this would be an indication for immunoglobulin.

Royal College of Obstetricians and Gynaecologists. Chickenpox in Pregnancy. Green-top Guideline 13. London: RCOG, 2007.
StratOG.net. Maternal Medicine: Infectious Diseases. London: StratOG, 2012. www.rcog.org.uk/stratog

11. C >0.3 g

Urinary protein excretion of >0.3 g in 24 hours indicates a significant level of proteinuria. This may be found in conditions such as pre-eclampsia or pre-existing renal disease. Severe proteinuria may not always be associated with significantly raised blood pressure and may be due to long-standing renal damage and should be investigated.

12. A Normal rise, cannot exclude ectopic pregnancy

When serum β-human chorionic gonadotrophin (β-hCG) is 1500 IU/L it is unlikely that an intrauterine pregnancy will be seen on transvaginal ultrasound scan. Serum β-hCG monitoring is used to aid the management and diagnosis of women in early pregnancy with symptoms of suggestive of early miscarriage or ectopic pregnancy when scanning is unlikely to yield little useful information. A normal rise in serum β-hCG is that of at least 66% every 48 hours. Although a normal rise over 48 hours is suggestive of a normal pregnancy it remains a pregnancy of unknown location until there has been a confirmatory scan. A β-hCG that is falling may indicate both a failing intrauterine or failing ectopic pregnancy. A suboptimal rise in β-hCG, i.e. a rise that is <66% over 48 hours, increases suspicion of an ectopic pregnancy; however, it does not rule out the presence of an intrauterine pregnancy.

Royal College of Obstetricians and Gynaecologists. The Management of Early Pregnancy Loss. Green-top Guideline 25. London: RCOG, 2006.

13. C Reduced sperm count, with all other parameters normal

The World Health Organization (WHO) has recently redefined the normal reference ranges for semen analysis. A minimum of 15 million sperm/mL is acceptable as per the WHO. This man's sperm count is only 12 million sperm/mL and therefore is considered to be suboptimal. A minimum of 4% of semen with normal morphology is acceptable. The lowest acceptable volume of the ejaculate is 1.5 mL. The total motility of a sample refers to the percentage of both progressive and non-progressive forms. The WHO considers 40% to be the minimum acceptable percentage for total motility. For the most accurate results analysis should be performed within 60 minutes of production.

Cooper TG, Noonan E, von Eckardstein S, et al. World Health Organization reference values for human semen characteristics. Hum Reprod Update 2010; 16(3):231–245.

14. A Abnormal result, consider immediate delivery of baby

Fetal blood sampling (FBS) is a means of assessing fetal well-being when there are concerns raised when using electronic fetal monitoring during labour. The results of fetal blood samples are used to assess fetal hypoxia in the presence of an accompanying pathological cardiotocograph (CTG). The normal fetal blood pH range is 7.25–7.35. If a sample within this range in the presence of a pathological CTG then a further FBS sample should be taken within 1 hour if the CTG remains pathological. When the pH obtained is between 7.21 and 7.24 the result is classified as borderline and a repeat sample should be taken within 30 minutes if the CTG remains pathological. A sample with a pH of 7.20 or less is considered abnormal and therefore immediate delivery of the baby should be considered.

National Institute for Health and Clinical Excellence. Intrapartum Care. Clinical Guideline CG55. London: NICE, 2007.

15. C Suspicious CTG with one non-reassuring feature

Cardiotocographs (CTGs) record a number of parameters which together can be used to interpret fetal well-being, which include the baseline fetal heart rate, the beat-to-beat variability, the presence and type of decelerations, the presence of accelerations and the number of contractions in 10 minutes. The classification of CTGs is based on the presence of reassuring, non-reassuring and abnormal parameters as recommended by NICE (National Institute of Health and Clinical Excellence) in the UK. See **Table 10.1** for classification of CTGs.

A CTG can be classified as:

*   **Normal:** only reassuring features are present
*   **Suspicious:** the presence of a single non-reassuring feature
*   **Abnormal:** the presence of a single abnormal feature or the presence of two non-reassuring features

National Institute for Health and Clinical Excellence. Intrapartum Care. Clinical Guideline CG55. London: NICE, 2007.

16. D 3.5–5.0 mmol/L

The normal range for potassium in an adult human is 3.5–5.0 mmol/L. This value may vary between hospitals. Hypokalaemia is a common abnormality in hyperemesis gravidarum as a result of persistent vomiting and should be corrected to avoid dangerous hypokalaemia.

17. D Less than half the myometrial depth invaded

Endometrial cancer is classified according to the extent of tumour invasion.

Stage I: limited to uterus

*   a: limited to endometrium
*   b: less half myometrial depth
*   c: greater than half myometrial depth

Stage II: tumour in uterine body and cervix

Stage III: extended to uterine serosa, peritoneal cavity +/– lymph nodes

Stage IV: extended outside the pelvis, may involve bladder or bowel

18. C Paget's disease

Lactate dehydrogenase is a plasma enzyme that may be raised in the following conditions:

- Active liver disease
- Haemolysis
- Pulmonary embolism
- Myocardial infarction

It is not associated with Paget's disease; alkaline phosphatase is raised in Paget's disease.

19. A Alpha-fetoprotein

Alpha-fetoprotein is increased in hepatocellular cancer and active liver disease. CA 15-3 is a non-specific tumour marker which may be raised in breast cancer. Carcinoembryonic is generally increased in abdominal and gastric cancers. It may also be increased in cirrhosis.

Neurone-specific enolase is raised in small cell cancer of the lungs.

20. C <4 mm

Bleeding after the menopause is a common presentation and should initially be investigated using transvaginal ultrasound scan. An endometrial thickness of ≥4 mm is abnormal and should be followed up with endometrial sampling, which may be via pipelle biopsy or hysteroscopy. The majority of women with postmenopausal bleeding are found to have atrophic endometrium, however there may be polyps, hyperplasia or malignant change.

Bakour SH, Timmermans A, Willem B, et al. Management of women with postmenopausal bleeding: evidence-based review. The Obstetrician & Gynaecologist 2012; 14(4):243–249.

21. E Obstetric cholestasis

Obstetric cholestasis is a condition that is unique to pregnancy. It is characterised by pruritus, abnormal liver enzymes and raised bile acids. It should be considered a diagnosis of exclusion. There is thought to be a genetic link and a predisposition to the cholestatic effect of increased circulating oestrogen.

Treatment is to control the symptoms with antihistamines and ursodeoxycholic acid. There should be increased fetal surveillance and consideration of delivery from 37 weeks' gestation as there is an association with intrauterine fetal death after 37/40 weeks.

Royal College of Obstetricians and Gynaecologists. Green-top guideline 43. London: RCOG, 2011.

22. C 2/3 thickness of squamous epithelium affected

Cervical intraepithelial neoplasia (CIN) is the term given to describe the histological changes associated with dysplasia that may occur in the cervix. CIN is considered the precursor of cervical cancer. The grading of CIN is based on the thickness of the squamous epithelium affected (from the basal layer of the transformation zone upwards). CIN I is the mildest form, only affecting the bottom third of the basal layer, CIN II affects the bottom two-thirds of the squamous epithelium, whereas CIN III is the most severe form of CIN and refers to changes affecting more than two-thirds to full thickness of the epithelium (**Table 10.3**).

Table 10.3 Cervical intraepithelial neoplasia (CIN) categories and histology	
Grade	**Thickness of squamous epithelium affected**
CIN I	Basal 1/3
CIN II	Bottom 2/3
CIN III	> 2/3 to full thickness

23. E Repeat smear in 6 months

Borderline nuclear changes on cervical screening are suggestive of cervical intraepithelial neoplasia (CIN) II to III affecting some of the cells sampled. It is appropriate for this woman to have a repeat smear test in 6 months time. If she was to have a total of three consecutive smears with the same result she would need to be referred with colposcopy. A similar recall of 6 months would also be appropriate for a result showing inflammatory changes on smear. The standard recall for a normal smear test result is 3 years. More severe changes smear, i.e. mild, moderate or severe dyskaryosis indicate the need for colposcopy.

24. C Third degree tear – class A

This woman has sustained a third degree perineal tear. This means that the tear is severe enough as to involve the anal sphincter. Third degree tears can be graded A–C, according to the extent of trauma to the external and internal anal sphincters. In a third degree A tear < 50% of the thickness of the external anal sphincter has been damaged. A third degree B tear describes a tear damaging more than 50% of the thickness of the external anal sphincter. When the internal anal sphincter has been damaged (to any extent) the tear is classified as a third degree C tear. A fourth degree tear involves damage to the anal epithelium, in addition to any third degree tear. A first degree tear is considered to be a minor injury to the perineal skin or vaginal epithelium. This superficial injury typically does not require any repair. A second degree tear is one where the vaginal/perineal muscles are torn, whilst maintaining the integrity of the anal sphincter.

Sultan AH, Kettle C. Chapter 2: Diagnosis of Perineal Trauma. In: Sultan AH, Thakar R, Fenner DE (eds). Perineal and Anal Sphincter Trauma. London: Springer-Verlag, 2009.

25. B Placenta praevia

Placenta praevia is a common cause of antepartum haemorrhage. It is classified as either minor placenta praevia or major placenta praevia. Minor placenta praevia is described as placenta which has inserted into the lower segment of the uterus, but does not cover the cervical os. Major placenta praevia (previously classified as grade III and grade IV) describes placental position when the placenta covers the cervical os. Risk factors for placenta praevia include previous caesarean section, multiple pregnancy and maternal age. The majority of antepartum haemorrhages are idiopathic. Other causes include placental abruption, vasa praevia and local cervical or vaginal pathologies.

26. E ≥22 cm

Polyhydramnios is an overall increase in liquor volume. It may be diagnosed if the deepest pool of fluid seen on ultrasound scan is deeper than 8 cm or if the overall amniotic fluid index (AFI) is > 22 cm. Causes of polyhydramnios include diabetes, fetal anomalies causing problems swallowing and idiopathic causes.

Chapter 11

Immunology

Questions: MCQs

Answer each stem 'True' or 'False'.

1. **Antibodies:**
   A   Are polypeptides
   B   Consist of two heavy and two light chains
   C   The antigen binding site is on the variable region
   D   The antibody binding site occurs on the light chain
   E   The largest antibody is IgG

2. **Concerning hypersensitivity:**
   A   Type II hypersensitivity is antibody dependent
   B   Type I hypersensitivity is associated with IgM activation
   C   The Arthus reaction is an example of type II hypersensitivity
   D   The Mantoux test is an example of type IV hypersensitivity
   E   Haemolytic disease of the newborn is an example of type II hypersensitivity

3. **Concerning complement:**
   A   The classical activation pathway is independent of antibody involvement
   B   The spleen is the main site of complement production
   C   Complement is a form of cytokine
   D   C3 is cleaved to C3a
   E   The alternative activation pathway requires binding of mannose-binding lectin

4. **Natural killer cells:**
   A   Are part of the acquired immune system
   B   Detect changes in the major histocompatability complex
   C   Release perforins
   D   Require antibody stimulation
   E   Have strong cytotoxic properties

Questions: SBAs

For each question, select the single best answer from the five options listed.

5. Haemolytic disease of the newborn (Rhesus incompatibility) occurs as a result of which of the following classes of hypersensitivity reaction?

    A IgE mediated
    B Immune complex mediated
    C Type I
    D Type II
    E Type IV

6. Which of the following gives the structure of the antibody IgG?

	Structure	Properties
a	Dimer	Main immunoglobulin found in secretions, e.g. saliva, and mucosal surfaces
b	Monomer	Antigen receptor on B cells
c	Monomer	Main mediator of allergic reaction
d	Monomer	Only immunoglobulin to cross the placenta
e	Pentamer	First immunoglobulin to be produced; expressed on surface of B cells

7. What is the common step to all complement activation pathways?

    A Activation of C1 to antibody-antigen complexes
    B Cleavage of C3 into C3a and C3b
    C Formation of the mannose-binding lectin complex
    D Formation of the IgG antibody-antigen complex
    E Formation of the IgM antibody-antigen complex

8. A 32-year-old woman presents to hospital 5 days postemergency caesarean section, complaining of a painful scar. On examination, there is erythema at one of the scar edges and some purulent discharge. She is started on antibiotic treatment for a wound infection.

    Which of the following local changes can be seen in this type of acute inflammatory process?

    A Fibroblast infiltration
    B Haemostasis
    C High concentration of monocytes
    D Decreased vascular permeability
    E Vasoconstriction

9. A female baby is born via spontaneous vaginal delivery at term. As she is born in an urban area with high levels of tuberculosis she is given the BCG (Bacillus Calmette–Guerin) vaccination before she is taken home by her parents.

What type of vaccine is the BCG vaccine?

A   Conjugate vaccine
B   Killed (inactivated) vaccine
C   Live (attenuated) vaccine
D   Subunit vaccine
E   Toxoid vaccine

10. Which of the following is an example of a disease caused by type III hypersensitivity?

A   Asthma
B   Autoimmune haemolytic anaemia
C   Eczema
D   Multiple sclerosis
E   Systemic lupus erythematosus

11. Which of the following is most important in the adaptive immune system?

A   Complement
B   Macrophages
C   Natural killer cells
D   Neutrophils
E   T-helper cells

12. One of the known benefits of breastfeeding is its role in supporting the infant's immune system.

Which of the following antibodies is secreted in large amounts in breast milk?

A   IgA
B   IgD
C   IgE
D   IgG
E   IgM

Answers

1. A **False**

    B **True**

    C **True**

    D **False**

    E **False**

    Antibodies, also known as immunoglobulins, are glycoproteins, produced by activated B cells. In humans there are five classes of antibodies, namely IgA, IgD, IgE, IgG and IgM. Antibodies consist of two identical heavy polypeptide chains and two identical light chains, which both contain a variable and a constant region. The antigen binding site is made up of the variable regions of the light and the heavy chain. The largest antibody is IgM, which is a pentamer, consisting of five joined IgG units (**Figure 11.1**).

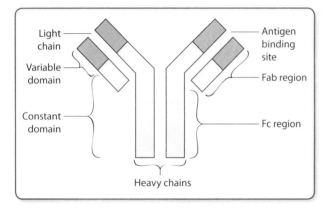

Figure 11.1 Immunoglobulin G.

2. A **True**

    B **False**

    C **False**

    D **True**

    E **True**

    Hypersensitivity reactions are categorised according to the type of immune response and traditionally are known as types I, II, III and IV. Type I hypersensitivity reactions may also be referred to an immediate hypersensitivity; here the associated allergen binds with IgE antibodies which are present on the surface of mast cells. This leads to the activation of the mast cells leading them to degranulate and release histamine into the circulation. This kind of reaction is typical in atopy and at the extreme, anaphylaxis following exposure to allergens, e.g. peanuts. Type II hypersensitivity is antibody dependent, whereby IgG and IgM antibodies are stimulated by an allergen, which then activates the classical pathway of the complement cascade. In haemolytic disease of the newborn maternal IgG crosses the placenta and attacks fetal red blood cells. Other conditions associated with type II hypersensitivity include pernicious anaemia and Goodpasture's disease. Type III hypersensitivity is associated with the deposition of immune complexes (i.e. antibody-antigen complexes) in tissues. The Arthus reaction is an example of type III hypersensitivity where there is localised vasculitis due to immune complex deposition typically after booster immunisation with toxoid vaccines such as tetanus. Type IV hypersensitivity is a delayed cell-mediated response to an antigen. T cells are key to this reaction, and having been presented a specific antigen by cells such as macrophages, they both secrete interleukins and activate macrophages to produce cytokines. The Mantoux reaction is a form of type IV hypersensitivity where there is localised induration of the skin at the site of tuberculin injection.

3. A False

    B False

    C False

    D True

    E False

Complement describes around 20 glycoproteins, the majority of which are produced by the liver. The complement cascade is activated via three pathways. The classical pathway requires binding of the complement C1 to an antibody molecule (either IgM or IgG) which has been activated by an antigen to begin the cascade. The alternative pathway begins with the activation of the complement protein C3; this pathway does not require the presence of antibodies. The third pathway is the mannose–lectin activation pathway, whereby carbohydrate residues on the surface of pathogens activate circulating mannose-binding lectin (produced by the liver), which then form a type of protease that is able to cleave complement and begin the complement cascade. C3 is one of the complement proteins and as part of the cascade (instigated by all three of the activation pathways), is cleaved to form C3a.

4. A False

    B True

    C True

    D False

    E True

Natural killer cells are a form of lymphocyte and are part of the innate immune system. They are activated in several ways, e.g. in response to the presence of cytokines released by infected cells, after antibody stimulation and also when there is failure by cells to normally express the class 1 major histocompatibility complex (as occurs in infected cells). They have strong cytotoxic activity and their main role is in the destruction of cancerous cells or cells infected with viruses. Natural killer cells kill by releasing perforin and granzyme from their cytoplasms which lead to apoptosis in their target cells.

5. D Type II

Rhesus (Rh) D antigen is carried on erythrocytes. If a child is born to a Rh negative mother and the father is Rh positive, he or she may express Rh D on their erythrocytes. If fetal erythrocytes pass into the maternal circulation or if Rh D positive blood is transfused into the mother, then sensitisation may occur; the mother produces antibodies. In subsequent pregnancies fetal erythrocytes may cross the placenta and stimulate a memory response, leading to the production of IgG antibodies which destroy fetal erythrocytes. Anti-D immunoprophylaxis, using anti-D immunoglobulin, during pregnancy and in the immediate postnatal period prevents the development of maternal anti-D antibodies.

6. D

Monomer	Only immunoglobulin to cross the placenta

Immunoglobulins, also known as antibodies, are formed by B cells. There are five different classes of human immunoglobulin, which differ in both their structure and function. Immunoglobin (IgG) is the predominant immunoglobulin found in serum and is the only form of immunoglobulin that is able to cross the placenta and therefore result in immunity in the fetus. It is also the longest living antibody class, with a half life of around 3 weeks. There are four IgG subclasses. Named IgG 1–4, this class of immunoglobulin is the predominant form involved in the secondary immune response. IgG antibodies are good at fixing complement, as well as opsonising targets, such as bacteria, for phagocytosis by cells such as macrophages.

Cookson S, Sargent I. Chapter 19: Basic Immunology. In: Fiander A, Thilganathan B (eds). Your Essential Revision Guide MRCOG Part 1. London: RCOG Press, 2010.

7. B Cleavage of C3 into C3a and C3b

The complement system consists of around 20 proteins, which are produced in a cascade and aim to attack pathogens. Although the complement cascade forms part of the innate immune system, it can also be activated by the adaptive immune system. Traditionally the complement cascade is described as being activated by three different pathways. The classical complement pathway occurs in response to activation of the complement protein C1 to antigen-antibody complexes. The alternative activation pathway does not rely on the presence of activated antibody complexes and instead starts with the activation of the complement protein C3. The third activation pathway is the lectin activation pathway. Mannose-binding lectin is produced by the liver. It forms a complex with a further protein called MASP. When the lectin binds to a pathogen containing mannose, the MASP protein converts the C3 complement protein to C3b and the cascade begins. Despite three different activation pathways, the common step in all is the cleavage of the complement protein C3 to C3a and C3b (**Figure 11.2**).

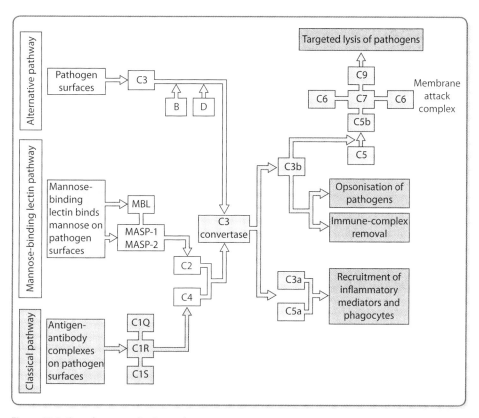

Figure 11.2 Complement activation pathways.

8. B Haemostasis

After an insult, the processes involved in acute inflammation are aimed at removing the source of the trauma and encouraging healing. Acute inflammation is associated with a series of vascular changes which aim to bring key components of the inflammatory response to the site of injury. Vasodilation occurs rapidly after an insult in response to mediators such as histamine. This leads to increased blood flow to the traumatised area, with associated hyperaemia. Vascular permeability also increases, allowing the passage of proteins, leucocytes and fluid from the vasculature into the surrounding tissues. The movement of protein-rich fluid out of the vasculature is associated with increased hydrostatic pressure. With a reduction in intravascular volume there is an element of haemostasis, also contributing to local hyperaemia. Both fibroblast infiltration and a high concentration of monocytes are typical of chronic inflammation rather than acute.

9. C Live (attenuated) vaccine

Attenuated vaccines contain live but attenuated organisms. That is, they lack the ability to be pathogenic, but will initiate an immune response. Examples of live (attenuated) vaccines are MMR (mumps, measles, rubella), polio (Sabin) and Bacillus Calmette–Guérin. Killed (inactivated) vaccines are generally considered more stable and safer than live vaccines. However, as the immune response to killed vaccines is generally weaker than to live vaccines, adjuvants such as aluminium hydroxide are added to the killed vaccine in order to precipitate an improved immune response. Examples of killed (inactivated) vaccines include the hepatitis A, pertussis, influenza and polio (Salk) vaccines. Toxoid vaccines confer immunity by the administration of inactivated toxin. Examples include the tetanus and diphtheria vaccines which are often given in combination. Subunit vaccines use specific antigens, in order to elicit an appropriate immune response. The hepatitis B vaccine is one such subunit vaccine.

10. E Systemic lupus erythematosus

Type III hypersensitivity is also known as immune complex hypersensitivity. It refers to a failure of immune complex clearance leading to their deposition in tissues. In this form of hypersensitivity, there is a failure to clear antibody-antigen complexes (usually IgG). These complexes initiate the complement cascade, activate neutrophils and macrophages and lead to platelet aggregation. This inflammatory reaction may lead to a vasculitis in the surrounding tissues. This complex deposition may have a systemic effect or localised to an organ. Systemic lupus erythematosus is an example of a condition in which there is multiple organ immune complex deposition leading to manifestations such as arthritis, rashes, lupus nephritis and myocarditis. Type III hypersensitivity is also responsible for conditions such as serum sickness, poststreptococcal glomerulonephritis, rheumatoid arthritis, extrinsic allergic alveolitis and the Arthus reaction, whereby there is immune complex deposition and a localised vasculitis at the site of an injection, e.g. after a tetanus vaccination.

11. E T-helper cells

The innate immune system provides immediate and non-specific response to attack, whereas the adaptive immune system provides a more complex and specific response to antigens and generates immunological memory. Central to the rapid response (within hours) of the innate immune system is the complement cascade. Complement are a group of proteins, mainly made by the liver, that provide immune defence by marking antigens for destruction by other cells (through opsonisation), recruiting other elements of the innate immune system, e.g. macrophages and neutrophils, assisting antibodies (part of the acquired immune system) and also by aiding the removal of immune complexes. Natural killer cells are part of the innate immune system and provide a non-specific response. This response is particularly strong against tumour cells and viruses due to their cytotoxic activity. Programmed cell death takes place in target cells as a result of the release of cytotoxic granules, e.g. perforin. T-helper cells are a specialised type of lymphocytes and therefore part of the adaptive or acquired immune system; in particular they play an important role in activating B-lymphocytes.

12. A IgA

Antibodies, or immunoglobulins, are glycoproteins produced by B cells as part of the acquired immune system. The 'default' form of antibody is IgM, however each form of antibody has a specialised function, and therefore they are differentially distributed in line with their role in immunity (**Table 11.1**). The key to the acquired immune system is the ability of B cells to switch class of antibody production in response to the attacking antigen. IgA has key role in mucosal immunity and is therefore the predominant antibody present in bodily secretions such as saliva, colostrum, tears and is found in high concentrations in the respiratory, reproductive and gastrointestinal tracts. Key to its functionality in inferring immunity to the neonate is IgA's resistance to stomach acid; this enables the capacity for IgA to be secreted in breast milk and benefit the infant from its mother's immunological memory.

Table 11.1 Antibodies and their properties

Antibody	Properties	Additional properties
IgA	Protects mucosal surfaces	Secreted in breast milk, tears, saliva, etc.
IgD	Role uncertain	Found in serum
IgE	Activates mast cells	Involved in allergic response and anaphylaxis
IgG	Fixes complement Opsonising properties	Crosses placenta
IgM	Fixes complement Opsonising properties	Default antibody, i.e. first made

Chapter 12

Microbiology

Questions: MCQs

Answer each stem 'True' or 'False'.

1. The following are Gram-positive bacteria:
   - A *Campylobacter jejuni*
   - B *Clostridium difficile*
   - C *Escherichia coli*
   - D *Listeria monocytogenes*
   - E *Staphylococcus aureus*

2. Group B β-haemolytic *Streptococcus* infection can cause:
   - A Chorioamnionitis
   - B Glomerulonephritis
   - C Necrotising fasciitis
   - D Neonatal sepsis
   - E Toxic shock syndrome

3. Concerning *Neisseria*:
   - A *N. meningitidis* is a Gram-positive cocci
   - B Infection with *N. gonorrhoeae* may cause a suppurative urethritis in males
   - C *N. gonorrhoeae* is a commensal of the genital tract
   - D *N. gonorrhoeae* thrives in conditions with low levels of carbon dioxide
   - E Species are cultured on chocolate agar

4. The following are DNA viruses:
   - A Hepatitis A
   - B Hepatitis B
   - C HIV
   - D Human herpesvirus 8
   - E Varicella zoster virus

5. Regarding varicella zoster:
   - A Distribution of lesions is myotomal
   - B The use of antivirals prevents infection
   - C It is an RNA virus
   - D Maternal exposure at term infers minimal risk to the fetus
   - E Varicella zoster immunoglobulin G (VZV–IgG) should be given to exposed pregnant women who are antibody negative

6. The following diseases/conditions are paired with their causative agent:
   A   Human herpesvirus 4: mononucleosis
   B   *Treponema pallidum pallidum*: bejel
   C   *Gardnerella vaginalis*: bacterial vaginosis
   D   *Trypanosoma brucei*: sleeping sickness
   E   *Toxoplasma gondii*: dengue fever

7. Regarding interventions to reduce the risk of surgical site infections:
   A   There is no convincing evidence that prophylactic antibiotics reduce postoperative incidence of surgical site infection
   B   Hair removal should be performed with clippers rather than a razor
   C   Antibiotics should be given intravenously no more than 60 minutes prior to surgery
   D   Blood sugars should be kept <12 mmol/L in patients with diabetes
   E   Use of prophylactic antibiotics increases the risk of *Clostridium difficile* infection

8. Concerning cytomegalovirus infection:
   A   It affects 0.5% of pregnancies
   B   Primary maternal infection may be treated with ganciclovir
   C   Has an incubation period of 3 weeks
   D   Affected individuals are always symptomatic
   E   Previous infection provides effective immunity

9. Bacterial toxins:
   A   Exotoxins are released from cell wall during bacterial cell death
   B   Exotoxins are released by Gram-positive and Gram-negative bacteria
   C   Endotoxins are a feature of Gram-positive bacteria
   D   Lipid A is responsible for the systemic features of endotoxic shock
   E   Gastrointestinal symptoms of cholera are caused by an endotoxin

10. Molluscum contagiosum:
   A   Is a fungal infection
   B   May be sexually transmitted
   C   Only affects the skin
   D   Lesions appear 6 months after infection
   E   Can be treated with cryotherapy

11. Mycobacteria:
   A   Are obligate anaerobic bacteria
   B   *Mycobacteria avium* complex are found in patients with pre-existing lung conditions
   C   *M. leprae* is effectively treated with amikacin
   D   *M. kansasii* can be found in indwelling central venous lines
   E   Are non-motile

Questions: SBAs

For each question, select the single best answer from the five options listed.

12. A 50-year-old woman has ongoing pelvic pain; she has had a coil in situ for the last 8 years. She has a pelvic mass; histological sampling of the mass at laparoscopy shows a suppurative and granulomatous inflammatory process with the presence of sulphur granules.

    Which is the most likely causative agent?

    A   *Actinomyces israelii*
    B   *Chlamydia trachomatis*
    C   *Gardnerella vaginalis*
    D   *Neisseria gonorrhoeae*
    E   *Neisseria meningitidis*

13. An 18-year-old woman presents to a sexual health clinic requesting a sexually transmitted infection screen; she is asymptomatic, however she is concerned as her new boyfriend is complaining of dysuria, penile discharge and scrotal pain.

    What is the most likely cause of his symptoms?

    A   *Actinomyces israelii*
    B   *Candida albicans*
    C   *Chlamydia trachomatis*
    D   *Toxoplasma gondii*
    E   *Treponema pallidum pallidum*

14. A 35-year-old man presents at a sexual health clinic with a new painless round lesion on his penis; he also has non-tender inguinal lymphadenopathy.

    What is the most likely causative agent of his symptoms?

    A   *Chlamydia trachomatis*
    B   *Neisseria gonorrhoeae*
    C   *Treponema pallidum carateum*
    D   *Treponema pallidum pallidum*
    E   *Treponema pallidum pertenue*

15. A 63-year-old man with an open fracture of the femur develops the rare complication of gas gangrene and requires leg amputation.

    What is the most likely causative agent?

    A   *Clostridium botulinum*
    B   *Clostridium perfringens*
    C   *Clostridium tetani*
    D   *Escherichia coli*
    E   *Klebsiella pneumoniae*

16. A 28-year-old primiparous woman who is 16 weeks pregnant reports mild dysuria; otherwise she is well. Urine dipstick shows leucocytes ++ and is positive for nitrites. She is prescribed appropriate antibiotics.

    What is the most likely causative organism of her urinary tract infection?

    A   *Citrobacter freundii*
    B   *Escherichia coli*
    C   *Klebsiella pneumoniae*
    D   *Proteus mirabilis*
    E   *Staphylococcus saprophyticus*

17. Which of the following is the causative agent of Kaposi's sarcoma?

    A   HIV
    B   Human herpesvirus 4
    C   Human herpesvirus 8
    D   Human T-lymphotrophic virus 1
    E   All of the above

18. A 32-year-old primiparous school teacher is 16 weeks pregnant. She is seen in the antenatal clinic, where she reports a maculopapular rash and coryzal symptoms. The general practitioner has already sent serology and you review the result.

    Rubella IgG: positive
    Rubella IgM: negative
    Parvovirus B19 IgG: negative
    Parvovirus B19 IgM: positive

    What is the most likely diagnosis?

    A   Non-immunity to parvovirus B19
    B   Non-immunity to rubella
    C   Recent infection with rubella
    D   Recent infection with parvovirus B19
    E   None of the above

19. A 35-year-old multiparous woman has presented to labour ward in spontaneous labour. You see from her antenatal notes that she is HIV positive. She is currently using highly active antiretroviral therapy and has a viral load of 43 copies/mL.

    Which of the following is associated with increased risk of vertical transmission of HIV?

    A   Co-existent Group B *Streptococcus* carriage
    B   Chorioamnionitis
    C   Paternal HIV-infection
    D   Post-dates gestation
    E   Vaginal examination during labour

20. Antenatal screening of a 25-year-old patient is suggestive of hepatitis B infection. The results of her serology are as follows:

HBsAg	Positive
HBeAg	Positive
Anti-HBeAb	Negative
Anti-HBsAb	Negative
Total anti-HBc	Positive (IgM anti-core Ab negative, IgG anti-core Ab positive)

Which of the following is most likely to represent her hepatitis B status?

A   Acute infection (recent)
B   Acute infection (resolving)
C   Chronic infection (high infectivity)
D   Chronic infection (low infectivity)
E   Following vaccination

21. A 23-year-old woman attends antenatal clinic at 22 weeks' gestation. This is her second pregnancy and she is very concerned as during her first pregnancy she had an 'infection', which led to the permanent disability of her child. He is deaf, with delayed development and is small for his age. He became jaundiced shortly after birth.

What was the most likely cause of her son's condition?

A   Cytomegalovirus
B   Herpes
C   Parvovirus B19
D   Rubella
E   Varicella zoster

22. A 38-year-old woman from Sri Lanka attends her general practitioner at 10 weeks' gestation. She is complaining of fever and has pains in her joints. She developed a rash yesterday. On examination, she has a temperature of 38.1°C, postauricular lymphadenopathy and a maculopapular rash over her torso. Rubella is diagnosed.

What is the most likely fetal abnormality to occur as a result of this acute infection?

A   Cerebral palsy
B   Failure to thrive
C   Limb hypoplasia
D   Microcephaly
E   Sensorineural hearing loss

23. A 15-year-old girl attends the genitourinary medicine clinic complaining of vaginal itching and green vaginal discharge. She is sexually active with her 17-year-old boyfriend and uses the oral contraceptive pill. Speculum examination reveals haemorrhages on her cervix. A urine pregnancy test is negative.

Considering the most likely diagnosis, what is the most appropriate first line antibiotic?

A   Azithromycin 1 g once only
B   Doxycycline 100 mg twice daily + metronidazole 400 mg three times daily + ofloxacin 400 mg twice daily for 7 days
C   Doxycycline 100 mg twice daily for 14 days + metronidazole 400 mg three times daily for 7 days
D   Metronidazole 400 mg three times daily for 5 days
E   Tinidazole 2 g once only

24. Which of the following is an obligate anaerobic organism?

A   *Bacteroides*
B   *Escherichia coli*
C   *Listeria*
D   *Mycobacteria*
E   *Pseudomonas*

25. A 23-year-old woman attends her general practitioner complaining of numbness and tingling in both feet. She recently started treatment for pulmonary tuberculosis.

Which drug is most likely to be responsible for these symptoms?

A   Ethambutol
B   Isoniazid
C   Pyrazinamide
D   Rifampicin
E   Streptomycin

26. A 38-year-old woman is readmitted via the emergency department 10 days postemergency caesarean section complaining of vaginal bleeding, abdominal pain and foul-smelling vaginal discharge. Abdominal examination reveals suprapubic tenderness and the uterus is palpable 2 cm below the umbilicus. You suspect endometritis.

Which of the following is the most likely causative organism?

A   *Chlamydia trachomatis*
B   Group B *Streptococcus*
C   *Mycoplasma genitalia*
D   *Neisseria gonorrhoea*
E   *Ureaplasma*

27. A woman presents at 28 weeks' gestation with vomiting, headache, night sweats and abdominal pain. She has recently returned from the African country of Mali. Urgent blood films show the presence of *Plasmodium falciparum*, with a parasitaemia of 3%. After a diagnosis of malaria has been made she is treated with intravenous quinine.

The presence of which haematological characteristic is associated with increased incidence of malaria?

A   Haemoglobin C
B   Beta-thalassaemia
C   Duffy antigen
D   Glucose-6-phosphate dehydrogenase deficiency
E   Sickle cell trait

Answers

1. A False

    B True

    C False

    D True

    E True

    The ability to Gram-stain bacterium allows classification into two major groups, Gram-positive and Gram-negative. A bacterium which has peptidoglycan in its cell wall will take up Gram-stain and therefore is considered Gram-positive. In addition to Gram-staining, further simple classification of bacterium is based on appearance, whether as cocci (i.e. spherical shaped), bacilli (i.e. rod shaped) and a further classification of coccobacillus (intermediate shape) (**Table 12.1**).

Table 12.1 Classification of bacteria		
	Bacilli	**Cocci**
Gram-positive	*Listeria* species e.g.	*Staphylococcus* species, e.g.
	• *L. monocytogenes*	• *S. aureus*
	Clostridium species, e.g.	*Streptococcus* species, e.g.
	• *C. botulinum*	• *S. pneumoniae*
	• *C. difficile*	• *S. pyogenes*
	Actinomyces species, e.g.	*Enterococcus* species, e.g.
	• *A. Israelii*	• *E. faecalis*
	Mycobacterium species, e.g.	
	• *M. tuberculosis*	
Gram-negative	*Escherichia* species, e.g.	*Neisseria* species, e.g.
	• *E. coli*	• *N. gonorrhoeae*
	Enterobacter species e.g.	• *N. meningitidis*
	• *Proteus mirabilis*	
	Klebsiella species, e.g.	**Coccobacilli:**
	• *K. pneumoniae*	*Bordetella* species, e.g.
	Salmonella species, e.g.	• *B. pertussis*
	• *S. enterica*	*Brucella* species
	Shigella species, e.g.	*Haemophilus* species, e.g.
	• *S. dysenteriae*	• *H. influenzae*
	Campylobacter species, e.g.	
	• *C. jejuni*	
	Legionella species, e.g.	
	• *L. pneumophila*	

2. A True

    B False

    C False

    D True

    E False

    Group B β-haemolytic *Streptococcus* (GBS), also known as *Streptococcus agalactiae*, is a common commensal in the gastrointestinal tract and is also part of normal vaginal flora in around one-third of women. Although maternal vaginal carriage is not itself harmful there is the risk of transmission to the baby with the potential to cause neonatal sepsis once membranes rupture. GBS may also be associated with chorioamnionitis.

    GBS infection in infants is classified as having early onset (i.e. it occurs within the first week of life) and late onset (occurs from the first week to the first few months of life). Early-onset disease typically manifests as pneumonia, septicaemia and meningitis, with the latter being more common when there is late-onset disease. It is not current practice within the UK to routinely screen pregnant women for GBS. Nevertheless, if GBS has been detected during the current pregnancy, standard practice is the administration of intrapartum antibiotic therapy (a typical regimen being 3 g intravenous penicillin G, followed by 1.5 g every 4 hours in labour).

    Royal College of Obstetricians and Gynaecologists. Prevention of Early Onset Group B Streptococcal Disease. Green-top Guideline 36. London: RCOG 2003.

3. A False

    B True

    C False

    D False

    E True

    Neisseria are from the genus of aerobic Gram-negative cocci. *Neisseria gonorrhoeae* and *N. meningitidis* are both human pathogens. Both species prefer a moist environment with 5–10% levels of carbon dioxide.

    Neisseria meningitidis is a commensal of the nasopharynx in around 10% of the population, with higher carriage rates amongst teenagers. It is transmitted via droplet spread of respiratory secretions and can lead to bacteraemia and meningitis, with rarer manifestations including arthritis and osteomyelitis. Bacteriological diagnosis of meningococcal meningitis requires culturing cerebrospinal fluid from a lumbar puncture.

    Neisseria gonorrhoea causes the sexually transmitted disease gonorrhoea. It can be asymptomatic in up to 50% of women, and can lead to pelvic inflammatory disease.

    Symptomatic individuals with gonorroheoa may present with lower abdominal pain, increased or altered vaginal discharge or dysuria.

British Association for Sexual Health and HIV. Management of Gonorrhoea in Adults, 2011. www.bashh.org
Health Protection Agency. Meningococcal Infection Factsheet. London: HPA, 2011. www.hpa.org.uk

4. A False

    B True

    C False

    D True

    E True

Viruses contain either DNA or RNA as their genetic material, which may be either
single-stranded (ss) or double-stranded (ds) (**Table 12.2**). Further classification
of their genetic material is dependent on the 'sense' of the strands, i.e. whether
positive-sense or negative-sense.

Table 12.2 Classification of DNA and RNA viruses

RNA viruses (ss or ds)	DNA viruses (ss or ds)
Hepatitis A, C, D, E (ss)	Herpes simplex 1 and 2 (ds)
HIV (ss)	Varicella zoster (ds)
Human T-lymphotrophic virus (ss)	Cytomegalovirus (ds)
Rubella (ss)	Hepatitis B (ds)
Japanese B Virus (ss)	Human papillovirus (ds)
Respiratory syncytial virus (ss)	Epstein–Barr (ds)
Rotavirus (ds)	Parvovirus B19 (ss)

ss = single-stranded, ds = double-stranded

5. A False

    B False

    C False

    D False

    E True

The varicella zoster virus (VZV) is a double-stranded DNA virus and is a member of the
herpesviridae family. First exposure to the virus results in chickenpox, which manifests
around 2 weeks after exposure as a widespread vesicular rash and is often associated
with pyrexia and malaise. After the initial exposure the virus lays dormant in the
sensory root ganglia until it is reactivated, often after many years. Reactivation results
in shingles; here the reactivated virus travels down the nerve root it has infected and
causes inflammation. A characteristic rash and neuralgia is found with a dermatomal
distribution representing the affected nerve root. Antivirals such as acyclovir may be

given after 20 weeks' gestation if the rash has been present for < 24 hours. If VZV is contracted by a pregnant woman who has not been exposed to the virus previously then she should urgently receive varicella zoster immune globulin. If exposure is close to delivery there is a 50% chance that the fetus will become infected with VZV as there is insufficient time for passive immunity to develop.

Royal College of Obstetricians and Gynaecologists. Chickenpox in Pregnancy. Green-top Guideline 13. London: RCOG, 2007.

6. A True

    B False

    C True

    D True

    E False

Mononucleosis is caused by the Epstein–Barr virus, which is also known as human herpesvirus 4. Bejel is caused by the spirochete *Treponema pallidum endemicum* and should be distinguished from yaws which is caused by *Treponema pallidum pertenue*, pinta caused by *Treponema pallidum carateum* and syphilis caused by *Treponema pallidum pallidum*. Bacterial vaginosis is caused by a variety of bacterium including *Gardnerella vaginalis*, *Bacteroides* and *Mycoplasma*. Sleeping sickness, also known as African trypanosomiasis is caused by the transmission of the protozoal *Trypanosoma brucei* via the tsetse fly. Dengue fever is caused by Dengue virus. *Toxoplasma gondii* causes toxoplasmosis, which typically affects rodents and cats, but may lead to fetal abnormalities such as intracranial calcification, chorioretinitis and miscarriage if contracted for the first time during pregnancy.

7. A False

    B True

    C False

    D False

    E True

Preoperative antibiotic prophylaxis is now common practice. In order to be the most effective, the antibiotic given needs to have the relevant spectrum of activity to cover the organism(s) that may be found at the operative site. Removing hair with a shaver leads to abrasions which may increase the chance of infection. Intraoperative blood sugars should be kept below 11 mmol/L in patients with any type of diabetes mellitus. The use of any prophylactic antibiotics, particularly more than one dose, increases the risk of *Clostridium difficile*.

8. A True

    B False

    C True

D False

E False

Cytomegalovirus (CMV) is a herpesvirus and is the most common cause of congenital infection. Previous infection does not offer immunity, as both primary and recurrent infection during pregnancy may lead to congenital infection. The virus is spread through contact with infected body fluids. Both primary and recurrent infections are often asymptomatic. Any symptoms that are experienced are usually vague and include lethargy and fever. If conception occurs within 6 months of the primary infection, then the risk of placental transmission is higher. The fetus may be affected by infection in any of the trimesters. Most babies who have been congenitally infected show no signs or symptoms. However, those who are affected may have jaundice, thrombocytopaenia, microcephaly, and motor disorders. The main neurological sequelae are deafness and learning disabilities. There is no CMV vaccine and antiviral drugs are not currently licensed for use to treat CMV infection during pregnancy. Ganciclovir is sometimes used to treat infection in babies and toddlers to help prevent hearing loss associated with contracting CMV at this age.

9. **A False**

   B True

   C False

   D True

   E False

Toxins are produced by both Gram-positive and Gram-negative bacteria. Exotoxins are produced by both Gram-positive and Gram-negative bacteria, whilst endotoxins are constituents of the cell walls of Gram-negative bacteria. **Table 12.3** gives further details.

Table 12.3 Exotoxins and endotoxins		
	Exotoxin	**Endotoxin**
Producing bacteria	Gram-positive Gram-negative	Gram-negative
Release	Extracellular, released	Structural molecule of Gram-negative bacterial cell wall, released on cell death
Examples of action	Tetanus toxins Cholera symptoms E. coli Shigella	Lipopolysaccharide Lipid A
Antigenicity	Susceptible to antibodies Destroyed by heating	Limited effect of antibodies

10. A False

   B True

   C False

   D True

   E True

Molluscum contagiosum is viral infection caused by the molluscum contagiosum DNA poxvirus. It is usually a disease of the skin, but occasionally affects mucous membranes. The lesions are painless and have a pearly-white appearance with a dimpled centre. They are usually < 5 mm in diameter. It is spread through direct contact and the fluid from the vesicles is infectious. Although most common amongst children, it can also be sexually transmitted and may be mistaken for genital warts. Individuals are infectious, whereas the lesions are present. Molluscum is self clearing, but treatment may be expedited with cryotherapy or topical treatments, such as benzoyl peroxide. Most cases are cleared within 6–9 months. There is no immunity to the virus and it does not lie dormant within the body.

Health Protection Agency. Factsheet on Molluscum contagiosum. Essex: HPA, 2011. www.hpa.org.uk

11. A False

   B True

   C False

   D True

   E True

Mycobacteria are non-motile, obligate aerobic bacteria which are generally considered to be Gram-positive. They are a group of bacteria subdivided into several complexes and are generally associated with immunosuppressed individuals. Diagnosis is performed via auramine staining and confirmatory testing is carried out with Ziehl–Neelsen stain which stains mycobacteria pink. *Mycobacterium avium* complex is associated with people with pre-existing lung conditions, including chronic obstructive pulmonary disease, smoking and granulomatous disease. *Mycobacterium leprae* (Hansen's disease) causes classic symptoms leading to leprosy and systems affected include skin, peripheral nerves and eyes. Dapsone is used to treat leprosy.

12. A *Actinomyces israelii*

The Gram-positive bacteria *Actinomyces israelii* is a commensal of the colon, mouth and vagina. It is the commonest cause of actinomycosis, a chronic, suppurative and granulomatous inflammatory infection. The majority of cases of actinomycosis affect the cervicofacial area, classically presenting as painless facial lumps; however, thoracic, abdominal and pelvic forms do occasionally occur. Diagnosis of pelvic actinomycosis is usually made from histological samples taken during surgery and has been associated with intrauterine contraceptive devices which have been in situ for long periods of time. The presence of sulphur granules is characteristic of actinomyces infection.

13. C *Chlamydia trachomatis*

The boyfriend's symptoms are suggestive of a urethritis, which from the list of given options, the cause is most likely to be *Chlamydia* infection. It is caused by *Chlamydia trachomatis*, a Gram-negative intracellular bacterium which infects squamocolumnar epithelial cells. *Chlamydia* infection is often asymptomatic, especially in women. Women may notice postcoital or intermenstrual bleeding, dysuria and low abdominal pain, whereas men may experience dysuria, penile discharge and scrotal pain. *Chlamydia* infection is the commonest cause of pelvic inflammatory disease and may go on to cause subfertility and increased risk of ectopic pregnancy. Treatment regimens for uncomplicated *Chlamydial* infection include azithromycin, doxycycline and erythromycin.

British Association for Sexual Health and HIV. National Guideline for the Management of Genital Tract Infection with *Chlamydia trachomatis*. London: BASHH, 2006. www.bashh.org

14. D *Treponema pallidum pallidum*

Syphilis is caused by the spirochete *Treponema pallidum pallidum*. Primary syphilis typically presents with a painless genital ulcer (a chancre) alongside inguinal lymphadenopathy, occurring 10–90 days after infection. Secondary syphilis develops within 2 years of infection and tertiary syphilis after this period. Screening tests for syphilis include the venereal disease research laboratory (VDRL) carbon antigen test and the rapid plasma regain test, both of which can give false positives. More specific tests for syphilis include fluorescent treponema antibody absorption test; however, these tests can give a positive result when there is infection from other treponema, such as the causative agents of yaw, bejel and pinta. Syphilis in pregnancy is associated with stillbirth, preterm delivery and congenital defects.

Kingston M, French P, Goh B, et al. UK National Guidelines on the Management of Syphilis 2008. International Journal for STD & AIDS 2008;19:729–740.

15. B *Clostridium perfringens*

Gas gangrene is most commonly caused by *Clostridium perfringens*; however, it can also be caused by other species of anaerobic bacteria including *Clostridium septicum*, *Klebsiella pneumoniae* and *Escherichia coli*.

Exotoxins produced by the bacteria lead to necrotic tissue damage and sepsis often requiring amputation of the affected tissue. Gas gangrene was historically associated with war injuries, where open wounds were exposed to these soil-loving bacterium. Today, risk factors for the development of gas gangrene include trauma such as open fractures and burns, alongside malignancy of the gastrointestinal tract, diabetes mellitus, chronic alcohol abuse and as a rare post-surgical complication.

16. B *Escherichia coli*

Uncomplicated urinary tract infections (UTIs) are common in women, particularly during pregnancy. The most common causative organism of uncomplicated urinary tract infection is *Escherichia coli*, a gastrointestinal commensal. Suitable antibiotics for the treatment of a proven *E. coli* UTI in pregnancy include cefalexin and nitrofurantoin (should be avoided at term due to risk of neonatal haemolysis). *Klebsiella pneumoniae*, *Proteus mirabilis*, *Citrobacter freundii* are also Gram-negative commensals of the gastrointestinal tract and therefore may all cause infection of the urinary tract, particularly in women due to the close proximity of the anus and the urethra.

Staphylococcus saprophyticus is a common cause of urinary tract infection in sexually active women.

17. C Human herpesvirus 4

Kaposi's sarcoma is caused human herpesvirus 8; although not always coexistent with HIV infection, Kaposi's sarcoma is considered an AIDS-defining illness, whereby reduced immunosurveillance can result in its characteristic lesions of the skin, respiratory and gastrointestinal tract. Human herpesvirus 4, more commonly known as the Epstein–Barr virus, is the causative agent of infectious mononucleosis; it is also associated with several forms of lymphoproliferative neoplasias, e.g. Burkitt's lymphoma, nasopharyngeal carcinoma and Hodgkin's lymphoma.

18. D Recent infection with parvovirus B19

Both parvovirus 19 and rubella infection may present with a rash. If contracted in pregnancy both viruses have implications for the fetus, and therefore rapidly establishing the immune status of the mother is vital as this will guide the further management of the pregnancy. It is important to send urgent serology requesting specific IgG and IgM status for each virus. The presence of IgG suggests previous exposure to an antigen, whether in the form of a vaccine or through contracting the virus. Development of IgM is an acute event and occurs after exposure to the antigen. In this patient, the serology results for rubella suggests either previous exposure or immunisation to rubella, without any evidence of acute infection.

Specific parvovirus B19 serology indicated recent infection with parvovirus B19. Parvovirus B19 has been implicated with pregnancy loss and in ongoing pregnancies with fetal hydrops and anaemia.

Health Protection Agency. Guidance on Viral Rash in Pregnancy: Investigation, Diagnosis and Management of Viral Illness Rash, or Exposure to Viral Rash Illness, in Pregnancy. London: HPA, 2011. www. hpa.org.uk

StratOG.net. Maternal Medicine: Infectious Diseases. London: StratOG 2012. www.rcog.org.uk/stratog

19. B Chorioamnionitis

The risk of vertical transmission of HIV is highest at delivery. In non-breastfeeding untreated European women vertical transmission of HIV occurs in around 20% of cases. Use of highly active anti-retroviral therapy (HAART) has reduced vertical transmission in treated women to < 2%. Nevertheless, the management of the delivery and postnatal period requires planning and a multidisciplinary team approach. Prematurity, chorioamnionitis, prolonged rupture of membranes and breastfeeding all increase the risk of transmission. Elective caesarean section is the recommended mode of delivery for certain cases, i.e. HIV positive women not using HAART, women with a viral load above 50 copies/mL or if there is coexistent hepatitis C. A planned vaginal delivery may be suitable for women with viral loads < 50 copies/mL who are using HAART.

Royal College of Obstetricians and Gynaecologists. Management of HIV in Pregnancy. Green-top Guideline 39. London: RCOG, 2010.

20. C Chronic infection (high infectivity)

Hepatitis B is a double-stranded DNA virus. The virus is responsible for causing jaundice, hepatitis, cirrhosis and an increased risk of hepatocellular carcinoma. The virus may be spread via sexual intercourse, exposure to infected blood (i.e. shared needles) or vertically from mother to child. The presence of HBs-antigen (HBsAg) indicates infection; HBsAg is typically present for the first 6 months after infection; however, if it persists beyond this then infection is considered chronic. The presence of HBeAg shows viral replication and therefore high infectivity. Anti-HBc is produced soon after infection (initially as IgM, then as IgG) and indicates previous or ongoing infection. Anti-HBsAb indicates previous exposure and is positive after vaccination and in cases where infection has been cleared by the immune system with subsequent immunity. In this patient there is evidence of chronic infection with ongoing high infectivity. The baby will likely need immunising against hepatitis B and specific immunoglobulin at birth and the neonatologist should be informed.

Centres for Disease Control & Prevention. Interpretation of Hepatitis B Serologic Test Results. Altanta: CDC, 2012. http://www.cdc.gov
StratOG.net. Maternal Medicine: Infectious Diseases. London: StratOG 2012. www.rcog.org.uk/stratog

21. A Cytomegalovirus

Cytomegalovirus (CMV) is the most common congenital infection. Pregnant women often do not realise they have the infection as it is frequently asymptomatic. Approximately 5–10% of congenitally infected babies have symptoms apparent at birth which, if present, is a poor prognostic sign. Ten per cent of babies affected at birth die and one-third develop cerebral palsy. Of the babies who are not symptomatic at birth, approximately 1 in 6 are deaf, 1 in 10 have developmental delay and 1% suffer from retinitis.

Bhide A, Papageorghiou AT. Managing primary CMV infection in pregnancy. BJOG 2008;115:805–807.

22. E Sensorineural hearing loss

Rubella causes most problems if it is contracted during the first trimester, leading to miscarriage in up to 20% of cases. If miscarriage does not occur, there is a strong possibility that the fetus will be affected in some way. Approximately, 70% will suffer sensorineural hearing loss, 50% suffer retinopathy and eye abnormalities and 40% may suffer from congenital heart abnormalities, such as a patent ductus arteriosus and ventricular septal defects. This woman should have her serology sent urgently.

The virus is excreted in pharyngeal secretions during the incubation period for up to 7 days before the appearance of the rash.

23. D Metronidazole 400 mg three times daily for 5 days

Trichomonas vaginalis is a sexually transmitted infection of the lower genital tract caused by a protozoa. Symptoms include itching and inflammation of the vulva and vagina. There is often purulent vaginal discharge and the cervix may have the classic haemorrhages giving it the classic description of a 'strawberry cervix'. Swabs should be sent for culture and other sexually transmitted diseases should always be considered. *Trichomonas* is a rare cause of pelvic inflammatory disease, however contact tracing is necessary. First line treatment is metronidazole, either 2 g as a single dose or 400 mg three times a day for 5 days. Sexual intercourse should be avoided until treatment is completed in the patient and also the partner, if necessary. This patient should be advised that while the oral contraceptive pill is effective for preventing pregnancy, barrier methods should also be used to prevent sexually transmitted infections. Treatment with metronidazole would be safe in pregnancy.

StratOG.net. Sexual and Reproductive Health: Sexually Transmitted Infections (including HIV). London: StratOG 2012. www.rcog.org.uk/stratog

24. A *Bacteroides*

Obligate anaerobes are organisms that live and thrive in the absence of oxygen; they will die in the presence of oxygen. Examples include bacteroides, *Clostridium* and *Actinomyces*. By contrast, a facultative anaerobe is able to alter its function depending on the presence or absence of oxygen. Examples include *Staphylococcus aureus*, *E. coli* and *Listeria*.

25. B Isoniazid

Tuberculosis (TB) has a prevalence in the UK of 15–50/100,000 population, depending on the location. The highest levels are currently in London. The disease most commonly affects the lungs and 60% of infected individuals having pulmonary involvement. TB may affect other organs including the genitourinary tract, which may present with a pelvic mass or chronic pelvic inflammatory disease. This occurs as a result of haematogenous spread from the primary location. Treatment of TB involves 6 months of medication with rifampicin, isoniazid and pyrazinamide. Ethambutol has recently been added to address the issue of resistance. Side effects of the medication include:

- Rifampicin: orange urine and tears, hepatotoxicity
- Isoniazid: hepatotoxicity, peripheral neuropathy (may be reduced by administration of pyridoxine)
- Pyrazinamide: hepatotoxicity, gout
- Ethambutol: optic neuritis

National Institute for Health and Clinical Excellence. Tuberculosis. Clinical Guideline CG117. London: NICE, 2011.

26. E *Ureaplasma*

Endometritis may be acute or chronic. In this case, the patient has an acute endometritis after caesarean section. Causes to be considered include retained products of conception and ascending infection from the lower genital tract, with prolonged rupture of membranes being a particular risk factor. Acute endometritis from an obstetric cause is most often polymicrobial, involving vaginal commensals. These bacteria include *Ureaplasma*, *Gardnerella* and group B *Streptococcus*. Other bacteria implicated in endometritis are those associated with sexually transmitted infections including *Chlamydia* and gonorrhoea. Treatment includes initial resuscitation and swift administration of broad spectrum antibiotics. Other investigations include a full blood count, C-reactive protein, clotting profile and pelvic ultrasound.

Hay PE. Chapter 22: Infections in Obstetrics and Gynaecology. In: Fiander A, Thilganathan B (eds).Your Essential Revision Guide MRCOG Part 1. London: RCOG Press, 2010: 381.

27. C Duffy antigen

Beta-thalassaemia, like many other haemoglobinopathies, is known to confer an element of protection against malaria. The presence of the sickle cell trait is known to reduce the severity of malarial disease, with fewer hospital admissions and reduced parasite densities. This is due to the suboptimal conditions for the parasites caused by low oxygen concentrations in the serum of individuals with the trait. Individuals with haemoglobin C are also less likely to experience severe malaria, due to reduced ability of the parasite to reproduce. The absence of the Duffy factor provides immunity against *Plasmodium vivax*, as it is the Duffy antigen that parasites bind to.

An individual with glucose-6-phosphate dehydrogenase deficiency typically has an enhanced protection against malaria, in particular *Plasmodium falciparum*.

Royal College of Obstetricians and Gynaecologists. The Diagnosis and Treatment of Malaria in Pregnancy, Green-top Guideline 54B. London: RCOG, 2010.

Chapter 13

Pathology

Questions: MCQs

Answer each stem 'True' or 'False'.

1. Congenital absence of the uterus:
   A   Has an incidence of 1:1000 births
   B   Has a chromosomal pattern of 45XX
   C   Hirsutism is common
   D   Is known as Mayer–Rokitansky–Küster–Hauser syndrome
   E   The ovaries are normally affected

2. Choriocarcinoma:
   A   Is a malignant condition
   B   Is more common in women over 40 years old
   C   Can follow a normal pregnancy
   D   Most commonly metastasises to the lungs
   E   Syncytiotrophoblasts are filled with eosinophilic cytoplasm

3. Systemic effects of inflammation:
   A   Cytokines act on the bone marrow to reduce production of leucocytes
   B   Fever is mediated by tumour necrosis factor and interleukin-1
   C   Fever is partly mediated by prostacyclins
   D   Fibrinogen is an acute phase protein
   E   Tumour necrosis factor is a cytokine implicated in the process of septic shock

4. Uterine fibroids:
   A   Are a risk factor for ovarian cancer
   B   Are usually benign in nature
   C   Are also known as leiomyomas
   D   Consist predominantly of fibrous tissue
   E   Can be treated by uterine artery embolisation

5. The following neoplasms are paired with the appropriate causative viruses.
   A   Burkitt's lymphoma and Epstein–Barr virus
   B   Cervical cancer and human papillomavirus 2
   C   Kaposi's sarcoma and human herpesvirus 8
   D   Hepatocellular carcinoma and hepatitis
   E   Testicular cancer and human T-lymphotrophic virus-1

6. **The following tumours are paired with their causative carcinogens:**
   A   Mesothelioma and asbestos
   B   Vaginal clear cell carcinoma and aflatoxin B1
   C   Leukaemia and benzene
   D   Bladder cancer and aniline dye
   E   Bowel cancer and nickel

7. **The following tumours are hormone dependent:**
   A   Ductal carcinoma of the breast
   B   Endometrial cancer
   C   Malignant melanoma
   D   Adenocarcinoma of the prostate
   E   Adenocarcinoma of the pancreas

8. **The following premalignant conditions are paired with their sequelae:**
   A   Leukoplakia and oral cancer
   B   Ulcerative colitis and colorectal cancer
   C   Actinic keratosis and basal cell carcinoma
   D   Atrophic gastritis and oesophageal cancer
   E   Cervical intraepithelial neoplasia and cervical cancer

9. **Sarcomas:**
   A   Are slow growing
   B   Include gastrointestinal stromal tumours
   C   Can metastasise to the lungs
   D   Originate from embryonic ectoderm
   E   Respond poorly to chemotherapy

10. **Pheochromocytomas:**
    A   Are corticosteroid producing tumours
    B   High levels of serum metanephrine can be diagnostic
    C   May present with severe hypertension and palpitations
    D   Originate from chromaffin cells
    E   Commonly develop in the renal cortex

11. **Conn's syndrome:**
    A   Is associated with excess aldosterone
    B   Is caused by a squamous cell carcinoma of the adrenal glands
    C   Is characterised by profound hypotension
    D   Can cause hyperkalaemia
    E   Responds to spironolactone

12. **The following conditions are linked to abnormalities in DNA repair:**
    A   Bloom's syndrome
    B   Cockayne's syndrome
    C   Neurofibromatosis

D   Noonan's syndrome
E   Xeroderma pigmentosum

13. **Regarding genetically inherited predispositions to tumour development:**

A   Li–Fraumeni syndrome is caused by a defect in *p16*
B   The *BRCA1* gene is inherited via autosomal recessive inheritance
C   Inheritance of the *RB* gene is linked to bilateral retinoblastomas
D   Neurofibromatosis type 1 is inherited on chromosome 11
E   Hereditary non-polyposis colonic cancer is a risk factor for development of endometrial cancer

14. **Osteoporosis:**

A   Can be diagnosed when the bone mineral density T score is >1.5 standard deviations from the mean
B   Is more common in patients with Turner's syndrome
C   There is with increased osteoclast activity
D   Sufferers have a normal Z score
E   Can be coexistent with increased parathyroid hormone activity

15. **Risk factors for osteoporosis include:**

A   Caffeine intake
B   Increased body mass index
C   Hyperparathyroidism
D   Kallmann's syndrome
E   Smoking

16. **Apoptosis is characterised by:**

A   Apoptotic bodies
B   Cell swelling
C   Karyorrhexis
D   Pyknosis
E   Release of inflammatory mediators

17. **Necrosis:**

A   Caseous necrosis can occur in the presence of *Mycobacterium tuberculosis*
B   Is a natural sequelae of the cell cycle
C   Leads to the release of inflammatory mediators
D   Is reversible
E   Involves nuclear changes including karyolysis

18. **The following can give a positive direct Coombs test:**

A   Cephalosporins
B   Cyclosporin administration
C   Haemolytic disease of the newborn
D   Methyldopa
E   *Mycoplasma pneumonia*

19. **Concerning inherited coagulation abnormalities:**
    A   Christmas disease is caused by abnormalities in factor IX
    B   Factor V Leiden is an autosomal recessive condition
    C   Haemophilia A is linked with excessive levels of factor VIII
    D   Protein C deficiency causes increased thrombus formation
    E   von Willebrand's disease is an autosomal dominant condition

20. **Concerning hyperplasia:**
    A   It can be reversible
    B   It occurs in the adrenal cortex of sufferers of Cushing's syndrome
    C   It occurs in the uterus during pregnancy
    D   It should be treated the same as a malignancy
    E   It is associated with an increase in cell size

21. **Concerning cellular function:**
    A   Atrophy can be reversible
    B   Dysplasia is irreversible
    C   Metaplasia is the conversion of differentiated tissue into undifferentiated tissue
    D   Hypertrophy is the increase in cell number
    E   Neoplasia represents malignant change

22. **Metaplasia:**
    A   Is synonymous with heteroplasia
    B   In the cervix it describes the change from columnar to transitional epithelium
    C   Is the change of one differentiated cell type to another
    D   Can be reversible
    E   Represents malignant change

23. **Concerning shock:**
    A   There is metabolic alkalosis
    B   Hypoxia is characteristic
    C   Capillary permeability is reduced
    D   Hypokalaemia occurs
    E   There may be coagulopathy

Questions: SBAs

For each question, select the single best answer from the five options listed.

24. A 27-year-old nulliparous woman and her husband have a series of routine investigations to investigate primary subfertility. She has a hysterosalpingogram which shows she has a bicornuate uterus.

    Which obstetric phenomenon is of increased prevalence in women with a bicornuate uterus?

    A   Breech presentation
    B   Stillbirth
    C   Postpartum haemorrhage
    D   Placenta praevia
    E   Placenta accreta

25. A 31-year-old nulliparous woman has heavy bleeding at 8 weeks' gestation. An early pregnancy scan is suggestive of a molar pregnancy, and no fetus is observed.

    What is the typical genotype of a complete molar pregnancy?

    A   45 XO
    B   46 XX
    C   46 XXX
    D   69 XXY
    E   92 XXXY

26. In addition to mast cells, which of the following cells produces histamine?

    A   Basophils
    B   Erythrocytes
    C   Macrophages
    D   Monocytes
    E   Neutrophils

27. Within what timeframe from injury do macrophages replace neutrophils in cutaneous wound healing?

    A   1–2 hours
    B   6–12 hours
    C   18–24 hours
    D   48–92 hours
    E   7–10 days

28. A 40-year-old primiparous woman is admitted to the labour ward at 36 weeks' gestation with severe pre-eclampsia and presumed renal involvement. Her blood pressure on arrival is 184/95 mmHg. Her urine contains protein +++. Her serum creatinine is 92 μmol/L and serum urea 5.3 mg/dL. She has an emergency caesarean section.

Which of the following best describes the renal pathology of pre-eclampsia?

A   Atheromatous plaques
B   Glomerular capillary endotheliosis
C   Glomerular hypertrophy
D   Mesangial cell hypertrophy
E   Tubular vacuolization

29. A 45-year-old woman is seen in the gynaecology outpatients' clinic with a history of severe menorrhagia. She has a body mass index of 42. An endometrial biopsy is taken at hysteroscopy which shows evidence of simple endometrial hyperplasia.

Which of the following describes the type of cellular change that occurs in hyperplasia?

A   Increase in the number of cells
B   Increase in the number of mitotic figures
C   Increase in the number of nuclei in each cell
D   Increase in the size of cells
E   Increase in the thickness of the cell

30. A 50-year-old woman is admitted to hospital following a myocardial infarction. She remains hypotensive for several days. Her serum lactate becomes elevated and her serum urea nitrogen and creatinine are also increased. Microscopic urinalysis reveals granular and hyaline casts.

Which of the following renal pathologies is most likely to be the cause?

A   Acute tubular necrosis
B   Chronic pyelonephritis
C   Minimal change glomerulonephritis
D   Nodular glomerulosclerosis
E   Renal vein thrombosis

31. A 43-year-old woman was diagnosed at 15 years of age with type 1 diabetes mellitus. Her disease has been poorly controlled. She develops a non-healing ulcer of her foot at age 35 years. By 40 years of age, she has an increasing serum urea and a urinalysis shows a specific gravity of 1.012, pH 6.5, 1+ protein, no blood, 1+ glucose, negative leukocyte esterase, negative nitrite, and no ketones.

Which of the following renal diseases is she most likely to have?

A   Crescentic glomerulonephritis
B   Hyperplastic arteriolosclerosis
C   Nodular glomerulosclerosis
D   Papillary necrosis
E   Pyelonephritis

32. A 59-year-old man presents with a 1-week history of frank haematuria. On physical examination, there are no abnormal findings. Urinalysis confirms the presence of blood, but no proteinuria or glucosuria. Urine culture is negative. A cystoscopy is

performed, and a 3 cm exophytic mass is seen in the dome of the bladder. A biopsy of this mass is performed and microscopic examination reveals fibrovascular cores covered by a thick layer of transitional cells.

Which of the following risk factors is most likely to have led to development of this lesion?

A   Chronic use of nonsteroidal anti-inflammatory drugs
B   Cigarette smoking
C   Diabetes mellitus
D   Recurrent urinary tract infection
E   Obesity

33. A 30-year-old woman has had increasing malaise with fever, abdominal pain, and weight loss of 3 kg over the past 3 weeks. On physical examination, her blood pressure is 160/110 mmHg. She has a stool positive for occult blood. Urinalysis reveals haematuria. She has no serum antineutrophil cytoplasmic autoantibodies and her antinuclear antibody test is negative. Aneurysmal arterial dilations and occlusions are seen in the medium-sized renal and mesenteric arteries with angiography. She improves with corticosteroid therapy.

Which of the following is the most likely diagnosis?

A   Benign nephrosclerosis
B   Nodular glomerulosclerosis
C   Polyarteritis nodosa
D   Systemic lupus erythematosus
E   Wegener granulomatosis

34. A 55-year-old woman is admitted to the emergency department 1 week after a work-related crush injury. On physical examination, she is febrile and appears dehydrated. After catheterisation, she passes a small amount of very dark urine. The urine dipstick test for blood is positive but no red blood cells are seen on microscopy. Her serum biochemistry shows:

Creatinine = 120 μmol/L
Serum potassium = 5.7 mmol/L
Creatinine kinase = > 50,000 U/L

Which of the following is the most likely diagnosis?

A   Poststreptococcal glomerulonephritis
B   Renal infarction
C   Renal papillary necrosis
D   Rhabdomyolysis
E   Ureteral lithiasis

35. Which of the following is characteristic of the cellular changes seen in dysplasia?

A   Absence of mitotic figures on microscopy
B   Decreased mitotic activity
C   Hyperchromatism

    D Irreversibility

    E Uniformity in cell shape

36. Which of the following vulval skin disorders is associated with the highest risk of developing malignant disease?

    A Contact irritant dermatitis

    B Lichen planus

    C Lichen sclerosus

    D Squamous cell hyperplasia

    E Psoriasis

37. A 75-year-old woman presents to her general practitioner (GP) with increasing abdominal girth, reduced appetite and increasing shortness of breath. Her GP, suspicious of malignancy, performs laboratory investigations and refers her for an urgent review to the local hospital.

The results of her laboratory investigations are as follows:

Tumour marker	Result	Reference range
CA 19-9 (U/mL)	34	0–40
CA-125 (U/mL)	812	0–35
Carcinoembryonic antigen (µg/L)	1.2	0–2.5
A-Fetoprotein U/mL	1.4	0–5

From the tumour marker levels given what is the most likely primary tumour?

    A Colorectal cancer

    B Hepatocellular cancer

    C Lung cancer with abdominal metastases

    D Pancreatic cancer

    E Primary peritoneal cancer

38. Which of the following paraneoplastic syndromes is paired with a recognised causal malignancy?

    A Acanthosis nigricans and bowel cancer

    B Carcinoid and uterine cancer

    C Cushing's syndrome and small cell lung cancer

    D Dermatomyositis and renal cancer

    E Syndrome of inappropriate antidiuretic hormone secretion and fibroma

39. Which of the following is a risk factor for the development of ovarian cancer?

    A Early menopause

    B History of breastfeeding

    C Nulliparity

    D Oral contraceptive use

    E Physical activity

40. A grand multiparous woman has a postpartum haemorrhage soon after delivery. She is tachycardic, hypotensive, with a capillary refill time of 3 seconds and she appears confused. She has grade IV haemorrhagic shock.

    What do you think is the estimated blood loss thus far based on clinical findings?

    A   500 mL
    B   750 mL
    C   1000 mL
    D   1300 mL
    E   2000 mL

41. A 39-year-old woman has a forceps delivery. She is diagnosed as having a fourth degree tear of the perineum, which is repaired in theatre. She is readmitted 5 days later with wound dehiscence and it is noted that faecal matter is draining per vaginam. She has a temperature, is tachycardic and is feeling unwell. She is in septic shock soon after arrival.

    Which of the below pathogens is the most likely causative agent?

    A   *Actinomyces israelii*
    B   *Clostridium perfringens*
    C   *Staphylococcus aureus*
    D   *Listeria monocytogenes*
    E   *Escherichia coli*

Answers

1. A False

    B False

    C False

    D True

    E False

    Mayer–Rokitansky–Küster–Hauser (MRKH) syndrome occurs in approximately 1 in 5000 females. The cause is unknown and it is not known to have a genetic inheritance. Women affected have a female chromosomal pattern of 46XX and normally-functioning ovaries. MRKH syndrome occurs as a result of abnormal development of the Müllerian system which forms the uterus, fallopian tubes and upper part of the vagina. There is a spectrum of abnormalities ranging from absence of the proximal two-thirds of the vagina to more significant genital abnormalities including absence of the uterus. It is not associated with hirsutism, but may be found alongside abnormalities of the skeleton, kidneys and other organs.

2. A True

    B True

    C True

    D True

    E True

    Choriocarcinoma is a malignant form of gestational trophoblastic disease which most commonly occurs after a complete molar pregnancy. It is more common at extremes of fertility: teenagers and those over 40 years of age. Pathology reveals sheets of syncytiotrophoblasts and cytotrophoblasts with evidence of necrosis, haemorrhage and intravascular growth. Treatment is carried out at specialist units and often requires chemotherapy, however overall survival is good if metastasis has not yet occurred.

3. A False

    B True

    C False

    D True

    E True

    Inflammation occurs in response to tissue injury. Acute inflammation occurs immediately and may last hours or days, whereas chronic inflammation can potentially last for months and years. In response to insult, a series of cellular and chemical mediators become part of response aimed at removing the cause of the trauma and bringing about tissue healing. Cytokines are cell-derived polypeptides, predominantly produced by macrophages and lymphocytes as part of the inflammatory response. A form of cytokines called colony stimulating factors act on the bone marrow to increase the production of leucocytes. Fever is mediated by tumour necrosis factor (TNF) and interleukin-1 (both cytokines), causing damage to the heat regulating system.

4. A False

B True

C True

D False

E True

Uterine fibroids, also known as leiomyomas, are benign growths of smooth muscle which arise from the myometrium of the uterus. They can be classified according to their location. Women with fibroids may complain of menorrhagia, dysmenorrhoea, and problems with urinary frequency and hesitancy. In severe cases fibroids may be associated with anaemia and urinary retention. Reduced fertility may be associated with fibroids; the possible link between fibroids and recurrent miscarriage remains unclear. Fibroids are more common in women of Afro–Caribbean origin and in obese women. Treatment options include hormone therapy such as gonadotropin-releasing hormone analogues to cause preoperative shrinkage, myomectomy, uterine artery embolisation and hysterectomy. Rarely fibroids may undergo malignant change and become leiomyosarcomas (**Figure 13.1**).

National Institute for Health and Clinical Excellence. Heavy Menstrual Bleeding. Clinical Guideline CG44. London: NICE, 2007.

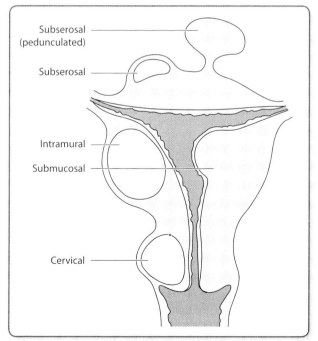

Figure 13.1 Location of uterine fibroids.

Subserosal (pedunculated)

Subserosal

Intramural

Submucosal

Cervical

5. A True

    B False

    C True

    D True

    E False

Epstein–Barr virus, also known as human herpesvirus 4, causes infectious mononucleosis and is also associated with the development of neoplasms such as Burkitt's lymphoma, Hodgkin's disease and nasopharyngeal carcinoma. The primary cause of cervical cancer is infection by subtypes of the human papilloma virus (HPV). By far the majority of cervical cancers are caused by the HPV subtypes 16 and 18. Kaposi's sarcoma, an AIDs-defining illness, is caused by infection with human herpesvirus 8. Hepatocellular carcinoma is associated with infection by hepatitis viruses B and C, although it may also be caused by carcinogens such as aflatoxin B1 and may also be the sequelae of alcoholism and haemochromatosis.

6. A True

    B False

    C True

    D True

    E False

Vaginal clear cell carcinoma is a rare form of tumour associated with exposure to diethylstilbestrol during fetal development. Several forms of leukaemia, i.e. acute myeloid leukaemia and chronic lymphocytic leukaemia have been associated with exposure to myelotoxic agents such as benzene. Exposure to aniline dye (also known as benzidine) in factory workers is classically associated with the subsequent development of bladder cancer. Similarly associated with bladder cancer is β-naphthylamine, a carcinogen which is a constituent of cigarette smoke. A low-fibre diet, high levels of processed meats and smoking are just a few of the risk factors associated with the development of bowel cancer.

Chapter 25: Gynaeclogical Neoplasia. In: Fiander A, Thilganathan B (eds).Your Essential Revision Guide MRCOG Part 1. London: RCOG Press, 2010: 404.

7. A True

    B True

    C False

    D True

    E False

Tumours may express receptors for certain hormones and therefore be considered as hormone-dependant. Ductal carcinoma of the breast may be oestrogen receptor-positive and can respond to oestrogen antagonist drugs such as tamoxifen. Endometrial cancer may be considered a consequence of the effects of unopposed oestrogen. Adenocarcinoma of the prostate is a hormone-dependent tumour which may respond to antiandrogens and gonadotropin-releasing hormone analogues.

8. A True

B True

C False

D False

E True

Actinic keratosis is associated with squamous cell carcinomas. Atrophic gastritis, a condition associated with chronic inflammation of the stomach, may develop into gastric adenocarcinoma. Leukoplakia is characterised by white patches of skin in the oral cavity, mainly occurring in tobacco users; sufferers may go on to develop oral cancer. Barrett's oesophagus, a condition where the squamous epithelium of the oesophagus is replaced by columnar epithelium as a consequence of chronic reflux oesophagitis, is considered as premalignant for oesophageal cancer. Cervical intraepithelial neoplasia (CIN) is the premalignant condition associated with cervical cancer and detection of CIN is the basis of cervical screening programmes.

9. A False

B True

C True

D False

E False

Sarcomas are relatively rare fast growing connective tissue tumours. They originate from embryonic mesoderm. The commonest form of childhood cancer, these malignant tumours may rapidly metastasise to sites such as the lungs. Sarcomas may be found in soft tissues, in bone or in the form of gastrointestinal stromal tumours. The commonest form of sarcoma is gastrointestinal stromal tumours (GISTs). Other examples of sarcomas include osteosarcoma, malignant schwannoma and chondrosarcoma. Low-grade tumours may be effectively surgically excised, however higher-grade forms may respond to both radiotherapy and chemotherapy. GISTs tend to respond better to the drug imatinib (a protein kinase inhibitor) rather than traditional radio- and chemotherapy.

10. A False

B True

C True

D True

E False

Phaeochromocytomas are neuroendocrine tumours of chromaffin cells. The majority of these tumours occur in the chromaffin cells of the renal medulla, although they may also develop elsewhere and be found retroperitoneally, in the organ of

Zuckerkandl (located at the bifurcation of the aorta), the neck and at other sites. Pheochromocytomas secrete catecholamines, i.e. adrenaline and noradrenaline, and are associated with high blood pressure (which may be malignant) and symptoms such as palpitations, anxiety and headaches. Diagnosis may be made on the finding of high levels of metanephrine in blood. High levels of urinary adrenaline, noradrenaline, vanillylmandelic acid and homovanillic acid may also aid diagnosis. The treatment of choice is surgical resection.

11. A True

    B False

    C False

    D False

    E True

Conn's syndrome, a form of primary hyperaldosteronism, describes a series of symptoms related to the excess production of aldosterone. Hypertension, hypokalaemia and alkalosis may all be present. It may be caused by an aldosterone-producing adenoma of the adrenal glands (Conn's tumour) or hyperplasia of the adrenal glands or may be idiopathic. Aldosterone's action is at the distal tubule and collecting duct of the kidneys, where it promotes the reabsorption of sodium ions and water and the subsequent excretion of sodium ions. Excess aldosterone therefore leads to abnormally low levels of potassium and volume expansion with hypertension and its inevitable sequelae, e.g. heart failure. Treatment options include surgery and the usage of aldosterone-antagonists such as spironolactone.

12. A True

    B True

    C False

    D False

    E True

Xeroderma pigmentosum and Cockayne's syndrome are both conditions where there is autosomal recessive inheritance of a defect in DNA repair. Such conditions, which also include Bloom's syndrome, Fanconi's anaemia and Rothmund–Thomson syndrome, are associated with accelerated ageing and with a higher risk of developing certain forms of cancer. For example, individuals with xeroderma pigmentosum are prone to skin cancers such as malignant melanoma due to a defect in the ability to correct DNA damage caused by ultraviolet light. Cockayne syndrome is associated with premature ageing, photosensitivity and growth problems.

13. A False

    B False

    C True

    D False

    E True

The genetic predisposition to oncogenesis can be due to inheritance of a gene mutation leading to the absence of a tumour suppressor. For example, in inherited retinoblastoma there is a defect in the *RB* gene (a tumour suppressor gene) on chromosome 13. Other forms of inheritable predisposition to malignancy may be due to the inheritance of genes that lead to defects in DNA repair. For example, the transmission of mutated forms of any of the hereditary non-polyposis colonic cancer (HNPCC) genes via autosomal dominant inheritance leads to increased cancer susceptibility. These mismatch repair genes include *MLH1*, *MSH2*, and *MSH6*. Inheritance of mutated forms of these genes is associated not only with colon cancer, but also other cancers including endometrial, ovarian, central nervous system and urinary tract malignancies.

Li–Fraumeni syndrome is an autosomal dominant disorder where there is an inherited mutation in the tumour suppressor gene *p53*, leading to increased malignancies, such as breast cancer and sarcomas, in affected individuals.

Neurofibromatosis type 1 is caused by a mutation in a tumour suppressor gene in chromosome 17; transmitted via autosomal dominant inheritance, this condition is associated predominantly with benign tumour growth.

Increased breast and ovarian cancer are associated with the transmission of mutated forms of the *BRCA1* and *BRCA2* genes via autosomal recessive inheritance.

14. **A** False

    B True

    C True

    D False

    E True

Osteoporosis is a condition whereby there is reduced bone mineral density and deterioration of bone architecture with a subsequent increased risk of fractures. The World Health Organisation has defined osteoporosis as a bone mineral density (T score) that is > 2.5 standard deviations from the mean peak bone mass. Osteoporosis may occur secondary to other pathologies, e.g. in hyperparathyroidism and renal failure. Osteoporosis is also more prevalent in states when there is hypogonadism, e.g. in Turner's syndrome. Treatments for osteoporosis include modification of reversible risk factors, such as smoking, and medications such as bisphosphonates and calcium supplementation.

15. **A** False

    B False

    C True

    D True

    E True

Osteoporosis is a condition associated with significantly reduced bone density. Osteoporosis is more common in women and affects large numbers after the menopause. Risk factors for osteoporosis include: having a low body mass index, smoking, calcium deficiency, excess alcohol intake, minimal exercise, family history and corticosteroid usage. Osteoporosis is also common in states of hypogonadism, e.g. in individuals with Kallmann's syndrome. Prevention of osteoporosis is possible by early recognition of modifiable risk factors such as smoking and low levels of weight-bearing exercise. Individuals with osteoporosis may benefit from the usage of bisphosphonates and calcium supplementation.

16. A True

    B False

    C True

    D True

    E False

Apoptosis is also known as programmed cell death. Essential for normal physiology, apoptosis usually confers a biological benefit, such as tissue differentiation in embryogenesis and the sloughing off of the endometrium during menstruation. Apoptosis differs from necrosis, which is cell death following a form of trauma. In apoptosis there are a series of sequential changes in the cell and its organelles. During this energy-dependant process there is cell shrinkage followed by a series of changes in the nucleus which include pyknosis, which refers to nuclear shrinkage and condensation of chromatin, and karyorrhexis, which is the fragmentation of the nuclei. In apoptosis there is formation of cytoplasmic blebs called apoptotic bodies. Markers are expressed on the cell's surface to encourage phagocytosis. The whole process occurs without the release of inflammatory markers.

17. A True

    B False

    C True

    D False

    E True

Necrosis refers to the irreversible death of cells due to injury. There are a series of changes that occur within necrotic cells. These sequential microscopic changes include cytoplasmic eosinophilia, pyknosis (cell shrinkage), karyorrhexis (breakdown of the nucleus) and karyolysis (complete dissolution of the nucleus secondary to the action on DNAase). Necrosis is associated with the release of inflammatory mediators. There are several types of necrosis, which are specific to the type of cell trauma and the tissues involved; these include coagulative necrosis, caseous necrosis and colliquative necrosis. In caseous necrosis a cheese-like matter is formed at the site of necrosis following infection with *Mycobacterium tuberculosis*. Necrosis is not an inevitable event in the cell cycle.

18. A True

    B False

    C True

D True

E True

The Coombs test is used to detect serum antibodies directed against red blood cells. The direct Coombs test detects the presence of antibodies or complement on the red blood cell surface. The indirect Coombs test detects the presence of unbound antibodies in the blood, which react in vitro against certain antigens. Haemolytic disease of the newborn is an example of alloimmune haemolysis. Warm antibody autoimmune haemolysis may occur in conditions such as systemic lupus erythematosus. Cold antibody autoimmune haemolysis may occur in conditions such as atypical pneumonias caused by bacterium mycoplasma, infectious mononucleosis and paroxysmal cold haemoglobinuria. Administration of methyldopa can cause a drug-induced, immune-mediated haemolysis and therefore gives a positive direct Coombs test. Usage of cephalosporins can also give a positive direct Coombs test.

19. A True

B False

C False

D True

E True

Protein C deficiency and factor V Leiden are both congenital conditions associated with increased thrombus formation. Haemophilia A and haemophilia B (also known as Christmas disease) are both sex-linked inherited disorders. Haemophilia A is caused by a mutation in the factor VIII gene on the X-chromosome, with subsequent factor VIII deficiency; haemophilia B is associated with factor XI deficiency due to a gene mutation. Both haemophilias are associated with impaired clotting. In von Willebrand's disease there may be either a deficiency, or abnormality in the function of von Willebrand Factor (vWF). vWF promotes platelet adhesion and sufferers may experience varying levels of bleeding problems.

20. A True

B True

C True

D False

E False

Hyperplasia is the increase in the number of cells in a tissue and is easily confused with hypertrophy, which is the increase in the size of cells. Hyperplasia can have physiological benefit and may occur naturally in tissues, e.g. in the smooth muscle of the pregnant uterus and in female breast tissue during puberty. In some circumstances hyperplasia may be considered pathological, such as hyperplasia of the adrenal cortex in Cushing's syndrome, of the endometrium (due to unopposed oestrogen) and in benign prostatic hypertrophy.

21. A True

    B False

    C False

    D False

    E False

Atrophy, (a diminution of the size of the cell, organ or part) and dysplasia may both be reversible. Metaplasia is the conversion of a full differentiated cell type into another differentiated cell type. Neoplasia refers to the abnormal proliferation of cells. Neoplastic change may be malignant in nature, e.g. in breast cancer. However, there are also benign neoplasms, e.g. uterine fibroids. Hypertrophy refers to the potentially reversible increase in cell size, not number.

22. A False

    B False

    C True

    D True

    E False

Metaplasia represents the benign change from one form of differentiated type of cell to another type of differentiated cell. Metaplasia typically occurs in response to an irritant stimulus, whereby the cell type of a tissue changes in order to cope better with the stresses of the irritant. This change in cell phenotype may be reversible, especially when the 'stressful stimulus' is removed. Examples of metaplastic change include the change from columnar epithelium to squamous epithelium in the transition zone of the cervix, and the conversion of the squamous epithelium to transitional epithelium in cases of Barrett's oesophagus, which occur due to chronic acid exposure. Although metaplastic change in itself is benign, persistent exposure to irritants may eventually lead to dysplasia and potentially neoplastic change. Heteroplasia describes the abnormal growth of cells in the wrong location in the absence of any stimulus.

23. A False

    B True

    C False

    D False

    E True

Shock describes a state of acute circulatory failure leading to compromised organ perfusion. Shock has various aetiologies and can occur secondary to anaphylaxis, hypovolaemia, sepsis, obstruction and also cardiogenic causes. Regardless of the cause, there are a number of characteristic features of shock which reflect the role of the nervous and immune systems to compensate for this compromised state. These features include tachycardia, hypotension, oliguria, reduced capillary refill time and reduced levels of consciousness.

Central to the management of all forms of shock is the maintenance of optimal tissue perfusion and ventilation through the administration of oxygen and intravenous fluids. Further management is dependant on the likely cause of the shock, i.e. administration of intravenous antibiotics for septic shock.

24. A Breech presentation

A bicornuate uterus has an incidence of 0.1–0.5%. It is caused when the müllerian (paramesonephric) ducts incompletely fuse during embryonic development. This results in two separate, but communicating, endometrial cavities. The extent to which there is incomplete fusion of the müllerian ducts can result in varying degrees of abnormality. This varies from uterus didelphus where there are two entirely separate uterine cavities and a septate uterus where there is essentially a single uterine cavity interrupted by a thin septum. The presence of a bicornuate uterus is associated with recurrent miscarriage, breech presentation and preterm delivery. **Figure 13.2** shows structural abnormalities of the uterus.

Royal College of Obstetricians and Gynaecologists. Query Bank: Recurrent miscarriage and bicornuate uterus. London: RCOG, 2010. http://www.rcog.org.uk/womens-health/clinical-guidance/recurrent-miscarriage-and-bicornuate-uterus-query-bank

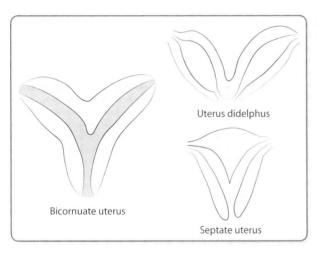

Figure 13.2 Structural abnormalities of the uterus.

Uterus didelphus

Bicornuate uterus

Septate uterus

25. B 46 XX

Gestational trophoblastic disease describes a variety of conditions ranging from complete and partial molar pregnancies to malignant choriocarcinoma. Histologically there is cystic swelling of chorionic villi.

A complete molar pregnancy is usually caused by a single sperm combining with an egg which is devoid of DNA. The genotype is usually diploid 46 XX, as a result of mitosis of the fertilising sperm. Occasionally the genotype is 46 XY.

A partial molar pregnancy is usually caused by two sperm or one which duplicates and has a triploid genotype 69 XXY, or quadraploid XXXY. Gestational trophoblastic disease is a premalignant condition. Overall approximately 1–2% of hydatiform pregnancies develop into choriocarcinoma and complete moles are more likely to do so. They are diagnosed histologically by cystic swelling of chorionic villi and marked trophoblastic proliferation.

Royal College of Obstetricians and Gynaecologists. The Management of Gestational Trophoblastic Disease. Green-top Guideline 38. London: RCOG, 2010.

26. A Basophils

Histamine (5-hydroxytryptamine) is a significant contributor to the immediate response in acute inflammation and is a vasoactive amine. It is predominantly produced by local mast cells, but also by basophils and platelets. Histamine is typically stored in mast cell granules and released during a process called degranulation following mast cell activation. This activation may occur in response to stimuli, such as mast cell antibody binding, following complement activation and in direct response to injury. The main action of histamine is vascular dilatation, however it is also involved in increasing vascular permeability.

27. D 48–92 hours

The process of cutaneous wound healing occurs with initial inflammation, followed by proliferation and then maturation. Healing by primary intention follows surgical incision closed by suturing. The initial surgical incision causes platelets to rapidly gather to form a clot which instigates the inflammatory response. Healing by secondary intention occurs when there is a traumatic wound causing large loss of cells and tissues. Neutrophils appear with 24 hours of the insult. Fibroblasts proliferate in the first 24–72 hours forming granulation tissue which fills the wound within 1 week. Neutrophils are replaced by macrophages within 48–96 hours. Leucocyte infiltration and increased vascularity is present for up to 14 days.

28. B Glomerular capillary endotheliosis

Pre-eclampsia is a complex condition which affects many body systems, including the kidneys, and affects both function and morphology. It leads to the glomerulus becoming hypertrophied with reduced perfusion as a result of hypertrophy of intracapillary cells. The reactive changes of the kidney are described as glomerular capillary endotheliosis. The extent to which the kidneys are affected varies according to the location of the lesion but in severe cases may involve the whole of the renal cortex.

29. A Increase in the number of cells

Hyperplasia is an increase in the number of cells as a response to a specific stimulus. Hypertrophy is an increase in the size of the cells. Hyperplasia is often benign, as in benign prostatic hyperplasia, but can sometimes manifest as a premalignant condition. The microscopic and macroscopic appearance of the cells remains the same, but there are an increased number of them present. Other examples of cellular hyperplasia include the growth of glandular breast tissue during pregnancy, endometrial hyperplasia and the hyperplasia of the adrenal cortex seen in Cushing's disease (**Figure 13.3**).

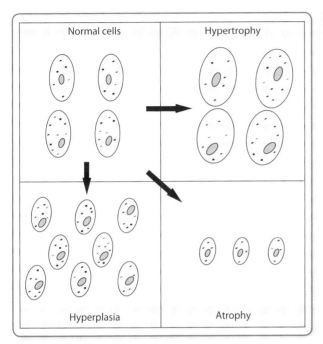

Figure 13.3 Hypertrophy, hyperplasia and atrophy.

30. A Acute tubular necrosis

Acute tubular necrosis (ATN) is the commonest cause of acute renal failure, and is a renal cause (as opposed to prerenal and postrenal causes). Acute tubular necrosis can be caused by a variety of insults including ischaemia, infection, toxins and drugs. Typically, ATN is characterised by injury to the tubular epithelial cells of the renal parenchyma leading to necrotic lesions and the formation of epithelial casts. Initially, ATN may present with a slightly reduced urine output, followed by profound oliguria, metabolic acidosis, uraemia and hyperkalaemia. When recovery begins there is a polyuria and an associated osmotic diuresis. Appropriately managed (i.e. using dialysis if needed), ATN can be reversible and there can be complete recovery if the cause is removed.

31. C Nodular glomerulosclerosis

Nodular glomerulosclerosis, also known as diabetic nephropathy, is a common complication of diabetes mellitus. The disease is characterised by thickening of the glomerulus basement membrane, mesangial sclerosis and glomerulosclerosis. These features are the sequelae of the known end-organ damage associated with diabetes mellitus as a consequence of microvascular disease and chronic hyperglycaemia.

This form of nephropathy is typically diagnosed in individuals with known diabetes mellitus, non-healing ulcers, proteinuria and retinopathy. The diagnosis is characterised by a progressively declining glomerular filtration rate, long-standing albuminuria and hypertension. The mainstay of treatment is improved glycaemic control, management of hypertension (often with the use of ACE inhibitors), dietary protein restriction and in some cases renal dialysis.

32. B Cigarette smoking

Cigarette smoking is known to be the greatest risk factor for the development of bladder cancer, and is thought to be associated with around 50% of cases. The disease is also more common in individuals who have worked in industrial settings and been exposed to carcinogens, such as aniline dyes. Exposure to cyclophosphamide is a further risk factor. An exophytic mass is a lesion that grows out of the surface of an organ. In this patient the mass represents a transitional cell carcinoma of the bladder. The patient has frank haematuria, which is the most common presenting symptom of this tumour of the urothelium. Management strategies of transitional cell carcinoma of this kind include bladder resection, cystectomy, chemotherapy and radiotherapy.

Scottish Intercollegiate Guidelines Network. Management of Transitional Cell Carcinoma of the Bladder. A national clinical guideline 85. Edinburgh: SIGN, 2005.

33. C Polyarteritis nodosa

Polyarteritis nodosa (PAN) is a systemic vasculitis of unknown aetiology which affects the small and medium-sized arteries. Necrotising transmural inflammation is typical in affected vessels. There is associated microaneurysm formation, tissue infarction and necrosis. Lesions can affect the gastrointestinal tract, the kidneys, the heart and the liver. There may be resultant hypertension due to renal involvement, melaena due to gastrointestinal lesions alongside abdominal pain, malaise, fever and weight loss. PAN affects men more then women and typically presents in young adulthood. Diagnosis is usually made by renal biopsy or by mesenteric angiography. Although the aetiology of PAN is uncertain there appears to be an association with chronic hepatitis B infection, with around 30% of individuals with PAN having hepatitis B antibody complexes present in affected arteries. Corticosteroids and cyclophosphamide form the mainstay of treatment.

34. D Rhabdomyolysis

This woman's urinalysis shows myoglobinuria, which typically follows significant trauma to muscle tissue. Although its presence may have minimal sequelae in severe cases, there may be rhabdomyolysis. Myoglobin is normally renally-excreted, but in excessive amounts it causes obstruction of the distal tubule and acute renal failure. In rhabdomyolysis there is excessive release of the intracellular contents of muscle cells leading to hyperkalaemia and metabolic acidosis. Hypocalaemia may also occur. In severe cases there may be disseminated intravascular coagulation.

35. C Hyperchromatism

Dysplasia is a term used to describe abnormal development of immature cells in a tissue, whereby there are abnormalities in the cellular architecture and appearance. Dysplastic cells can be thought of as showing some of cellular changes that occur in cancer cells. These atypical features infer malignant potential although not all dysplastic tissue will go on to become malignant. In dysplastic cells a series of visible characteristic changes occur which include:

- Increased mitotic activity
- Hyperchromatism: prominent cell nucleus due to increased chromatin
- Nuclear pleomorphism: abnormalities in the shape and size of the nucleus
- Anisocytosis: increased cell size
- Poikilocytosis: unusually shaped cells

Dysplasia may be reversible if in its early stages, especially if any causative stimulus is removed. A potentially reversible form of dysplasia is present in CIN I, where dysplastic changes are only seen in the basal third of the squamous epithelium; in these cases there is high likelihood of reversible changes and monitoring may be appropriate.

36. C Lichen sclerosus

All options given are non-neoplastic skin conditions of the vulva. Vulval cancer is a rare form of cancer (1.7/100,000 women) usually affecting women around 70–80 years old; the majority of cases are squamous carcinomas (90%). Risk factors for the development of vulval cancer include: smoking, chronic skin conditions such as lichen sclerosus, vulval intraepithelial neoplasia (VIN), Paget's disease and the presence of melanoma in situ.

Lichen sclerosus is an inflammatory condition affecting the anogenital area; the majority of sufferers are postmenopausal women. Patients often present with itching. Treatments include use of potent topical corticosteroids. Five–seven per cent of women may go on to develop vulval cancer. Vulval cancer spreads by direct extension to surrounding structures, local lymph nodes and by the blood stream.

Royal College of Obstetricians and Gynaecologists. Management of Vulval Cancer. London: RCOG, 2006. Royal College of Obstetricians and Gynaecologists. The Management of Vulval Skin Disorders. Green-top Guideline 58. London: RCOG 2011.

37. E Primary peritoneal cancer

Primary peritoneal cancer (PPC), like ovarian cancer, is associated with high serum levels of the tumour marker CA-125. PPC is a rare cancer of the peritoneum. Like ovarian cancer, many patients have few symptoms until relatively late in the disease's progression. Invasion to the peritoneum is not uncommon in ovarian cancer, however there is often minimal or no ovarian involvement when there is a primary peritoneal cancer. PPC has an association with transmission of the oncogene *BRCA1* and *BRCA2*. Treatment of PPC, like ovarian cancer, includes surgical interventions such as total abdominal hysterectomy, bilateral oophorectomy and omentectomy, as well as chemotherapy and radiotherapy. It is important to remember that whilst tumour markers can aid diagnosis they are limited in their specificity and sensitivity; they are especially useful for monitoring disease progression pre- and post-treatment (**Table 13.1**).

Table 13.1 Tumour markers and associated malignancies

Tumour markers	Associated malignancies
CA 19-9	Colorectal cancer
	Pancreatic cancer
CA-125	Ovarian cancer
	Primary peritoneal cancer
CA 15-3	Breast cancer
Carcinogenic embryonic antigen	Colorectal cancer
Alpha-fetoprotein	Pancreatic cancer
	Germ cell tumours
Human chorionic gonadotrophin	Gestational trophoblastic disease
	Germ cell tumours
Prostate specific antigen	Prostate cancer

38. C Cushing's syndrome and small cell lung cancer

Paraneoplastic syndromes are groups of symptoms which may present in patients with malignancy; they are not directly caused by the tumour itself. Paraneoplastic syndromes may present as pathologies of the endocrinological, dermatological, rheumatological, haematological, renal, gastrointestinal and neuromuscular systems (**Table 13.2**).

Table 13.2 Paraneoplastic syndromes and their associated malignancies

	Paraneoplastic syndrome	Associated malignancies
Endocrine	Syndrome of inappropriate antidiuretic hormone secretion	Lung cancer
		Tumours of central nervous system
	Cushing's syndrome	Small cell lung cancer
Dermatological	Acanthosis nigricans	Uterine cancer
	Dermatomyositis	Breast cancer
Haematological	Polycythaemia	Renal cancer
		Hepatocellular cancer
	Lambert–Eaton myasthenic syndrome	Small cell lung cancer

39. C Nulliparity

There are a series of risk factors for ovarian cancer. The main risk factors for the development of ovarian cancer are increasing age, the presence of gene mutations such as *BRCA* and *HNPCC* and a family history of the disease. Several additional risk factors relate to ovarian activity, i.e. ovarian cancer appears to be less common in women who have interrupted ovulation during their reproductive years. The malignancy is more common in women who have an early menarche and a late menopause. Women who have had no pregnancies are at a greater risk of developing ovarian cancer; the more children a woman has had the lower the risk. Protective factors include those who have used the contraceptive pill and those with a history of breastfeeding.

40. E 2000 mL

This patient is obviously compromised by her blood loss and needs rapid fluid resuscitation and is likely also to need blood products. Haemorrhagic shock can be classified according to the amount of blood lost and the subsequent derangement in vital signs as the body tries to compensate for the blood loss. In addition to tachycardia, hypotension and tachypnea, there may be altered consciousness and reduced urine output reflecting reduced organ perfusion. This patient's condition is suggestive a massive loss of blood volume, equivalent to around 2000 mL. This is classified as class IV haemorrhagic shock:

- Class I haemorrhage: up to 15% blood volume, up to around 750 mL blood loss
- Class II haemorrhage: 15–30% blood volume lost
- Class III haemorrhage: 30–40% blood volume lost
- Class IV haemorrhage: over 40% blood volume lost

41. E *Escherichia coli*

Most cases of septic shock are caused by infection with Gram-negative bacteria, although Gram-positive bacterium, viruses and fungi can be causative agents. *E. coli* is the only Gram-negative bacteria of the options given and therefore the most likely cause of this patient's life-threatening condition. Gram-negative bacilli release endotoxins which are bacterial wall lipopolysaccharides (LPS). LPS can lead to the systemic activation of macrophages, neutrophils, natural killer cells and the widespread release of cytokines and inflammatory mediators such as tumour necrosis factor and interleukins. The consequences of this immune system activation include vasodilation, increased vascular permeability and endothelial injury. Inflammatory mediators may activate the coagulation system leading to deranged clotting and in extreme cases disseminated intravascular coagulation. Untreated, septic shock may lead to death.

Chapter 14

Pharmacology

Questions: MCQs

Answer each stem 'True' or 'False'.

1. **Pharmacokinetics:**
   A   Lipid soluble drugs are easily absorbed
   B   Bioavailability is the proportion of drug that reaches its target
   C   Fat soluble drugs can have a prolonged duration of action
   D   There are two phases of elimination of drugs from the kidney
   E   Phase II liver metabolism often involves cytochrome P450 enzymes

2. **The following are enzyme inducers:**
   A   Griseofulvin
   B   Rifampicin
   C   Grapefruit juice
   D   Phenytoin
   E   Fluconazole

3. **Considering the mechanism of pain:**
   A   Prostaglandins directly cause pain
   B   Bradykinin is a potent cause of pain
   C   5HT is a transmitter of inhibitory neurons
   D   Adenosine has a role in regulating pain
   E   Glutamate is an inhibitory amino acid

4. **Opioid drugs:**
   A   Leads to an increase in vasopressin release
   B   Cause pupillary dilation
   C   Morphine can cause hypotension associated with a reflex tachycardia
   D   Cannot cross the placenta
   E   Codeine is a more effective analgesic than dihydrocodeine

5. **Anaesthetic agents:**
   A   Halothane is an inhalational agent
   B   Nitrous oxide causes an increase in sympathetic nervous system activity
   C   Halothane can cause liver toxicity
   D   Isoflurane causes cardiac vasodilation
   E   Malignant hyperthermia is a side-effect of halogenated anaesthetic agents

6. **Clomifene citrate:**

   A   Can cause ovarian hyperstimulation
   B   Is an antioestrogen
   C   Can cause visual blurring
   D   Is taken during the luteal phase of the menstrual cycle
   E   Can be used for up to 18 months in women with anovulatory menstrual cycles

7. **Cyproterone acetate:**

   A   Is an antiandrogen
   B   Irreversibly inhibits spermatogenesis
   C   Is used to treat hirsutism
   D   Promotes cortisol synthesis
   E   Is linked to increased risk of thrombosis

8. **Mifepristone:**

   A   Is an antiprogestogenic steroid
   B   Is a folate antagonist
   C   Can be used for emergency contraception
   D   Decreases myometrial sensitivity to prostaglandins
   E   Can be used in the medical management of ectopic pregnancy

9. **The following are cytotoxic antibiotics:**

   A   Doxorubicin
   B   Fluorouracil
   C   Bleomycin
   D   Dactinomycin
   E   Vinblastine

10. **The following teratogens are correctly paired with the abnormalities they cause:**

    A   Ramipril: polyhydramnios
    B   Phenytoin: spina bifida
    C   Diethylstilbestrol: vaginal clear cell adenocarcinoma
    D   Warfarin: hydrocephalus
    E   Danazol: masculinisation of the female fetus

Questions: SBAs

For each question, select the single best answer from the five options listed.

11. Which of the following normal physiological changes seen in pregnancy are associated with a slower drug metabolism?

   A   Delayed gastric emptying
   B   Increased body fat volume
   C   Increased cardiac output
   D   Increased glomerular filtration rate
   E   Increased third space volume

12. A 17-year-old girl discovers she is pregnant despite taking the oral contraceptive pill. She has recently been prescribed a new medication by her general practitioner.

   Which of the following drugs is most likely to have interacted with the efficacy of her contraception?

   A   Carbamazepine
   B   Cimetidine
   C   Erythromycin
   D   Metronidazole
   E   Sulphamethoxazole

13. Which of the following forms part of phase 2 reactions in drug metabolism?

   A   Conjugation
   B   Cyclisation
   C   Hydrolysis
   D   Reduction
   E   Oxidation

14. A 23-year-old woman is admitted to hospital as she is acutely unwell, having admitted to taking an overdose. On examination, her temperature is 38.6°C, blood pressure 105/68 mmHg, heart rate 96 beats per minute, and respiratory rate 12 breaths per minute. Her arterial blood gas test shows respiratory alkalosis.

   What is the most likely drug overdose?

   A   Amitriptyline
   B   Aspirin
   C   Cocaine
   D   Tramadol
   E   Zopiclone

15. A 27-year-old woman attends antenatal clinic at 14 weeks' gestation. This is her second pregnancy and she suffered a pulmonary embolism during her first pregnancy, 3 years ago. Her thrombophilia screen, taken prior to pregnancy, is negative.

What is the most appropriate course of action at this point?

A   Monitor closely for signs of thromboembolic event
B   Start prophylactic dose low-molecular weight heparin (LMWH) immediately
C   Start prophylactic dose LMWH at 24 weeks' gestation
D   Start treatment dose LMWH at 24 weeks' gestation
E   Urgent referral to haematology department

16. Which of the following is a recognised side effect of heparin usage?

A   Hirsutism
B   Hyperaldosteronism
C   Hypokalaemia
D   Osteomalacia
E   Thrombocytopaenia

17. A 37-year old-woman is requesting analgesia following a caesarean section. You notice that she has von Willebrand disease and wonder how this may affect her coagulation profile.

Which of the following is most likely to represent a patient with von Willebrand disease?

Activated partial thromboplastin time			
	Prothrombin time	Bleeding time	Platelet count
A	Unaffected	Prolonged	Prolonged	Unaffected
B	Unaffected	Prolonged	Unaffected	Unaffected
C	Prolonged	Mildly prolonged	Unaffected	Unaffected
D	Prolonged	Prolonged	Prolonged	Decreased
E	Unaffected	Unaffected	Prolonged	Decreased

18. A 32-year-old woman suffers a 1500 mL postpartum haemorrhage 15 minutes after delivery. She is given several drugs to contract the uterus and the bleeding stops. One hour later, she is found to have blood pressure of 178/110 mmHg.

Which drug is most likely to be responsible for this clinical finding?

A   Carboprost
B   Ergometrine
C   Misoprostol
D   Oxytocin
E   Ritodrine

19. A 2-year-old child has been investigated by the ear, nose and throat specialists for sensorineural hearing loss. Following a series of investigations he is found to have a defect of the 8th cranial nerve.

Which of the following medications did his mother take during her pregnancy?

A   Chloramphenicol
B   Co-trimoxazole
C   Doxycycline
D   Erythromycin
E   Streptomycin

20. A 27-year-old woman is treated for severe bronchitis at 38 weeks' gestation. Her baby, born at 41 weeks' gestation, has neonatal haemolysis.

Which drug taken by the mother for bronchitis is the cause of the baby's neonatal haemolysis?

A   Amoxicillin
B   Chloramphenicol
C   Co-trimoxazole
D   Doxycycline
E   Erythromycin

21. A 35-year-old woman, with a history of previous multiple pulmonary embolisms, is now 8 weeks pregnant.

Which is the anticoagulant of choice during her pregnancy?

A   Aspirin 300 mg
B   Heparin infusion
C   Low-molecular weight heparin
D   Warfarin
E   None of the above

22. A 25-year-old nulliparous woman, with a lifelong history of tonic clonic seizures, sees her neurologist as she wishes to start a family. In addition to her current anticonvulsant therapy which additional drug is now required?

A   A second anticonvulsant
B   Ferrous sulphate
C   Folic acid
D   Low-molecular weight heparin
E   Vitamin K

23. A 23-year old woman is 8 weeks pregnant. She has persistent itchy, thick, white vaginal discharge. A high vaginal swab has identified the presence of yeast species. She has already tried topical clotrimazole cream which has provided no relief of her symptoms.

Which is the most appropriate treatment for vaginal candidiasis unresponsive to clotrimazole cream?

A   Clotrimazole pessary
B   Metronidazole 400 mg orally
C   Fluconazole 400 mg orally
D   Hydrocortisone 0.5% cream
E   Trimovate creams

Answers

1. A True
    B False
    C True
    D False
    E False

    Pharmacokinetics refers to the processes of drug absorption, distribution and elimination. Drug distribution is dependent on the bioavailability and volume that the drug is distributed in.

    Lipid soluble drugs are easily absorbed as they cross membranes easily. Bioavailability refers to the amount of drug which enters the circulation before any change occurs to it. Fat soluble drugs are more widely distributed and often have a prolonged duration of action as they are stored in the fat tissue.

    Elimination of drugs occurs via the kidneys and liver. In the presence of liver or kidney dysfunction, the drug dosage may need altering.

    Hepatic elimination occurs in two phases:

    - **Phase I:** reduction, oxidation or hydrolysis which changes the drug to an active, inactive or toxic state
    - **Phase II:** drugs become more soluble by conjugation, e.g. with glucuronate, and they can then be excreted in urine

2. A True
    B True
    C False
    D True
    E False

    Enzyme inducers:

    - Griseofulvin
    - Phenytoin
    - Phenobarbitone
    - Rifampicin
    - Carbamazepine
    - Ethanol

    Enzyme inhibitors:

    - Metronidazole
    - Ciprofloxacin
    - Fluconazole
    - Erythromycin

- Ethanol (acute)
- Cimetidine
- Amiodarone
- Ketoconazole

3. A False

   B True

   C True

   D True

   E False

Pain is a subjective sensation. Prostaglandins enhance the pain sensation produced by other chemicals, e.g. serotonin; however, they are not themselves a direct cause of pain. By blocking potassium channels, prostaglandins make nerve terminals more sensitive to pain. Bradykinin is a peptide which acts as a potent mediator of pain. Prostaglandins work together with with bradykinin to increase its action at nerve terminals. 5-HT (serotonin) is a transmitter of inhibitory neurons. Glutamate is an excitatory amino acid. It is released from primary afferent neurons and is responsible for fast synaptic transmission and slow receptor-mediated responses. Adenosine has a role in both activation and inhibition of pain transmission.

4. A True

   B False

   C False

   D False

   E True

Opioid drugs affect many body systems and at a cellular level and exert their actions via G-protein coupled receptors which inhibit adenylate cyclase and reduce cAMP content. They cause an opening of potassium channels and thereby affect the neuronal excitability. Morphine may cause hypotension which is not usually accompanied with a reflex tachycardia. Other effects of opioid analgesics include respiratory depression, papillary constriction and vomiting (stimulation of the chemoreceptor trigger zone). Morphine and other opioid drugs cause an increase in vasopressin (antidiuretic hormone) release. Opioid drugs readily cross the placenta and this is the mechanism by which newborns can be affected by administration of pethidine, if given soon before delivery. Codeine is a more potent analgesic than dihydrocodeine.

5. A True

   B True

   C True

   D True

   E True

Examples of inhalational anaesthetic agents are given below.

Halothane

Widely used, side effects include cardiac arrhythmias (ventricular extrasystole) and liver toxicity. It is not analgesic and is not commonly used in obstetrics as it tends to relax the uterus.

Nitrous oxide

An odourless gas with low potency, therefore it is not used as a sole anaesthetic agent. It is an effective analgesic agent at doses too low to cause unconsciousness, and is used as an analgesic during labour.

Enflurane

Similar to halothane, but has quicker recovery as it is less fat soluble.

Isoflurane

Potent cardiac vasodilator and causes hypotension. This is the most widely used volatile anaesthetic.

Sevoflurane

A newer agent.

All halogenated anaesthetic agents may cause malignant hyperthermia.

6. **A** True

   B True

   C True

   D False

   E False

Clomiphene citrate, also known under the trade name Clomid, is commonly used to induce ovulation in the fertility of women with anovulatory cycles, e.g. in women with polycystic ovary syndrome. It may be used to induce ovarian hyperstimulation as part of in vitro fertilisation programmes. Traditionally considered as an antioestrogen, clomiphene blocks oestrogen receptors in the hypothalamus and the pituitary and thus acts by inhibiting the negative feedback that usually occurs at the hypothalamus. In the absence of raised oestrogen levels, the hypothalamus goes on to produce increased levels of follicle-stimulating and luteinising hormones which subsequently increase the chances of ovulation. Usually taken for 5 days from around day 2 of the menstrual cycle, i.e. during the follicular phase, clomiphene citrate will lead to successful conception in approximately 15% of women using it. Of these successful conceptions there is a higher level of miscarriage than naturally conceived pregnancies, alongside a higher rate of multiple pregnancies.

National Institute for Health and Clinical Excellence. Fertility Assessment and Treatment for People with Fertility Problems. Clinical Guideline CG011. London: NICE, 2004

7. A True

    B False

    C True

    D False

    E True

Cyproterone acetate is an antiandrogen, which also causes a negative feedback to hypothalamic receptors leading to reduced production of both gonadotrophins and testosterone. It is used in the treatment of advanced prostate cancer, in cases of severe male hypersexuality, for hirsutism and acne in women and to treat hot flushes, where other methods have failed. Cyproterone acetate may be combined with ethinylestradiol in the form of co-cyprindiol, trade name Dianette, for women with severe acne or hirsutism who also require contraception. This combination of cyproterone acetate with an ethinylestradiol is associated with an increased risk of thrombosis. During administration it is known to reversibly inhibit spermatogenesis. Known side effects include hepatotoxicity, gynaecomastia, low cortisol, low aldosterone and osteoporosis. Administration of cyproterone acetate requires close monitoring of liver function.

Anantharachagan A, Sarris I, Ugwumadu A. Revision Notes for the MRCOG Part 1. Oxford: Oxford University Press, 2011: 333.

8. A True

    B False

    C True

    D False

    E False

Mifepristone is an antiprogestogenic steroid which acts as a competitive progesterone receptor antagonist. It is used in the medical termination of pregnancy, where it acts to cause endometrial decidual degeneration, increase myometrial sensitivity to prostaglandins such as misoprostol (which are often given alongside the mifepristone), ripen the cervix and increase release of endogenous prostaglandins. Theoretically mifepristone can be used as an emergency contraceptive, where it is thought to both delay ovulation and prevent implantation.

9. A True

    B False

    C True

    D True

    E False

Cytotoxic antibiotics are used in the treatment of malignancy due to their ability to inhibit DNA and RNA synthesis. Doxorubicin inhibits both DNA and RNA synthesis and also interferes with the action of topoisomerase II action, which is highly active in rapidly replicating cells. Bleomycin is a metal-chelating glycopeptide antibiotic which damages cells via DNA strand breakage. It is able to also work on non-dividing cells and is used to treat malignancies such as testicular cancer. Dactinomycin incorporates itself into the DNA chain, where it prevents effective movement of RNA polymerase and subsequently inhibits transcription. Fluorouracil is not a cytotoxic antibiotic but an antimetabolite which is a uracil analogue. Vinblastine is a plant alkaloid which interferes with the microtubules of dividing cells and therefore inhibits mitosis.

10. A False

   B True

   C True

   D False

   E True

Ramipril taken during pregnancy has been associated with fetal renal failure, oligohydramnios and skull defects and therefore alternative antihypertensives should be given to pregnant women. Phenytoin is an antiepileptic drug which is an antagonist of folate; folate is essential for DNA synthesis. Use of phenytoin during pregnancy has been linked to defects in fetal neural tube development such as spina bifida, in addition to fetal hydantoin syndrome where developmental delay and deformities such as microcephaly have been reported. Stilbestrol, also known as diethylstilbestrol, was given to pregnant women up until the 1970s. Indications for its use included the prevention of miscarriage in those with a history of recurrent pregnancy loss. It was banned in the 1970s after exposure was associated with the subsequent development of vaginal clear cell adenocarcinoma and other abnormalities of the female genital tract in those exposed to the drug in utero. Warfarin is thought to be teratogenic if given in the first trimester. It is known to lead to abnormalities such as deformities of the fetal face and nose, axial skeletal abnormalities and mental retardation. Exposure in the third trimester is associated with abnormalities of the central nervous system such as seizures and cerebral haemorrhage at delivery. Danazol is a synthetic form of testosterone and causes virilisation of fetal genitals.

11. A Delayed gastric emptying

The natural physiological changes in pregnancy lead to a change in the pharmacokinetics of drugs. Pregnancy is associated with delayed gastric emptying, which subsequently increases the bioavailability of drugs that are slowly absorbed. Increased third space volume leads to a greater area of distribution and therefore a lower plasma concentration. An increase in renal blood flow means faster renal clearance. In pregnancy there is a reduction in circulating binding proteins including albumin, and this leads to an increase in free levels of drugs that are usually bound to albumin.

12. A Carbamazepine

Carbamazepine is an enzyme inducer. Drugs acting as enzyme inducers increase the action of the enzyme system and lead to increased metabolism and therefore clearance of the drug. In this case, the oral contraceptive pill has been less effective due to the co-administration of an enzyme inducer. The rest of the drugs on this list are enzyme inhibitors. Enzyme inhibitors increase the concentration and availability of other drugs as they prevent their metabolism.

Other enzyme inducers are rifampicin, ethanol and carbamazepine.

13. A Conjugation

The process of elimination of a drug from the body is an irreversible process and occurs via metabolism and excretion. Drug metabolism occurs via phase 1 and phase 2 reactions, which both normally take place in the liver. Phase 1 reactions include oxidation, reduction or hydrolysis, with the resulting products being more reactive. Phase 2 reactions generally involve conjugation, e.g. with amino acids, leading to inactivation of the drug. Some of the products are excreted in bile after the phase two reaction.

14. B Aspirin

A large dose of aspirin results in uncoupling of oxidative phosphorylation which leads to higher consumption of oxygen and increased carbon dioxide. The higher carbon dioxide results in stimulation of the respiratory centre, causing hyperventilation and a respiratory alkalosis. Higher doses of salicylates can cause respiratory depression and produce respiratory acidosis. Increased temperature may result from an increased respiratory rate. Aspirin is a non-steroidal anti-inflammatory and in normal doses is an effective antipyretic and analgesic.

Overdose of amitriptyline can cause nausea and vomiting, but may also have more serious side effects such as cardiac arrhythmia, agitation and unconsciousness.

Tramadol is an opioid and zopiclone is a benzodiazepine. Both of these medications would lead to respiratory depression, but are unlikely to lead to a respiratory alkalosis or hyperpyrexia.

15. B Start prophylactic dose low-molecular weight heparin (LMWH) immediately

Pulmonary embolism (PE) during pregnancy is responsible for the greatest number of maternal deaths in the UK (1.56/100,000 pregnancies). It is therefore essential that any woman who is clinically at risk of developing PE in pregnancy is recommended appropriate prophylaxis. The Royal College guideline recommends that antenatal thromboprophylaxis with LMWH is offered if there is a history of VTE in one of the following categories: recurrent, unprovoked, oestrogen-related, pregnancy-related, or associated with significant risk factors such as a documented thrombophilia.

In this case, the most appropriate answer is to start low-molecular weight heparin immediately. It should be started from the first trimester, however in cases where this has been missed; prophylactic dose should be commenced immediately. This patient should also be referred urgently to haematology, but this is not the *best* answer.

Bourjeily G, Paidas M, Khalil H, Rosene-Montella K, Rodger M. Pulmonary embolism in pregnancy. Lancet 2010;375(9713):500–12.
Royal College of Obstetricians and Gynaecologists. Reducing the Risk of Thrombosis and Embolism During Pregnancy and the Puerperium. Green-top Guideline 37a. London: RCOG

16. E Thrombocytopaenia

Heparin prevents coagulation via the activation of antithrombin III. Binding of heparin to the antithrombin III changes its conformation and thereby speeds up its rate of action. There are several potential side effects of heparin and these include:

- **Bleeding**: treated by stopping heparin therapy and treating with protamine
- **Thrombocytopaenia**: may be caused by IgM or IgG antibodies against circulating platelets
- **Hypoaldosteronism**: may be associated with hyperkalaemia, rather than hypokalaemia
- **Osteoporosis**: usually associated with long-term therapy. The mechanism of this is unknown

17.

A	Unaffected	Prolonged	Prolonged	Unaffected

B represents haemophilia, C represents warfarin, D represents disseminated intravascular coagulation while E represents thrombocytopaenia.

von Willebrand's disease is a common inherited haemostatic disorder, with an incidence of 1 in 10,000. It is autosomally inherited and is prevalent equally in males and females. There are several types of disease; the most common is type I which shows autosomal dominant inheritance. von Willebrand's disease is a deficiency in von Willebrand's factor, a protein which brings platelets into contact with damaged subendothelium, causing platelet adhesion and is essential for normal clotting. Patients often present with an abnormality of bleeding which may manifest as nose bleeds, abnormal menses or easy bruising. Females often present with menorrhagia. The overall platelet count is not affected. These patients should not be given non-steroidal anti-inflammatories due to the prolonged bleeding time. Clotting profile may demonstrate a raised activated prothrombin time (APTT); however, the international normalised ratio and platelets are usually normal.

18. B Ergometrine

Drugs that contract the uterus are as listed below.

- **Oxytocin**: is released from the posterior pituitary gland; can be given as an intravenous infusion to augment labour or postpartum to prevent or treat postpartum bleeding.

- **Ergometrine**: an ergot alkaloid; increases basal tone of the uterus. It has most effect on the uterus if it is not properly contracted. It has an effect of vasoconstriction. Side effects are vomiting via stimulation of the chemoreceptor trigger zone. It also causes a rise in blood pressure as a result of the vasoconstriction effect.
- **Misoprostol**: an artificial prostaglandin-1 (PGE-1) analogue. Often used with mifepristone for 1st and 2nd trimester abortions.
- **Carboprost**: an artificial prostaglandin (15-methyl PGF2α). Can be given intramuscularly or intrauterine.

Ritodrine is a β2-adrenoreceptor agonist which acts as a uterine relaxant. It may be used in threatened preterm labour; however, there are newer drugs such as atosiban which are more commonly used.

19. E Erythromycin

The aminoglycosides, such as gentamicin and streptomycin, are known to damage the fetal 8th cranial nerve and are ototoxic when given in the second and third trimesters. The greatest risk to the fetus occurs with streptomycin, which has been associated with an incidence of 8th cranial nerve damage of > 10%. Gentamicin may be required during pregnancy, e.g. in severe urinary tract infections and should be given cautiously if indicated. In addition to the risks to the fetus, the aminoglycosides are associated with both ototoxicity and nephrotoxicity in adults.

20. C Co-trimoxazole

Historically, sulphonamides such as sulfadiazine were thought to increase the risk of neonatal kernicterus via displacement of bilirubin from albumin binding sites; however, this is now thought to be an unsubstantiated concern. Both the sulphonamides and trimethoprim are thought to cause neonatal haemolysis and methaemoglobinaemia and therefore should be avoided in third trimester. Co-trimoxazole, a mixture of the sulphonamide sulphamethoxazole and trimethoprim, is therefore to be avoided in pregnancy. In addition to the risks associated with the administration of these antimicrobials in the third trimester, trimethoprim is known to be teratogenic during the first trimester of pregnancy due to its action as a folate antagonist.

21. C Low-molecular weight heparin

Appropriate anticoagulation in pregnancy is determined by gestation. Warfarin is teratogenic and should be stopped before 6 weeks' gestation; heparin does not cross the placenta and therefore in its low-molecular weight form is an appropriate alternative to warfarin. Warfarin is present in breast milk, however not at levels known to be harmful, whereas heparin is not excreted in breast milk. Aspirin is an antiplatelet medication which should be avoided in the third trimester.

Royal College of Obstetricians and Gynaecologists. Thrombosis and Embolism during Pregnancy and the Puerperium, Reducing the Risk Green-top Guideline 37a. London: RCOG, 2009.

22. C Folic acid

All anticonvulsant drugs are associated with an increased risk of teratogenesis. This is thought to be due their known inhibition of folate which is an essential cofactor involved in DNA synthesis. Although neural tube defects are the most well-known malformations associated with the use of anticonvulsants, other problems such as cardiac defects, orofacial clefts and fetal anticonvulsant syndrome have been reported. Folic acid (5 mg) supplementation is required for those women using anticonvulsants in pregnancy and ideally should be started prior to conception in order to reduce the risk of malformations, such as neural tube defects, associated with lowered serum folate levels. Vitamin K should be given to the neonate to prevent the increased risk of haemorrhage associated with anticonvulsants. A second form of anticonvulsant therapy should only be commenced with caution as the risk of teratogenesis increases with the number of anticonvulsants used.

23. A Clotrimazole pessary

Candidiasis is caused by the yeast *Candida albicans* in most cases. It is carried on the skin and in the gut. Vaginal candidiasis is common in pregnancy and this is partly due to the raised levels of oestrogen and a relative immunosuppressed state. It usually presents with vaginal itching and soreness and may be a recurrent infection. Diagnosis is confirmed by microscopy and culture of vaginal discharge. If a woman is asymptomatic with growth of *Candida* then there is no indication to treat the yeast. Symptomatic vaginal candidiasis may respond to clotrimazole in a pessary or cream form. Although used for resistant cases in non-pregnant women, oral antifungals should be avoided in pregnancy; fluconazole is known to cause congenital abnormalities when given at high doses over long periods.

Chapter 15

Mock paper 1

There are 30 multiple choice questions and 60 single best answer questions in this paper. The paper should be sat in exam conditions and completed in two and a half hours.

Questions: MCQs

Answer each stem 'True' or 'False'.

1. Concerning organs of the pelvis:
   A The ureter runs above the uterine vessels at the lateral vaginal fornix
   B The posterior wall of the vagina is longer than the anterior wall
   C The vulva derives some nerve supply from the anterior cutaneous nerve of the thigh
   D The labia minora contain no adipose tissue or hair follicles
   E The internal anal sphincter is supplied by sympathetic nerves to maintain a resting tone

2. With regard to the ischiorectal fossa:
   A The levator ani muscle is found at the apex
   B It has the obturator internus as its medial wall
   C It has the sacrotuberous ligament running posteriorly
   D It is found within the anal triangle
   E The external anal sphincter is found at the medial aspect

3. The rectum:
   A Commences at the level of the first sacral vertebrae
   B Is about 25 cm in length
   C Drains lymph to the preaortic nodes
   D Is lined by columnar epithelium
   E The posterior wall of the pouch of Douglas forms the anterior peritoneum of the upper two-thirds of the rectum

4. With regard to the uterus:
   A The ureter travels over the uterine artery
   B The uterine arteries are branches of the internal iliac vessels
   C Pain sensation from the uterine body is carried by the hypogastric nerve
   D It develops from embryonic mesoderm
   E In the newborn female the cervix forms the largest part of the uterus

5. **In the human pelvis:**
   A There are four pairs of sacral foramina
   B The acetabulum is formed from the joining of the ischium, ilium and pubis
   C The obturator foramen is formed from the fusion of the ilium and the pubic rami
   D The iliacus muscle originates at the iliac fossa
   E The pubic symphysis is a cartilaginous joint

6. **The femoral ring:**
   A Is bounded laterally by the lacunar ligament
   B Is bounded anteriorly by the inguinal ligament
   C Has its posterior border formed from the inferior ramus of the pubis
   D Is approximately 3 cm wide
   E Contains the femoral nerve

7. **Concerning parathyroid hormone related peptide:**
   A It regulates chondrocyte proliferation
   B It can be raised in some malignancies
   C Causes increased calcitriol levels
   D Has a role in the placental transport of calcium
   E Its levels are raised in hyperparathyroidism

8. **In cell signalling pathways, the following are second messengers:**
   A Acetylcholine
   B Adenosine triphosphate
   C Cyclic adenosine monophosphate
   D Inositol triphosphate
   E Nitric oxide

9. **The following substances can cause myometrial contraction:**
   A Nitrous oxide
   B Oxytocin
   C Prostaglandin F2α
   D Progesterone
   E Relaxin

10. **With regard to placental development:**
    A The syncytiotrophoblast is derived from the cytotrophoblast
    B Each placental lobule is derived from a single primary stem villus
    C Each cotyledon has 2–5 lobules
    D Chorion laeve forms no part of the placental
    E The maternal and fetal blood supply connect in the intervillous space

11. **Concerning fertilisation:**
    A Capacitation is a reaction of the ovum
    B Fertilisation leads to completion of the second mitotic division
    C Fertilisation leads to a haploid number of chromosomes

    D   The zona pellucida disappears at the stage of the morula

    E   On average, the fertilised ovum enters the uterus 3 days after fertilisation

12. Congenital adrenal hyperplasia:

    A   Is most commonly due to deficiency of enzyme 21 hydroxylase

    B   Has an incidence of 1 in 50,000 births

    C   Commonly has low levels of 17-OH progesterone

    D   Has high levels of urinary 17-ketosteroids

    E   Is autosomal recessive

13. Hirsutism:

    A   Is associated with polycystic ovary syndrome

    B   Is a recognised side effect of cyproterone acetate

    C   Can be pathognomonic of certain ovarian tumours

    D   Can be caused by hypothyroidism

    E   Can be treated by spironolactone

14. With regard to thyroid hormones:

    A   The majority of free T4 is carried in plasma bound to thyroxine-binding globulin

    B   The ratio of T3:T4 in blood is approximately 20:1

    C   Deiodinases are responsible for converting T3 to T4

    D   T3 and T4 are lipophilic molecules

    E   T4 is secreted by follicular cells of the thyroid

15. With reference to hormones:

    A   Luteinising hormone and follicle-stimulating hormone act through a cytokine cell surface receptor

    B   Seven transmembrane cell surface receptors have the hormone binding domain at the G terminus

    C   Growth factor receptors are linked to tyrosine kinase

    D   Hormones acting through nuclear receptors act in the nucleus to alter gene expression

    E   Glucocorticoid receptors are found in the nucleus

16. Vitamin D:

    A   Is a steroid hormone

    B   Undergoes 25-hydroxylation in the kidney

    C   Is stored in the liver

    D   Undergoes 1α-hydroxylation in the liver

    E   Its synthesis is influenced by cortisol

17. Concerning skewed data:

    A   Positively-skewed data has a left-hand tail

    B   Skewed data can be more easily interpreted using a logarithmic transformation

    C   May have a bimodal distribution

    D   Skewed data distribution is caused by extreme values

    E   Skewness can be measured using the Mann–Whitney U test

18. Concerning the epidemiology of pregnancy failure:

A   Paternal smoking is a risk factor for miscarriage
B   Recurrent miscarriage is the loss of any four consecutive pregnancies
C   Uterine anomalies are a risk factor for miscarriage
D   Recurrent miscarriage affects 5% of women
E   Chromosomal abnormalities exist in 20% of first trimester miscarriages

19. Concerning the epidemiology of infertility:

A   5% of the population experience delay in conceiving
B   8% of the population require assisted conception techniques
C   Male factors are implicated in 10% of couples with primary subfertility
D   The cause of primary subfertility for 20% of couples remains unexplained
E   Around 80 out of every 100 couples having regular intercourse will conceive within 1 year

20. Regarding p-values:

A   A *p*-value of > 0.05 typically indicates a significant difference
B   The *p*-value assumes that the null hypothesis is false
C   The *p*-value gives an estimate of how likely an event is to have occurred by chance
D   The *p*-value indicates the likelihood of a type 1 error
E   The significance level of a test should be determined before data collection

21. The following genetic disorders are correctly paired with the affected chromosome:

A   Cystic fibrosis: chromosome 7
B   Duchenne muscular dystrophy: X chromosome
C   Neurofibromatosis type 1: chromosome 22
D   Prader–Willi syndrome: chromosome 16
E   Sickle-cell disease: chromosome 11

22. Concerning amniocentesis and chorionic villus sampling (CVS):

A   Amniocentesis is associated with an increased risk of miscarriage of 5%
B   Amniocentesis can be linked with increased rates of fetal talipes if performed before 15 weeks
C   Chorionic villi sampling can be performed from 15 weeks' gestation
D   CVS can be performed transcervically
E   Maternal HIV infection is an absolute contraindication for CVS

23. The following are examples of autonomic dominant genetic disorders:

A   Cystic fibrosis
B   Tuberous sclerosis
C   Fragile X
D   Duchenne's muscular dystrophy
E   Tay–Sachs disease

24. Regarding Barr bodies:

A   They are present in all human somatic cells

B   They represent inactive X chromosomes
C   In Turner's syndrome cells have an extra Barr body
D   They are found in the cell nuclei
E   They may be stained

25. **The following genetic conditions are associated with infertility:**

A   Turner's syndrome
B   Klinefelter's syndrome
C   Cystic fibrosis
D   Down's syndrome
E   Neurofibromatosis

26. **Regarding α-thalassaemia:**

A   It is an autosomal recessive condition
B   Affected fetuses may have hydrops fetalis
C   Having two affected alleles is incompatible with life
D   Individuals with α-thalassaemia trait can benefit from oral ferrous sulphate
E   Haemoglobin H disease is a form of α-thalassaemia

27. **With regards to fetal circulation**

A   The oxygen saturation in the umbilical vein is 80–90%
B   Fetal cardiac output is greater than that of the adult
C   Fetal haemoglobin is comprised of two α chains and two δ chains
D   Fetal red blood cells have no ABO antigen until after birth
E   Approximately 30% of blood from pulmonary artery travels to the lungs

28. **Regarding creatinine:**

A   Serum levels increase during pregnancy
B   It is secreted by the proximal tubules
C   It is found in greater amounts in the renal artery compared to the renal vein
D   It is not typically secreted
E   Creatinine clearance values are greater than the glomerular filtration rate

29. **Regarding the renal system in pregnancy:**

A   Filtration fraction falls consistently throughout pregnancy
B   The amount of filtered sodium increases in 3rd trimester
C   Kidneys increase in length by approximately 1 cm
D   There is dilatation of the ureters
E   The glomerular filtration rate increases to 140–170 mL/min at term

30. **Concerning the progesterone only pill:**

A   Reliably prevents ovulation
B   Has little effect on endometrial thickness
C   Increases the viscosity of cervical mucus
D   Effectiveness may be reduced by concomitant use of antibiotics
E   Is suitable for breastfeeding mothers

Questions: SBAs

For each question, select the single best answer from the five options listed.

31. Which muscle lies within the rectus sheath and is supplied by the subcostal nerve?

    A   External oblique
    B   Internal oblique
    C   Pyramidalis
    D   Rectus abdominis
    E   Transversus abdominis

32. Which muscle enters the abdomen behind the medial arcuate ligament?

    A   External oblique
    B   Iliacus
    C   Psoas
    D   Pyramidalis
    E   Transversus abdominis

33. Which muscle forms part of the inguinal ligament?

    A   External oblique
    B   Iliacus
    C   Internal oblique
    D   Rectus abdominis
    E   Transversus abdominis

34. Which artery is the terminal branch of the internal thoracic artery?

    A   Inferior mesenteric artery
    B   Inferior phrenic artery
    C   Lumbar artery
    D   Superior epigastric artery
    E   Superior mesenteric artery

35. Which artery arises from the posterior trunk of the internal iliac artery?

    A   Inferior gluteal artery
    B   Middle rectal artery
    C   Superior gluteal artery
    D   Superior vesical artery
    E   Uterine artery

36. A 41-year-old woman complains of prolonged numbness in her leg 2 days after a normal vaginal delivery. She had an epidural for pain relief during labour.

    What is the nerve root origin of lateral cutaneous nerve of the thigh?

    A   L1
    B   L2

C L3
D L1 and L2
E L2 and L3

37. A 25-year-old woman has a routine smear test for the first time. She complains of discomfort during the procedure.

    Which nerve or nerve plexus carries afferent fibres from the cervix to the upper sacral nerves?

    A Inferior hypogastric plexus
    B Obturator nerve
    C Pelvic splanchnic nerves
    D Pudendal nerve
    E Superior hypogastric plexus

38. A 72-year-old woman is referred to the gynaecology outpatient clinic with a 2-day history of postmenopausal bleeding. She subsequently undergoes a hysteroscopy and endometrial biopsy as part of her investigation.

    Which of the following best describes the cells that line the uterus?

    A Columnar epithelium
    B Cuboidal epithelium
    C Pseudostratified columnar epithelium
    D Stratified squamous epithelium
    E Transitional cells

39. A 63-year-old woman is referred to the urogynaecology clinic with recurrent urinary tract infections and microscopic haematuria. A midstream urine sample is sent for cytology.

    Which cells line the distal half of the urethra?

    A Columnar epithelium
    B Epidermis
    C Secretory cells
    D Stratified squamous epithelium
    E Transitional cells

40. An 82-year-old woman undergoes a vaginal hysterectomy for treatment of her procidentia. You are revising the stages of the operation.

    Which ligament runs laterally from the body of the uterus, through the internal inguinal ring to the labium majus?

    A Broad ligament
    B Cardinal ligament
    C Iliolumbar ligament
    D Round ligament
    E Uterosacral ligament

41. Which of the following runs outside of the ischiorectal fossa?

    A Pudendal canal
    B Fat pad
    C Inferior rectal nerve
    D Middle rectal artery
    E Perineal branch of S4 nerve

42. Which of the following is correct regarding the embryological origin of the anal canal?

    A Above pectinate line: derived endoderm, superior rectal artery
    B Above pectinate line: derived ectoderm, superior rectal artery
    C Above pectinate line: derived ectoderm, columnar epithelium
    D Below pectinate line: derived ectoderm, superior rectal artery
    E Below pectinate line: derived endoderm, middle and inferior rectal artery

43. Prior to a forceps delivery, you wish to give a pudendal nerve block.

Where is the pudendal canal?

    A Lateral wall of ischiorectal fossa; above sacrotuberous ligament
    B Lateral wall of ischiorectal fossa; below sacrospinous ligament
    C Lateral wall of ischiorectal fossa; below sacrotuberous ligament
    D Medial wall of ischiorectal fossa; above sacrospinous ligament
    E Medial wall of ischiorectal fossa; below sacrotuberous ligament

44. A 24-year-old woman is catheterised prior to a diagnostic laparoscopy to investigate chronic pelvic pain.

The distal aspect of the female urethra is lined with which type of epithelial cells?

    A Ciliated
    B Simple cuboidal
    C Simple squamous
    D Stratified squamous
    E Transitional

45. A 26-year-old woman attends her general practitioner for her 6 week postnatal check. She has a central abdominal protrusion which is diagnosed as a divarication of the rectus muscle.

What is the nerve supply to the rectus abdominis muscle?

    A T2–T12
    B T7–T12
    C T12–L3
    D L2–L5
    E L5–S3

46. A 32-year-old woman attends the gynaecology outpatient clinic complaining of severe premenstrual symptoms and pelvic pain. Her 4-year-old son is also present and it is noticed that he has an abnormal gait, with slightly bent and shortened legs.

What is the most likely diagnosis of this child?

A   Congenital abnormality
B   Osteopetrosis
C   Perthes disease
D   Rickets
E   Scurvy

47. A 65-year-old man attends his general practitioner with a 3-month history of lower backache and fatigue.

Blood tests are as follows:

Urea	13.2 mmol/L
Creatinine	145 μmol/L
Potassium	5.9 mmol/L
Haemoglobin	9.8 g/dl
Mean corpuscular volume	82.2 fL/red cell
Calcium	2.65 mmol/L

What is the most likely diagnosis?

A   Bone metastases
B   Immobilisation
C   Multiple myeloma
D   Sarcoidosis
E   Thiazide diuretics

48. A 62 year-old woman is diagnosed with a glucagonoma.

Which one of the following metabolic conditions is most likely to result from this tumour?

A   Decreased lipolysis
B   Hyperglycaemia
C   Increased muscle protein synthesis
D   Increased liver glycolytic rate
E   Increased glycogenesis

49. A 42-year-old woman is day 3 after a total abdominal hysterectomy for menorrhagia and fibroids. She is acutely short of breath, with pain on inspiration.

Her observations are as follows:

SpO_2	93% on room air
Blood pressure	115/74 mmHg
Heart rate	105 beats per minute
Respiratory rate	22 breaths per minute

You perform an arterial blood gas. You are concerned she may have a pulmonary embolus.

Considering the most likely diagnosis, which is the most likely result?

A pH 6.9, pCO_2 7.5 kPa, pO_2 15.1 kPa, HCO_3 15.4 mmol/L, base excess -12 mmol/L
B pH 7.16, pCO_2 8.2 kPa, pO_2 8.8 kPa, HCO_3 21.2 mmol/L
C pH 7.36, pCO_2 5.6 kPa, pO_2 13.2 kPa, HCO_3 26 mmol/L
D pH 7.50, pCO_2 3.0 kPa, pO_2 9.2 kPa, HCO_3 25 mmol/L
E pH 7.52, pCO_2 6.0 kPa, pO_2 12.0 kPa, HCO_3 17 mmol/L, base excess +4.5

50. A 28-year-old woman is admitted to the high dependency unit following a caesarean section. She was diagnosed during pregnancy with acute fatty liver of pregnancy. She was started on a morphine infusion postoperatively and is receiving oxygen by mask. She is noted to be very drowsy. You perform an arterial blood gas.

What is the most likely finding in the case?

A pH 7.16, pCO_2 8.2 kPa, pO_2 15.3 kPa, HCO_3 21.2 mmol/L
B pH 7.2, pCO_2 4.8 kPa, pO_2 10.2 kPa, HCO_3 14 mmol/L
C pH 7.36, pCO_2 5.6 kPa, pO_2 13.2 kPa, HCO_3 26 mmol/L
D pH 7.52, pCO_2 6.0 kPa, pO_2 12.0 kPa, HCO_3 17, base excess +4.3 mmol/L
E pH 7.62, pCO_2 6.2 kPa, pO_2 12.2 kPa, HCO_3 15 mmol/L

51. A 23-year-old woman is admitted to hospital complaining of abdominal pain and vomiting. She is a type I diabetic and did not take her insulin today as she has been vomiting for 12 hours. On examination, she is tachycardic and feels cold and clammy. An arterial blood gas confirms your diagnosis of ketoacidosis.

Which of the following findings is most correct regarding diabetic ketoacidosis?

A High blood levels of fatty acids
B Hypoventilation
C Increased blood volume
D Low levels of lactate
E Respiratory acidosis

52. A 72-year-old woman is seen in the pre-assessment clinic prior to a hysteroscopy to investigate postmenopausal bleeding. She is taking aspirin and is asked to stop taking it 5 days prior to the procedure.

Which of the following prostanoids inhibits platelet aggregation?

A Prostacyclin PGI2
B Prostaglandin E2
C Prostaglandin D2
D Prostaglandin F2α
E Thromboxane TXA2

53. A 27-year-old woman is admitted to hospital with acute left iliac fossa pain, a positive pregnancy test and a haemoglobin level of 7.9 g/dL. She undergoes a diagnostic laparoscopy and is found to have an ectopic pregnancy.

Where is the most common site of fertilisation of the ovum?

A   Fimbria of the fallopian tube
B   Ampulla of the fallopian tube
C   Isthmus of the fallopian tube
D   Tubal ostia
E. Fundal endometrium

54. A 28-year-old woman is admitted to hospital with acute-onset right iliac fossa pain. She has low-grade pyrexia and is nauseous. Her blood tests reveal a C-reactive protein of 62 mg/dL and white cell count of 17.2×10^9/L. A diagnostic laparoscopy reveals a Meckel's diverticulitis.

Meckel's diverticulum is the persistence of which structure?

A   Urachal remnant
B   Vitellointestinal duct
C   Primitive streak
D   Paraxial mesoderm
E   Buccopharyngeal membrane

55. Which one of the following is a derivative of the urogenital sinus in male?

A   Vas deferens
B   Epididymis
C   Ejaculatory duct
D   Prostate
E   Seminal vesicle

56. A 56-year-old woman attends her general practitioner's surgery complaining of feeling unwell for the last couple of months. The general practitioner decides to do a range of blood tests, including thyroid function, liver function and calcium and vitamin D levels.

Which of the following is associated with hypercalcaemia?

A   Chvostek's sign
B   Numbness
C   Perioral tingling
D   Shortened Q–T interval and widened T wave on ECG
E   Trousseau's sign

57. After an uneventful pregnancy a baby is born via spontaneous vaginal delivery. Soon after birth the midwife asks the paediatric team to review the baby as she is uncertain of the infant's sex. Following a series of investigations the baby is found to have the genotype 46XX and is diagnosed with congenital adrenal hyperplasia (CAH).

CAH is most commonly associated with a deficiency of which enzyme?

A   5α-reductase
B   11β-hydroxylase
C   17α-hydroxylase

    D   21α-hydroxylase

    E   Aromatase

58. A 26-year-old woman complains of increased facial hair and thinks it may be caused by a new medication she was prescribed 3 months previously.

Which of the following drugs is known to cause hirsutism?

    A   Dianette

    B   Erythromycin

    C   Gentamicin

    D   Phenytoin

    E   Tacrolimus

59. Where is thyroid-stimulating hormone produced?

    A   Acidophils of the anterior pituitary gland

    B   Basophils of the anterior pituitary gland

    C   Chromophobes of the anterior pituitary gland

    D   Supraventricular nucleus of the hypothalamus

    E   Paraventricular nucleus of the hypothalamus

60. Which of the following is a symptom of hyperthyroidism?

    A   Diarrhoea

    B   Infertility

    C   Palpitations

    D   Weight loss

    E   All of the above

61. The majority of extracellular calcium is bound to which of the following:

    A   Albumin

    B   Bicarbonate

    C   Calcitriol

    D   Fibrinogen

    E   Phosphate

62. A 63-year-old man attends his general practitioner with a 2-month history of lower back pain associated with radiation of pain down the right leg and shortness of breath. He has also lost some weight. Blood tests reveal:

Calcium	2.72 mmol/L
Haemoglobin	10.4 g/dL
Mean corpuscular volume	83.6 fL

Which of the following is the most likely diagnosis?

    A   Bone metastases

    B   Immobilisation

    C   Osteoporosis

D   Multiple myeloma
E   Sarcoidosis

63. A junior doctor is asked to check the calcium levels on a patient 6 hours after a removal of her parathyroid gland.

Which of the following is a function of parathyroid hormone (PTH)?

A   In bone, PTH reduces osteoclast activity
B   PTH acts in the kidney to reduce bicarbonate excretion
C   PTH acts on the kidney to increase level of phosphate absorption
D   PTH acts to reduce serum levels of calcium
E   PTH acts via a G-protein coupled receptor

64. Calcium is transferred from maternal circulation to fetal circulation via which transport mechanism?

A   Active transport
B   Endocytosis
C   Exocytosis
D   Facilitated diffusion
E   Passive diffusion

65. Which of the following is true regarding maternal calcium homeostasis during pregnancy?

A   Increased calcitonin
B   Reduced 1,25 vitamin D3
C   Reduced bone turnover
D   Reduced calcium absorption
E   Reduced parathyroid hormone production

66. Which of the following gives the World Health Organisation's definition of neonatal mortality rate?

A   The number of deaths during the first 28 completed days of life per 1000 live births
B   The number of deaths during the first 28 completed days of life per 100,000 live births
C   The number of deaths during the first 365 completed days of life per 1000 live births
D   The number of deaths during the first 365 completed days of life per 10,000 live births
E   The number of deaths, including stillborn fetuses of more than 24 weeks' gestation, up to 28 completed days of life, per 1000 pregnancies

67. The quadruple test is a widely used screening test that aims to identify pregnancies with a high-risk of chromosomal abnormalities.

Which of the following gives the best definition of the test's specificity?

A   The proportion of women with a normal pregnancy who had a low-risk result
B   The proportion of women with an affected fetus who had a high-risk result
C   The proportion of women with a high-risk test result with an affected fetus
D   The proportion of women with a low-risk test result with a normal pregnancy
E   None of the above

68. The age of menarche was recorded for 100 women who attended a rapid access gynaecology clinic with suspected ovarian cancer. The data obtained showed a normal distribution.

    The following values were obtained.
    Mean = 13 years
    Standard deviation = 2 years

    What is the standard error of the mean for this sample?

    A   0.1
    B   0.2
    C   0.5
    D   1
    E   2

69. A research study is designed to look at the association between mothers who smoke during pregnancy and the subsequent growth of their children. The study population is all babies born in the Daisy Maternity Unit between 1975 and 1980. The babies were classified at birth as having being born to women who smoked during their pregnancies or not. All of the children have their height and weight measured every year from birth to the age of 20 years.

    What study design is being used?

    A   Case-control study
    B   Cohort study
    C   Cross-sectional study
    D   Double-blinded study
    E   None of the above

70. Which of the following best describes a type 1 error?

    A   The erroneous acceptance of the null hypothesis
    B   The erroneous rejection of the null hypothesis
    C   The inclusion of extreme outliers in a data set
    D   The occurrence of a γ error
    E   None of the above

71. Which of the following is a direct cause of maternal mortality?

    A   Diabetes
    B   Hormone-dependent breast cancer
    C   Obesity
    D   Community-acquired Group A streptococcal disease
    E   Suicide

72. Which of following statements defines the median in a data set?

    A   The median is the least frequently occurring value in a data set
    B   The median is the middle value in ranked set of data
    C   The median is the middle value in an unranked data set
    D   The median is the most frequently occurring value in a data set
    E   The median is the value obtained by dividing the sum of the data set by the number of values in the data set

73. A 28-year-old woman who is 13 weeks pregnant consents for routine antenatal screening. The results of her quadruple test show the fetus has a 1 in 58 chance of having trisomy 13.

    What is trisomy 13 commonly known as?

    A   Cri-du-chat syndrome
    B   Down's syndrome
    C   Edwards' syndrome
    D   Patau's syndrome
    E   Wolf–Hirschhorn syndrome

74. A 16-year-old boy is brought to his general practitioner by his parents. They are concerned that he appears to have developed breast tissue. On questioning, he feels self conscious about his appearance and feels his genitalia are smaller than individuals of his own age. On examination, he appears tall for his age, with objectively long arms and legs. Gynaecomastia is noted, alongside a fat distribution typically seen in females.

    What is the most likely genotype of this individual?

    A   45 XO
    B   46 XO
    C   46 XX
    D   46 XY
    E   47 XXY

75. A 40 year old primiparous woman has an elevated risk of trisomy 21 (1 in 50) at antenatal screening and opts for an amniocentesis at 15 weeks' gestation. The fetus is found to have the karyotype 46 XX/47 XX +21.

    What may this karyotype indicate?

    A   Trisomy 21
    B   Turner's syndrome
    C   Klinefelter's syndrome
    D   Mosaic for Down's syndrome
    E   None of above

76. A couple are seen for preconception counselling. The 26-year-old male partner is of above average height, with noticeably long arms. He is being monitored for worsening aortic root dissection and has had pleurodesis for recurrent

pneumothoraces. His vision is mildly impaired due to optic lens subluxation. The couple wishes to use preimplantation genetic screening techniques to prevent their children from inheriting their father's condition.

Which genetic condition does the male partner have?

A   Congenital contractual arachnodactyly
B   Ehlers–Danlos syndrome
C   Klinefelter's syndrome
D   Marfan's syndrome
E   Triple X syndrome

77. Which of the following conditions is transmitted via mitochondrial inheritance?

A   Alpha-thalassaemia
B   Colour blindness
C   Dermatomyositis
D   Duchenne muscular dystrophy
E   Leber's optic neuropathy

78. Which of the following genetic conditions occurs as a result of genomic imprinting?

A   Angelman's syndrome
B   Fragile-X syndrome
C   Friedreich ataxia
D   Patau's syndrome
E   All of the above

79. Which of the following hormones is not secreted by the human placenta?

A   Human chorionic gonadotrophin
B   Oestrogen
C   Oxytocin
D   Progesterone
E   Relaxin

80. At a term delivery, there is some concern about the placental structure.

Which of the following statements about the umbilical cord is correct?

A   At term the mean length is 70 cm
B   It is formed at 8 weeks' gestation
C   3% of cords have a single artery
D   Umbilical arteries arise from the internal iliac artery
E   Venous drainage is mainly to the inferior vena cava via the ductus arteriosus

81. Considering placental transport, which of the following are correctly paired?

A   Active transport: amino acids
B   Active transport: glucose
C   Facilitated diffusion: free fatty acids

D   Passive diffusion: glucose
E   Receptor mediated endocytosis: IgA

82. Which of the following is a systemic function of oestrogen?

A   Increases bone resorption
B   Increases cholesterol levels
C   Promotes atherosclerosis
D   Vasoconstriction
E   Vasodilation

83. A 22-year-old woman has undergone an endoscopic retrograde cholangiopancreatography after a missed miscarriage. The estimated blood loss was 1000 mL. You are called to see her as she is hypotensive and wish to administer intravenous fluids.

Which of the following is correct regarding 0.9% sodium chloride?

A   It contains 9 mmol/L sodium chloride
B   It contains 154 mmol/L sodium chloride
C   It contains 18 mmol potassium chloride
D   It is a better volume expander than Hartmann's solution
E   It is the first choice of fluid in the immediate postoperative period

84. Which of the following statements is correct in regard to the double Bohr effect?

A   The fetal side becomes acidotic
B   The fetus loses metabolites to the mother
C   Maternal and fetal oxygen dissociation curves move towards each other
D   The maternal oxygen dissociation curve shifts to the left
E   The maternal side has an increased pH

85. What is the structure of fetal haemoglobin?

A   Two alpha chains and two beta chains $(\alpha_2\beta_2)$
B   Two alpha chains and two delta chains $(\alpha_2\delta_2)$
C   Two alpha chains and two gamma chains $(\alpha_2\gamma_2)$
D   Two beta and two delta chains $(\beta_2\delta_2)$
E   Two beta and two gamma chains $(\beta_2\gamma_2)$

86. A 21-year-old woman is seen in the gynaecology clinic complaining of pain in the lower abdomen during the middle of her menstrual cycle.

A surge in which hormone around day 14 of the menstrual cycle leads to ovulation?

A   Follicle-stimulating hormone
B   Luteinising hormone
C   Oestradiol
D   Progesterone
E   Testosterone

87. During oogenesis, at what point is the second meiotic division is completed?

    A   At ovulation
    B   Immediately prior to the formation of the secondary oocyte
    C   Immediately prior to the formation of the primary oocyte
    D   At fertilisation
    E   None of the above

88. Which of the following structures communicates with the umbilical vein to form the ductus venosus?

    A   Aorta
    B   Inferior vena cava
    C   Left atrium
    D   Pulmonary artery
    E   Right atrium

89. Which of the following is a branch of the posterior division of the internal iliac artery?

    A   Inferior gluteal artery
    B   Internal pudendal artery
    C   Obturator artery
    D   Superior gluteal artery
    E   Uterine artery

90. After an elective caesarean section the anaesthetic team decide to administer a transversus abdominis plane block to provide analgesia. They use ultrasound to identify the layers of the abdominal wall.

    Which of these muscles is innervated by the femoral nerve?

    A   External oblique
    B   Iliacus
    C   Internal oblique
    D   Rectus abdominis
    E   Transverse abdominis

Answers

1. A False

   B True

   C False

   D True

   E False

   In the wall of the female pelvis the ureter forms part of the posterior boundary of the ovarian fossa, in which the ovary is situated. From here, it runs medially and anteriorly on the lateral side of the cervix and the upper part of the vagina to reach the fundus of the bladder. Here it is accompanied by the uterine artery for approximately 2.5 cm, which then crosses in front of the ureter and ascends between the two layers of the broad ligament.

   The labia minora are longitudinal cutaneous folds running obliquely downwards from the clitoris, between the labia majora. They contain both sweat and sebaceous follicles.

   The internal anal sphincter is an involuntary smooth muscle which receives parasympathetic supply from the inferior hypogastric plexus (S1, S2, S3) to maintain resting tone. Sympathetic supply is excitatory.

2. A True

   B False

   C True

   D True

   E True

   The ischiorectal fossa is a triangular space containing fat, found on either side of the anal canal below the pelvic diaphragm. The levator ani forms the apex, with the obturator internus muscle forming the lateral wall and the anal canal the medial wall. The sacrotuberous ligament and the gluteus maximus are found posteriorly. The perineal skin forms the base.

3. A False

   B False

   C True

   D True

   E True

   The rectum is approximately 15 cm long and starts at the level of the third sacral vertebra. It has an outer longitudinal and an inner circular layer of smooth muscle and is lined by columnar epithelium.

- **Artery:**
  - upper two-thirds – superior rectal artery
  - lower one-third – middle rectal artery
- **Vein:** superior rectal and middle rectal veins
- **Nerve:** inferior anal nerve
- **Lymph:** preaortic nodes, inferior mesenteric lymph nodes, pararectal nodes

4. A False

    B True

    C True

    D True

    E True

Nerve supply to the uterus is from the inferior hypogastric plexus which is derived from the sympathetic supply T10–T11. The pain from the uterus passes in the inferior hypogastric plexus, along with pain sensation from the superior region of the cervix. Pain from the inferior region of the cervix is via the pelvic splanchnic nerves. The blood supply to the uterus is from the uterine arteries and these arise from the anterior division of the internal iliac arteries. The ureter passes beneath the uterine artery.

5. A True

    B True

    C False

    D True

    E True

The sacrum is composed of five fused vertebra which provide four foramina. The innominate bone of the pelvis is made up of the ilium, ischium and pubis bones. They all contribute to the acetabulum which accommodates the femoral head to form the hip joint. The obturator foramen is closed by a fibrous membrane and is created by the ischial ramus together with the pubic bone. The obturator foramen contains the obturator artery, vein and nerve. The pubic symphysis is a cartilaginous joint that connects the superior rami of both pubic bones.

6. A False

    B True

    C False

    D False

    E False

Boundaries of the femoral ring are:

- Anteriorly: inguinal ligament
- Posteriorly: pectineus
- Medially: lacunar ligament
- Laterally: femoral vein fascia

7. A True

   B True

   C False

   D False

   E False

   Parathyroid hormone-related peptide (PTHrP) is a hormone, related to parathyroid hormone (PTH). It may be secreted by some cancers, including breast and squamous cell and is implicated in the hypercalcaemia of malignancy. It has a role in endochondral bone development and regulates chondrocyte proliferation. Being part of the PTH hormone family, PTHrP produces many of the same effects of PTH. It does not cause raised calcitriol levels and concentration is normal in hyperthyroidism.

8. A False

   B False

   C True

   D True

   E True

   Second messengers are intracellular molecules that relay signals from receptor proteins to intracellular receptors. The major types of second messenger systems are (1) the cyclic nucleotides, i.e. cyclic adenosine monophosphate (cAMP) and cyclic guanosine monophosphate (cGMP) (2) gases such nitric oxide and carbon monoxide (3) calcium ions and (4) the phosphoinositol system, i.e. inositol triphosphate and diacylglycerol. Second messengers are associated with increasing the signal strength of the first messenger, i.e. the hormone, which is detected by its receptor, and form part of a communication cascade. Acetylcholine is a neurotransmitter and acts as a first messenger and utilises second messengers such as cAMP and inositol triphosphate. Adenosine triphosphate is not a second messenger, but is a coenzyme used in cell signalling; it is converted to the second messenger cAMP by the action of adenylate cyclase.

9. A False

   B True

   C True

   D False

   E False

   Uterine activity is dependent on the balance between the myometrial relaxants and contractants. Oxytocin and prostaglandins – in particular prostaglandin F2α – both contribute to myometrial contractility. They act by increasing the intracellular calcium concentration via the action of phospholipase C and the subsequent stimulation of myosin light chain kinase and calcium-dependent protein kinase. The number of oxytocin receptors increases throughout pregnancy due to increased levels of oestrogen. These receptors contribute significantly to the relationship between oxytocin and prostaglandins. Contractility is enhanced by the ability of prostaglandin F2α to cause upregulation of oxytocin receptors in myometrial tissue and by the capacity of oxytocin to promote the synthesis of prostaglandins.

10. A True

    B False

    C True

    D True

    E False

Seven days after ovulation, the fertilised ovum trophoblast forms two distinct layers. There is an inner layer of mononuclear cytotrophoblastic cells and a layer on the outside of multinucleated syncytiotrophoblasts. The cotyledon is defined as the villous tree which arises from a single primary stem villous and each one contains 2–5 lobules. Each placental lobule is derived from a single secondary stem villus. The chorion is formed from two layers: the outer derived from trophoblast and the inner derived from mesoderm which is in contact with the amnion. The trophoblast forms the chorionic villi which invade the decidual tissue. The chorion laeve is in contact with the decidual capsularis tissue and forms no part in the formation of the placenta. The chorion frondosum is in contact with the placenta. The maternal and fetal blood supplies do not come into contact.

11. A False

    B False

    C True

    D True

    E False

Sperm entering the oocyte leads to completion of the second meiotic division. Capacitation involves release of lytic enzymes as the outer acrosomal membrane of the sperm fuses with cumulus cells of the ovum. It is thought that this process is essential to the process of fertilisation. It also prevents further sperm from penetrating the ovum. During the passage of the ovum from the ovary to the uterus, there is a temporary halt of movement at the ampulla of the fallopian tube. Because of this delay in motility, fertilisation often occurs at this location. Muscle activity of the fallopian tube aids the movement of the fertilised egg, which enters the uterus 5 days after fertilisation

12. A True

    B False

    C False

    D True

    E True

Congenital adrenal hyperplasia is an autosomal recessive condition and has an incidence of 1:10,000–1:18,000 births. The condition is caused by a deficient production of cortisol, however there are varying levels of severity. In the absence of the enzyme 21-hydroxylase, glucocorticoid precursors accumulate and are converted to androgenic steroids.

13. A True

    B False

    C False

    D True

    E True

Cyproterone is an antiandrogen which is used in the treatment of hirsutism and acts by blocking the androgen receptors. Cyproterone acetate is a synthetic derivative of 17-hydroxyprogesterone. Although a recognised sign in certain androgen producing ovarian tumours such as Brenner's tumour and arrhenoblastoma, hirsutism is not pathognomonic of these conditions.

Causes of hirsutism are as follows:

- Iatrogenic
- Drugs: danazol, testosterone
- Ovaries: polycystic ovarian syndrome, androgen secreting tumours
- Adrenal: congenital adrenal hyperplasia, acromegaly

14. A True

    B False

    C False

    D True

    E True

T3 and T4 are lipophilic tyrosine based hormones. T4 is produced by the follicular cells of the thyroid and converted to T3 within cells by deiodinases. T3 is more potent than T4, but it is present in a lower concentration in the blood. Most (99.5%) of the circulating thyroxine is bound to protein: 70% to thyroxine-binding globulin, 20% to albumin and 10% to transthyretin. 0.03% of T4 and 0.3% of T3 is free. Both T3 and T4 are lipophilic hormones and easily cross cell membranes. The synthesis of thyroid hormones involves several steps and takes place in the follicular cells of the thyroid. The thyroid hormones are produced from tyrosine, which occurs by deiodination.

15. A False

    B False

    C True

    D True

    E False

Peptide hormones act through cell surface receptors which are divided into four groups:

1. Seven-transmembrane domain
2. Single-transmembrane domain
3. Cytokine receptors
4. Guanylyl cyclase-linked receptors.

Seven-transmembrane receptors pass in and out of the cytoplasm, with a carboxy terminus linked to the G-protein transducer and the amino terminus linked to the hormone domain. The action of luteinising hormone and follicle-stimulating hormone is via this receptor. The growth factor receptors are linked to tyrosine kinase. Hormones acting through nuclear receptors include steroid and thyroid hormones. Nuclear receptors are found in the cytoplasm or the nucleus itself. Receptors in the cytoplasm include those for glucocorticoids and progesterone. Receptors in the nucleus include those for oestrogens and vitamin-D.

16. A True

B False

C False

D False

E True

Vitamin D is a steroid hormone and is synthesised from cholesterol. Ninety per cent is synthesised in the skin as a result of the action of UV light on 7-dehydrocholesterol to form cholecalciferol. Ten per cent is absorbed in the diet. Both forms are transported to the liver where they undergo 25-hydroxylation. From here it is stored in body fat as calcidiol (25-hydroxyvitamin D). Alpha1-hydroxylation occurs in the kidney and is tightly regulated by parathyroid hormone (**Figure 15.1**).

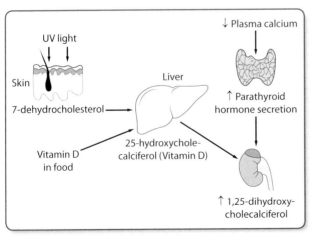

Figure 15.1 Synthesis of Vitamin D.

17. A False

   B True

   C True

   D True

   E False

Although some data may have a normal distribution, if there are extremes of values (also known as outliers) this may lead the distribution to be either negatively or positively skewed. In positively skewed data the extremes of values are found towards the right-hand of the distribution and the data can be described as having a right-hand tail. In negatively skewed data the extremes of values are found towards the left-hand of the distribution and the data distribution can be described as having a left-hand tail. Skewed data may have a unimodal and a bimodal distribution. In order to more easily analyse skewed data it can be partially normalised by logarithmic transformation (**Figure 15.2**).

Bland JM, Altman D. Statistics notes: transforming data. BMJ 1996;312:770.

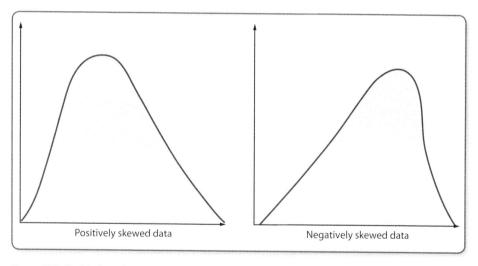

Figure 15.2 Positively and negatively skewed data.

18. A True

   B False

   C True

   D False

   E False

Miscarriage is common and in the first trimester occurs in approximately 1 in 5 pregnancies. Chromosomal abnormalities are a significant cause of loss and are present in > 50% of miscarried pregnancies. There are many risk factors for miscarriage including advanced maternal age, obesity, maternal and paternal smoking, dose-related caffeine intake, anatomical anomalies such as the presence of a uterine septum, thrombophilias (such as antiphospholipid syndrome), infection and endocrine causes such as diabetes. Recurrent miscarriage affects around 1% of woman and is defined as the loss of three consecutive pregnancies. Having had a previous pregnancy with a successful outcome does not mean a woman cannot go on to have recurrent miscarriages. Women with recurrent miscarriage need assessment regarding the presence of contributory risk-factors and management in a specialised clinic.

Royal College of Obstetricians and Gynaecologists. The Investigation and Treatment of Couples with Recurrent First-trimester and Second-trimester Miscarriage. Green-top Guideline 17. London: RCOG, 2011.

19. A False

    B True

    C False

    D True

    E True

Delay in conceiving is a common problem. Although the majority of couples will conceive within 1 year of having regular unprotected sexual intercourse, up to 1 in 7 couples will seek help regarding fertility. Of those seeking assistance many present with primary subfertility, i.e. the couple have never conceived a pregnancy. Other couples will present with secondary subfertility, i.e. they have previously conceived a pregnancy together, regardless of the outcome of the pregnancy (either a live birth or a miscarriage). Following investigation, the cause of primary subfertility is still unexplained for around 20% of couples. Male factors are attributed to around 20–30% of cases of couples with primary subfertility. Ovulatory and tubal dysfunctions are the other main contributors to subfertility. Around 8% of the population require the assistance of reproductive techniques such as ovulation induction, intrauterine insemination and in vitro fertilisation.

StratOG.net. Subfertility: Epidemiology, ethical and legal issues of subfertility. London: StratOG, 2012. www.rcog.org.uk/stratog.

20. A False

    B False

    C True

    D False

    E True

The p-value refers to the probability of detecting a significant finding in a study if the null hypothesis is true. The p-value assumes that the null hypothesis is true. The standard p-value used in most statistical analyses is 0.05 (however, a p-value of 0.01

or lower could be used). If the resultant *p*-value obtained from a study is < 0.05 then the null hypothesis can be rejected. That is, we can be 95% certain that the observed effect did not occur due to chance alone. Another way of describing this outcome is that the result was significant at the 5% level.

If, when using the same level of significance, the resultant *p*-value was greater than or equal to 0.05 then the null hypothesis can be accepted; i.e. the result is not significant at the 5% level. The inference here is that the effects observed in the study may have occurred due to chance alone.

It is important to remember that the chosen *p*-value is not entirely robust. For example, when a *p*-value of 0.05 is used 5% of the time the null hypothesis will be rejected incorrectly. The *p*-value cannot indicate the likelihood of a type 1 error.

Sedgwick P. Statistical question: P values. BMJ 2010;340:c2203.

21. A True

B True

C True

D False

E True

Cystic fibrosis is an autosomal recessive condition, which can be caused by a variety of different mutations affecting the *CFTR* gene found on chromosome 7. Neurofibromatosis type 1 is caused by a mutation of the *neurofibromin (NF) 1* gene of chromosome 17. The gene is transmitted by autosomal dominant inheritance, although in many cases the disease is caused by a random gene mutation. Neurofibromatosis type 2 is caused by a mutation of the *NF2* gene which is found on chromosome 22.

Prader–Willi syndrome is caused by either a loss or mutation of genes found on the proximal arm of chromosome 15. An example of genomic imprinting, it occurs through the loss of the paternally derived genes as a consequence of either deletion or due to maternal disomy of chromosome 15. Angelman syndrome is also example of genomic imprinting and arises when there is loss of the maternal component of chromosome 15. Sickle-cell disease is an autosomal recessive condition, caused by a mutation in the beta-globulin gene found on chromosome 11. Duchenne muscular dystrophy is X-linked recessive.

22. A False

B True

C False

D True

E False

Amniocentesis and chorionic villus sampling (CVS) are both invasive prenatal diagnostic tests. They can be used to provide a diagnosis if there is thought to be a raised risk of fetal abnormality. They are offered if there is a raised risk of aneuploidy detected at screening, if there is a family history of abnormality or if both parents are known to be carriers of a genetically transmitted condition. Amniocentesis can be performed from 15 weeks' gestation. Increased fetal talipes and respiratory problems have been reported in amniocentesis performed before 15 weeks. CVS involves sampling of placental chorionic villi either transabdominally or transcervically from 11 weeks' gestation. Both amniocentesis and CVS are associated with a 1% excess risk of miscarriage. Maternal HIV infection is not an absolute contraindication for either test, however it is ideally performed when the maternal viral load is undetectable.

Royal College of Obstetricians and Gynaecologists. Amniocentesis and Chorionic Villus Sampling. Green-top Guideline 8. London: RCOG, 2010.

23. A False

   B True

   C False

   D True

   E False

Tuberous sclerosis is an example of an autosomal dominant genetic disorder. In autosomal dominant conditions, inheritance of a copy of the defective chromosome leads to expression of the condition. Cystic fibrosis shows an autosomal recessive mode of inheritance, by which both parents must carry a copy of the defective gene for the condition to be expressed, with an estimated 1 in 4 offspring of two carriers expressing the condition, 2 in 4 neither carriers affected and 1 in 4 an unaffected carrier. Other autosomal recessive conditions include sickle-cell anaemia, β-thalassaemia and Tay–Sachs disease. Fragile X is inherited by X-linked dominant inheritance. Duchenne's muscular dystrophy shows an X-linked recessive inheritance.

24. A False

   B True

   C False

   D True

   E True

A Barr body is found in all somatic cells in females. Each Barr body represents an inactivated X chromosome. They may be stained and visualised at the periphery of nuclei halted at interphase. Individuals with Turner's syndrome typically have an absence of one of the X chromosomes and therefore are missing a Barr body, rather than having an additional copy. This monosomy is described as 45 X0.

25. A True

   B True

   C True

   D True

   E False

Females born with Turner's syndrome typically have primary amenorrhoea due to the presence of streak gonads and are unable to conceive. Some individuals do experience menarche, but often experience an early menopause. Rarely, women with Turner's syndrome are able to conceive without assisted reproductive techniques (ART). Individuals with Klinefelter's syndrome may have varying degrees of hypogonadism with associated low levels of testosterone and in some cases azoospermia. Androgen therapy may be required manage hypothalamic – pituitary axis dysfunction. Individuals with Klinefelter's syndrome do rarely conceive without the need for ART.

Cystic fibrosis in males is associated with absence of the vas deferens thus leading to azoospermic ejaculate. Women with cystic fibrosis may experience amenorrhoea secondary to malnutrition. Both Klinefelter's syndrome and mild forms of cystic fibrosis may be diagnosed late in life when a couple have been unable to conceive. Both males and females with Down's syndrome may be able to conceive, however fertility is often reduced.

26. A True

    B True

    C False

    D False

    E True

α-Thalassaemia is an autosomal recessive inherited haemoglobinopathy associated with defective synthesis of α-globin chains. The severity of the disease depends on how the number of genes for α-globin that are affected (four genes in total code of α-globin). When only one gene has a deletion an individual is considered an unaffected carrier. When two genes on a single chromosome (or a single gene on two chromosomes) are affected, the individual can be considered to have the α-thalassaemia trait. Those with the trait are typically unaffected, with some individuals affected by mild anaemia. Haemoglobin H disease is caused by deletion of three (of the four) α-globin genes. The minimal production of α chains leads to the excessive formation of tetrameric β-globin chains which have a very high affinity for oxygen and are therefore poor at delivering oxygen to tissues. Haemoglobin H disease is associated with severe anaemia and splenomegaly. The deletion of all four α-globin genes leads to formation of haemoglobin Bart's (due excessive delta tetramers) in the absence of any α-globin formation, with subsequent poor oxygen delivery. Affected fetuses develop hydrops fetalis, with few surviving to delivery. Advances in fetal medicine and in utero blood transfusion may lead to the survival of individuals with a condition that until recently was thought to be incompatible with life.

27. A False

    B True

    C False

    D True

    E False

Fetal circulation involves high venous return from the placenta, maintaining a right to left shunt through the foramen ovale. This enables oxygenated blood to be delivered to the heart and brain. Oxygen saturation of the umbilical vein is approximately 70–80%. Approximately 10% of blood from the pulmonary artery travels to the lungs. Fetal haemoglobin (HbF) is comprised of two α chains and two γ chains. HbF has a higher affinity for oxygen than adult haemoglobin. Ninety per cent of fetal haemoglobin is HbF up until the third trimester, when it begins to be replaced with adult haemoglobin.

Fetal red blood cells are larger than maternal cells, with a shorter life span and lower levels of carbonic anhydrase and 2,3-diphosphoglyceric acid. They have no ABO antigens until after birth.

28. A False

    B True

    C True

    D False

    E True

Creatinine is filtered by the kidneys with no tubular reabsorption. The levels of creatinine in the blood and urine can be used to determine the creatinine clearance rate which gives a value of glomerular filtration rate (GFR), a marker of renal function. The creatinine levels in general reflect the individual's muscle mass. Serum levels of creatinine only tend to rise once there is a significant damage to the nephrons and therefore creatinine is a poor indicator of early renal damage. In pregnancy, creatinine levels tend to decrease and therefore an increase above normal values may indicate significant renal dysfunction. Creatinine clearance is often a more useful measurement of renal function and is calculated by comparing the amount of creatinine in the urine and the blood, giving an overall indication of the GFR.

29. A False

    B False

    C True

    D True

    E True

The filtration fraction describes the ratio of the glomerular filtration to the renal blood flow. It is usually about 20% and represents the volume of fluid reaching the renal tubules. Filtration fraction of the kidneys only falls at the beginning of pregnancy, with the amount of sodium filtered by the kidneys remaining unchanged.

During pregnancy the kidneys do increase in size and generally increase in length by approximately 1 cm. The ureters dilate as a result of the effect of progesterone and the increasing weight of a gravid uterus.

The dilation of the ureters is one reason why urinary tract infections are increasingly common in pregnancy and symptoms may be more subtle.

At term, both the renal blood flow and the glomerular filtration rate are significantly increased, by up to 50%.

30. A False

   B False

   C True

   D False

   E True

Progesterone-only contraceptives are now widely used and may be taken in tablet form, intradermally or as a levonorgestrel-releasing intrauterine system. Although referred to as containing 'progesterone' they actually contain synthetic analogues of progesterone and more accurately should be described as 'progestogen-only contraceptives'.

The usage of continuous progesterone analogues provides reliable contraception; however, this success is not based on the reliable prevention of ovulation and overall only around 60% of cycles will be anovulatory. Much of its effect comes from increased viscosity of cervical mucus that is associated with high levels of progesterone. Thick cervical mucus prevents passage of sperm and therefore acts as a barrier to conception. These changes in cervical mucus last only for around 20 hours after administration and therefore influence the need to take the progesterone-only pill within a short time window, every 24 hours.

Under the influence of constantly raised levels of progesterone the endometrium remains thin, further creating a hostile environment for any potential embryo implantation. Unlike the combined oral pill, the uptake of this form of contraception is not influenced by normal bowel flora so it is not affected by concomitant use of antibiotics. As progesterone-only contraceptives do not contain oestrogens they are not associated with any detrimental effects on breastfeeding.

Faculty of Sexual Health & Reproductive Healthcare, Royal College of Obstetricians and Gynaecologists. Clinical Guidance: Progestogen-only Pills. London: FSRH, 2009.

31. C Pyramidalis

Pyramidalis is a triangular muscle which lies within the rectus sheath in front of the rectus abdominis. It is absent in 20% of people and is supplied by the subcostal nerve. The subcostal nerve is the anterior branch of the 12th thoracic nerve. It communicates with the iliohypogastric nerve and gives a branch to pyramidalis. It gives off a lateral cutaneous nerve supplying sensory innervation to the skin over the hip.

32. B Iliacus

Iliacus is separated from extraperitoneal tissue by the iliac fascia. It has a wide peripheral attachment to the iliac crest which it shares with the psoas muscle and descends to leave the abdomen behind the inguinal ligament. The iliacus muscle has innervation from the femoral nerve and lumbar plexus. The iliacus and psoas muscles act in synergy to flex the hip joint.

33. A External oblique

The external oblique arises from the outer surface and lower borders of the eight lowest ribs, passing downwards and backwards. The aponeurosis forms part of the inguinal ligament (see Figure 1.9).

34. D Superior epigastric artery

The superior epigastric artery is a terminal branch of the internal thoracic artery and forms an anastomosis with the inferior epigastric artery. It pierces the rectus sheath and anastomoses with the inferior epigastric artery at the level of the umbilicus. It supplies the anterior part of the abdominal wall and some of the diaphragm. It has a corresponding vein, the superior epigastric vein.

35. C Superior gluteal artery

The superior gluteal artery is one of three branches of the posterior division of the internal iliac artery, the other two being the iliolumbar and the lateral sacral arteries. The superior vesical artery continues as the obliterated umbilical artery after supplying the lower ureter and upper bladder. The uterine artery runs medially on levator ani, in front of the ureter and above the lateral vaginal fornix. Once it has supplied the ureteric and vaginal branches it ascends the side of the uterus to anastomose with the ovarian artery.

36. E L2 and L3

The lateral cutaneous nerve of the thigh is a cutaneous nerve originating from the lumbar plexus. It arises from the dorsal division of L2 and L3. It emerges laterally on the psoas muscle and after crossing the iliacus muscle, passes under the inguinal ligament and divides into anterior and posterior branches.

37. C Pelvic splanchnic nerves

Pelvic splanchnic nerves are autonomic nerves that arise from the ventral rami of S2–S4, providing parasympathetic innervation. This parasympathetic outflow supplies part of the gut, bladder, genitals and blood vessels in the pelvis, releasing acetylcholine at its terminals. They also carry visceral afferent fibres. The pelvic splanchnic nerves communicate with the inferior hypogastric plexus located at each side of the rectum and vagina. From here the nerves are distributed locally and up through the inferior hypogastric nerve and superior hypogastric plexus. Afferent fibres from the cervix travel within the pelvic splanchnic nerves to the dorsal roots of the upper sacral nerves.

38. A Columnar epithelium

The uterus is lined by endometrium. The endometrium consists of a single layer of columnar epithelial cells which rest on a layer of connective tissue (stroma). Secretory glands and spiral arteries extend from the surface of the endometrium to the base of the stroma.

39. D Stratified squamous epithelium

The urethra originates from endoderm and arises from the pelvic part of the urogenital sinus. The proximal half of the urethra is lined with transitional epithelium and the distal half is lined with stratified squamous epithelium.

40. D Round ligament

The uterosacral ligaments extend from the posterior cervix to the sacrum. As they pull the cervix backwards, they help to hold the uterus in an anteverted position, as well as providing support for the uterus and vagina. The round ligament is approximately 12 cm long and runs from the body of the uterus in front of and below the insertion of the fallopian tube to the internal inguinal ring. It traverses the inguinal canal and exits from the external inguinal ring, breaking up into strands at the labium majus. In the fetus the round ligament is surrounded by a peritoneal tube, the processus vaginalis. This is usually obliterated at birth, however, it occasionally persists and if this is the case it can be a site for hernia development. The broad ligament is a double fold of peritoneum, providing no role in the support of the uterus.

41. D Middle rectal artery

Contents of the ischiorectal fossa include:

- Inferior rectal nerve and vessels
- Pudendal canal and its contents
- Fat pad
- Perforating cutaneous branch of S2 and S3
- Perineal branch of S4
- Labial nerve and vein

42. A Above pectinate line: derived endoderm, superior rectal artery

The pectinate line lies at the junction of the upper two-thirds and the lower one-third of the anal canal. Embryologically this represents the junction of the hindgut and the proctodeum (**Table 15.1**).

Table 15.1 Anatomy and embryology of the anal canal		
	Above pectinate line	**Below pectinate line**
Epithelium	Columnar	Stratified squamous
Embryological origin	Endoderm	Ectoderm
Artery	Superior rectal artery	Middle and inferior rectal artery
Vein	Superior rectal vein	Middle and inferior rectal vein
Nerves	Inferior hypogastric plexus	Inferior rectal nerves

43. A Lateral wall of ischiorectal fossa; above sacrotuberous ligament

The pudendal canal is a tunnel of fascia which runs in the lower lateral wall of the ischiorectal fossa, just above the sacrotuberous ligament. It contains the pudendal nerve and the internal pudendal vessels. During a pudendal block, the pudendal nerve is infiltrated where it crosses the ischial spine. It is reached through the vagina and infiltrated medial to the ischial spine.

44. D Stratified squamous

The female urethra is lined by transitional epithelium proximal to the bladder and by stratified squamous epithelium in its distal portion. It is endodermal in origin from the urogenital sinus. It takes its blood supply from the inferior vesical artery and the internal pudendal artery with drainage to the vesical plexus. Lymphatic drainage is to the internal iliac lymph nodes.

45. B T7–T12

The rectus abdominis muscle originates at the pubis muscle and has its insertion into the costal cartilages of the 5th, 6th and 7th ribs and the sternum. It is contained within the rectus sheath which is made up of the aponeuroses of the external and internal oblique muscle and the transversus abdominis muscle. The external oblique is the most superficial aponeurosis to make up the rectus sheath and has the internal oblique beneath it to keep it separate from the rectus muscle. It is supplied by the inferior epigastric artery and has its nerve supply from the thoracoabdominal nerves, T7–T12.

46. D Rickets

This 4-year-old boy is suffering from rickets, which is caused by failure or delay to mineralise endochondral bone in the growth plate. The main cause is impaired metabolism or deficiency of vitamin D. His mother is complaining of premenstrual symptoms, combined with bony pain. These are symptoms of vitamin D deficiency in adults. Treatment for both of these patients would be to ensure adequate sunlight exposure and prescribe Vitamin D supplements. Vitamin D is required for adequate absorption of calcium and is synthesised in the skin following sunlight exposure and from the kidney.

Osteopetrosis, also known as marble bone disease, is caused by a deficiency of osteoclasts. There is hardening of the bones and an elevation in levels of alkaline phosphatase. Perthes' disease is a disease of the hip joint, caused by avascular necrosis of the femoral head and a reduction in blood supply. Scurvy is caused by a lack of vitamin C and symptoms may include gum disease, easy bruising and myalgia.

47. C Multiple myeloma

Multiple myeloma is a neoplastic expansion of plasma cells within the blood, with an incidence of 5/100,000. Proliferation of plasma cells interferes with normal production of blood cells within the bone marrow, resulting in anaemia, leucopenia and thrombocytopaenia. Presentation of this condition includes bone pain, pathological fractures and renal failure. Diagnosis is via electrophoresis of serum and/or urine, identifying a monoclonal paraprotein. Bence Jones proteins (immunoglobulin light chains) may be identified in the urine. Patients develop hypercalcaemia due to excessive tumour-induced osteoclast-mediated bone destruction, caused by cytokines expressed or secreted locally at myeloma cells. This leads to an efflux of calcium into extracellular fluid. Treatment is supportive, with correction of renal failure and hypercalcaemia.

48. B Hyperglycaemia

A glucagonoma is a tumour of the α cells of the pancreas. It is associated with excessive production of glucagon. Glucagon can be thought of as acting in opposition to insulin, therefore raising serum glucose levels through gluconeogenesis and lipolysis. This rare tumour is characterised by a state of extreme hyperglycaemia due to excessive levels of glucagon. Other manifestations include a characteristic rash and anaemia. Although incredibly rare, this tumour is more common in perimenopausal and postmenopausal women.

49. D pH 7.50, pCO_2 3.0 kPa, pO_2 9.2 kPa, HCO_3 25 mmol/L

This patient has an acute pulmonary embolus (PE). PE is a relatively common postoperative complication and clinical presentation includes chest pain, dyspnoea and haemoptysis. Signs and symptoms in this case are the acute dyspnoea and pain on inspiration. The low oxygen saturations and tachycardia would also be found in patients with acute PE. It usually occurs when thrombosis from a more distal vein breaks loose and embolises into pulmonary blood vessels. The arterial blood gas in a patient with a PE most commonly shows respiratory alkalosis. The low partial pressure of carbon dioxide is most likely caused by hyperventilation. In cases of massive PE, the infarcted or non-functioning areas of the lung may lead to increased pCO_2 values. Hypoxaemia occurs due to altered areas of perfusion and ventilation of the lung tissue (VQ mismatch). Although a pH of 7.2 is reasonable, this patient is extremely unlikely to have a pO_2 of 12.0 kPa, given oxygen saturation of 93%.

50. A pH 7.16, pCO$_2$ 8.2 kPa, pO$_2$ 15.3 kPa, HCO$_3$ 21.2 mmol/L

This patient has central respiratory depression due to opiate overdose. Fatty liver of pregnancy may be associated with an acid-base abnormality if it is severe. Symptoms include fatigue, nausea and vomiting, and upper abdominal pain, usually in the third trimester. The pattern on arterial blood gas usually shows a mixed metabolic and respiratory acidosis, reflected in the degree of acidosis.

The Henderson–Hasselbach equation describes the relationship of pH as a measure of acidity.

$$pH = pK_a + \log \frac{[A\text{-}]}{[HA]}$$

Where pK$_a$ is the acid dissociation constant.

51. A High blood levels of fatty acids

There are profound changes in the metabolism of fat during episodes of diabetic ketoacidosis. There are high blood levels of fatty acids and lactate. Blood pH may drop to below 7.0 and the kidney excretes hydrogen ions to compensate. The state of metabolic acidosis causes an activation of chemoreceptors in the brain which subsequently leads to hyperventilation. Patients are usually severely dehydrated due to a state of osmotic diuresis and hyperglycaemia. They are often hypoxic. Diabetic ketoacidosis is a medical emergency and should be treated promptly. Treatment involves controlled replacement of fluids, including correction of electrolyte imbalance. A sliding scale should also be in place until normal glucose control can be initiated.

52. A Prostacyclin PGI2

All of the options given are either prostaglandins, thromboxanes or prostacyclins. Classified together as prostanoids, which are a form of eicosanoids, these fatty acid derivatives are all formed from the conversion of arachidonic acid via the action of cyclooxygenase (COX). Prostacyclin PGI2 is formed from the conversion of arachidonic acid to prostaglandin H2 which is then converted to its final form by the action of prostacyclin synthase. Released by endothelial cells, prostacyclin PGI2 acts predominantly to inhibit platelet aggregation via activation of G-protein coupled receptors on the platelet surface, leading to production of cyclic adenosine monophosphate with subsequent inhibition of platelet activation. Prostcyclin PGI2 also acts as a vasodilator. Thromboxane TXA2 is a prothrombotic which is produced by activated platelets, which acts to promote platelet activation and vasoconstriction.

53. B Ampulla of the fallopian tube

The ovum is carried from the ovary into the fallopian tube following ovulation. It is picked up by the fimbriae and carried into the tube. Inside the fallopian tube the ovum is moved medially by the action of cilia lining the tube and muscular action. The ovum is halted at the fallopian ampulla for up to 36 hours and therefore fertilisation occurs at this location most frequently.

54. B Vitellointestinal duct

Meckel's diverticulum is an abnormality of the midgut. It occurs in 2–4% of the population and is a common anomaly of the digestive system. It is more common in males than females and is a persistence of the vitellointestinal duct. The vitellointestinal duct is present in early embryonic life and its function is to provide nutrition to the yolk sac. It usually regresses by the 7th week. A Meckel diverticulum is a blind ending tube and contains all the layers of gut that are present in the ileum. It is located approximately 50–60 cm from the ileocaecal valve. If this remnant becomes inflamed, it may produce a condition with a similar presentation to appendicitis. The mucosa is gastric in origin and may therefore produce gastric acid which may lead to ulceration and bleeding.

55. D Prostate

The mesonephric duct ultimately gives rise to several parts of the male urogenital tract, including the epididymis, the vas deferens and the seminal vesicle. The prostate is not derived from the mesonephric duct and develops from the urogenital sinus.

56. D Shortened Q–T interval and widened T wave on ECG

Hypercalcaemia may cause ECG changes, specifically a shortened QT interval and a widened T wave complex. Hypocalcaemia may lead to many classic signs and symptoms, one of which is a prolonged Q–T interval on ECG. Circumoral tingling and numbness, carpopedal spasm and depression are all symptoms of hypocalcaemia. Chvostek's sign may be positive, twitching of the face with tapping of the facial nerve. Trousseau's sign is a carpopedal spasm, which can be induced by inflating a BP cuff around the arm. Calcium levels may be misinterpreted if the albumin levels are abnormal and therefore calculation should always take this into account.

57. D 21α-hydroxylase

Congenital adrenal hyperplasia (CAH) is an autosomal recessive disorder which occurs as a result of a defect in the pathway of steroidogenesis in the adrenal gland. As a result of this, there is cortisol deficiency and increased androgen production. The majority of cases occur as a result in deficiency of the enzyme 21α-hydroxylase. CAH is rare and occurs in approximately 1 in 14,000 births. Presentation of this syndrome may include salt wasting if production of aldosterone is affected and hypoglycaemia may occur. Neonates may have ambiguous genitalia and, despite a 46 XX genotype, may appear male. Diagnosis is made via detection of 17-hydroxyprogesterone levels. It may also be necessary to perform a 24-hour urinary steroid analysis.

58. D Phenytoin

Hirsutism is the presence of hair on the body and face that grows in excess. It is usually in a male pattern of growth and is caused by an excess of testosterone. It is associated with polycystic ovarian syndrome and alopecia.

The Ferriman–Gallwey score may be used to grade hirsutism and uses a score of 0–4 ranging from no hair cover (0) to fully hair covered (4) in 9 areas of the body: upper lip, chest, chin, upper abdomen, lower abdomen, upper and lower back, upper arms and thighs. A score above 8 suggests possible androgen excess.

Other drug causes include danazol, progesterones (including the combined oral contraceptive pill), metoclopramide, methyldopa, anabolic steroids, reserpine, testosterone, cyclosporine, minoxidil and diazoxide.

59. B Basophils of the anterior pituitary gland

Thyroid-stimulating hormone (TSH) is produced by the basophils of anterior pituitary gland. High levels of T4 and T3 lead to a reduction in the production of both TSH and thyrotrophin-releasing hormone (TRH) via the feedback loop, as shown in **Figure 15.3**. The same mechanism means that high levels of TSH lead to a reduction in production of TRH. TRH is produced by the paraventricular nucleus of the hypothalamus (**Figure 15.3**).

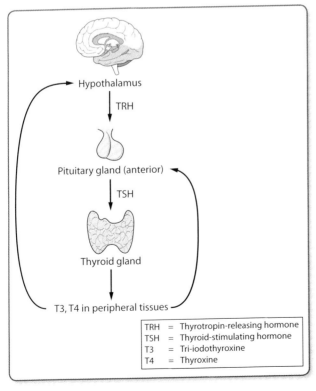

Figure 15.3 Hypothalamic–pituitary axis.

60. E All of the above

Hyperthyroidism produces a range of symptoms that occur as a result of increased production of thyroid hormones. Symptoms include diarrhoea, weight loss, increased appetite, psychosis, heat intolerance, oligomenorrhoea and infertility. In many circumstances, infertility may be how the disease is detected.

The most common cause of hyperthyroidism is Graves' disease, an autoimmune disease caused by thyroid autoantibodies against the TSH receptor.

61. B Bicarbonate

Calcium is essential for the regulation of the nervous and musculoskeletal systems and enzyme and hormone action. Calcium is an important intracellular messenger which has an essential role in the maintenance of cell membrane potential of nerve and cardiac cells and contractile muscle cells. It is absorbed by active transport in the duodenum. Total body calcium is about 1–2 kg with 99% held in the skeleton, 1% intracellular and 0.1% extracellular. Of the extracellular portion, approximately 55% is in the bound form. Most of this calcium is bound to plasma proteins, the majority of which is albumin. Extracellular calcium may also be bound to anions such as phosphate, lactate and bicarbonate.

The remaining extracellular calcium is in the ionised form, which is biologically active. The average level of calcium in plasma is 2.5 mmol/L, however levels range from 2.2–2.6 mmol/L. A level of > 2.6 mmol/L, taking into account corrected levels, would indicate a state of hypercalcaemia. In hypoalbuminaemia, there is less calcium in the bound state and therefore a higher level of total calcium.

62. A Bone metastases

Bone is the third most common site of metastases. Five cancers most frequently metastasising to bone are breast, lung, prostate, thyroid and kidney. Consequences include pain, pathological fractures and hypercalcaemia. Pain results from stretching of the periosteum and stimulation of nerves in the endosteum. Lytic lesions of bones lead to pathological fractures. Multiple myeloma is a cancer of plasma cells. Proliferation of plasma cells interferes with normal production of blood cells within the bone marrow, resulting in anaemia, leucopenia and thrombocytopaenia. Patients develop hypercalcaemia in this condition due to excessive tumour-induced osteoclast-mediated bone destruction, caused by cytokines expressed or secreted locally at myeloma cells. This leads to an efflux of calcium into the extracellular fluid.

63. E PTH acts via a G-protein coupled receptor

Parathyroid hormone (PTH) acts to increase circulating levels of calcium and phosphate. It acts via a G-protein coupled receptor. In the kidney, PTH acts proximally at the renal tubules to increase bicarbonate and phosphate excretion. At the distal renal tubule, calcium and hydrogen are reabsorbed in response to

PTH action. Alpha1-hydroxylation of vitamin D takes place in the kidney and this is enhanced by PTH action. PTH enhances the osteoclastic activity in bone, enhancing bone resorption.

PTH acts on many organ systems:

- **Bone:** increases release of calcium, indirectly stimulates osteoclasts, increased bone resorption.
- **Kidney:** enhances active reabsorption of calcium and magnesium from distal tubules, increases excretion of phosphate
- **Intestine:** increases absorption of calcium by increasing production of vitamin D.

64. A Active transport

Calcium and phosphate are transferred to the fetal circulation against a concentration by active transport. The fetus is relatively hypercalcaemic compared to the mother – 1:1.4 and contains approximately 21–33 g of calcium. Ossification occurs mainly in the third trimester, when the majority of the calcium accumulates. Active transport also facilitates the transfer of substances such as amino acids across the placenta. Substances such as oxygen and carbon dioxide travel via passive diffusion across a concentration gradient, whereas transport molecules aid the transfer of substances such as glucose in the form of facilitated diffusion.

65. A Increased calcitonin

During pregnancy and breastfeeding the female body has an increased requirement for calcium. The fetus is hypercalcaemic compared to the mother and most of the calcium reserve in the fetus is attained during the third trimester. Calcium is transferred to the fetus via active transport and the fetus is able to produce parathyroid hormone at around 12 weeks' gestation. During pregnancy, the mother has a reduced level of parathyroid hormone and an increased level of calcitonin in order to maintain an increased transfer of calcium to the fetus. There is an overall increase in bone turnover during the third trimester.

66. A The number of deaths during the first 28 completed days of life per 1000 live births

The World Health Organisation defines the neonatal mortality rate as the number of deaths during the first 28 completed days of life per 1000 live births in a given year or period. It considers the neonatal period to begin at birth and to carry on until 28 completed days of life. The definition includes babies who have shown any sign of life following delivery, even if this is only for a short period of time.

World Health Organization. Health Status Statistics: Mortality. Neonatal mortality rate (per 1000 live births). http://www.who.int

67. A The proportion of women with a normal pregnancy who had a low-risk result

Specificity of any test refers to its ability to correctly identify those individuals without any pathology so, in this case, it refers to the proportion of women who had a normal pregnancy and were given a correct low-risk result at screening. The specificity of a test should aim to be as high as possible, i.e. as close to 1 or 100% as possible. Similarly the sensitivity of a test should aim to be as close to 1 or 100% as possible. The sensitivity of a test refers its ability to correctly identify affected/high risk individuals. For this test it is the proportion of women with an affected fetus who were given a high-risk result at screening.

68. B 0.2

The standard error of the mean (SEM) is a measure of how close the sample mean lies from the mean of the true population. The larger the sample size (n), the smaller the SEM. Further, the smaller the resultant SEM, the more accurate an estimate the sample mean is of the true population mean. The SEM can be calculated using only the sample size and the standard deviation.

$SEM = \text{Standard deviation} \div \sqrt{n}$

Standard deviation $= 2$, $n = 100$

$SEM = 2 \div \sqrt{100} = 2 \div 10 = 0.2$

69. B Cohort study

The research study described has used a cohort study design. Cohort studies may either have a retrospective or prospective design. Within this design subjects from the exposure group (in this case maternal smoking) and the non-exposure group can be followed-up over a long period of time. This type of study is time-consuming as any differences between the two groups may take a long time to surface. Cohort studies may be subject to bias and confounding variables. They have the potential to provide an immense amount of detail about the study groups over a long period and therefore give the opportunity to realise unexpected outcomes. There is the potential to do retrospective cohort studies, based on hospital notes.

70. B The erroneous rejection of the null hypothesis

In order to understand type 1 and type 2 errors it is essential to understand what is meant by the null hypothesis. The null hypothesis must be defined before any statistical analysis takes place. The standard null hypothesis states that there is no difference between the sample groups being looked at. A type 1 error (also known as an α error) is said to have occurred in a study when the null hypothesis has been wrongly rejected. In simpler terms the study has reported a difference that does not exist.

A type 2 error (also known as a β error) is actually more common than a type 1 error and is said to have occurred when the null hypothesis has been accepted when there is, in fact, a difference between the sample groups being looked at.

71. D Community-acquired Group A streptococcal disease

The 8th report of the Confidential Enquiries into Maternal Deaths in the United Kingdom classified causes of maternal mortality as directly related, indirectly related or unrelated to pregnancy. Directly related causes of maternal mortality are those that result from obstetric complications. In the options A to E, the only cause directly related to pregnancy is community-acquired group A streptococcal disease. Genital tract sepsis, predominantly due to group A streptococcal disease, was given as the leading direct cause of maternal death in the report, and its incidence had increased since the previous triennial report. Causes of death that are indirectly related to pregnancy are those that are not caused by obstetric complications but were made worse by the physiological changes associated with pregnancy. These indirectly related causes may include conditions that were pre-existing or were diagnosed during pregnancy.

Within the UK, suicide is included as one of the indirectly related causes of maternal death because it is usually the result of puerperal psychosis. Other indirect causes include cardiac disease, diabetes and hormone-dependent cancers.

Centre for Maternal and Child Enquiries (CMACE). Saving Mothers' Lives: reviewing maternal deaths to make motherhood safer: 2006–2008. The Eighth Report on Confidential Enquiries into Maternal Deaths in the United Kingdom. BJOG 2011;118:1–203.

72. B The median is the middle value in ranked set of data

The median is one of the terms used to describe an 'average' of a set of data. The median is the middle value in a ranked data set. It should not be confused with the mode which refers to the most frequently occurring value in a data set. It also differs from the mean which is calculated by dividing the sum of a data set by the number of values in the data set. An advantage of using the median is that it is not influenced by outliers or skewed data, which can affect the mean of a data set. The median figure in a data set may be higher or lower than the mean.

73. D Patau's syndrome

Patau's syndrome is also known as trisomy 13. This condition is rarer than trisomy 18 or trisomy 21. Patau's syndrome occurs when there is an extra copy of chromosome 13. This extra chromosome usually arises after a non-disjunction event during meiosis, however it can also occur due a Robertsonian translocation. More rarely an individual may be mosaic for trisomy 13, i.e. only some of their cells will be trisomy 13, whereas other cells have a normal complement of chromosomes.

High-risk antenatal screening results may be suggestive of a trisomy, and can be confirmed by subsequent invasive testing, such as amniocentesis. An affected fetus generally has multiple organ system defects. Common abnormalities include microcephaly, polydactyly, bilateral cleft palate and cardiac defects. The majority of babies born with Patau's syndrome die in the first month of life. Few children survive infancy.

74. E 47 XXY

This boy has Klinefelter's syndrome, which is a relatively common disorder of the sex chromosomes. Around 1 in every 1000 male babies born have Klinefelter's syndrome. Affected individuals typically have the genotype 47 XXY, indicating that they have an extra X chromosome. This extra chromosome is present due a non-disjunction event in either spermatogenesis or oogenesis. Physical features associated with Klinefelter's syndrome include above average height, long arms and legs, gynaecomastia, a female body fat distribution and varying development of secondary sexual characteristics. Undiagnosed individuals typically present due to concern regarding gynaecomastia or unexplained infertility. Historically, individuals with Klinefelter's syndrome have been described as experiencing higher levels of behavioural difficulties and having lower IQs than average, although these stereotypes are probably unjustified.

75. D Mosaic for Down's syndrome

The karyotype given informs us that some of the fetus' cells are of the karyotype 46 XX, whereas other cells detected have an extra chromosome 21 and therefore contain 47 chromosomes (hence described as 47 XX + 21). This unusual finding is called mosaicism and refers to the existence of two different cell lines within an individual, each with a different number of chromosomes. Most commonly mosaicism is caused by a non-disjunction event which occurs during an early embryonic mitotic division and leaves some cells with an uneven number of chromosomes; i.e. some cells have a trisomy, whereas others have a normal number of chromosomes. The presence of mosaicism in fetuses is diagnosed by amniocentesis or chorionic villi sampling with analysis typically describing the percentage of cells with a normal karyotype versus those of a different cell line. Mosaicism is only found in 1% of cases of Down's syndrome. As the proportion of cells with trisomy 21 varies it is difficult to predict to what extent the individual will be affected.

76. D Marfan's syndrome

Marfan's syndrome is a connective tissue disorder is caused by a mutation in the FBN1 gene found on chromosome 15 that codes for the protein fibrillin-1. It is an autosomal dominant condition, however in some affected individuals the gene mutation has occurred de novo. The individual described has the characteristic appearance of someone with Marfan's syndrome. In addition to tall stature, long arms and digits, people with Marfan's syndrome may also have scoliosis and deformities of the chest wall. This individual has known aortic root dilation, a common finding in many affected individuals. Other cardiac sequelae include aortic dissection and mitral valve prolapse.

Congenital contractual arachnodactyly is an autosomal dominant condition causing skeletal abnormalities as a consequence of a mutation of the protein fibrillin-2. Ehlers–Danlos syndrome refers to heterogenous group of disorders associated with defects in collagen synthesis, the classical form of which is an autosomal dominant inherited condition.

77. E Leber's optic neuropathy

The mitochondria contain their own DNA (mtDNA) which is transmitted from a mother to her children. In humans there are 37 genes contained within mitochondrial DNA. Although both male and female offspring may be affected by any inherited mutations in mtDNA, only females can pass these defects onto the next generation. Leber's optic neuropathy is transmitted by mitochondrial inheritance. As mitochondria are key to cellular oxidative phosphorylation, mutations in mitochondrial DNA tend to manifest in systems heavily reliant on this process. Hence mitochondrial disease tends to manifest as a myopathy. Leber's optic neuropathy is one such condition and is caused by three known mutations of mitochondrial DNA. Colour blindness and Duchenne muscular dystrophy are both X-linked recessive conditions. Dermatomyositis is an autoimmune connective tissue disease. Alpha-thalassaemia is an autosomal recessive condition.

78. A Angelman's syndrome

Genomic imprinting refers to the loss of the either a maternal or paternal allele. It is known that maternally and paternally derived alleles are not the same and there can be devastating results if an allele is inactivated. Both Angelman's syndrome and Prader–Willi syndrome are examples of genomic imprinting with deleterious effects. In Angelman's syndrome there is loss of area of the long arm of the maternally derived chromosome 15, whereas Prader–Willi syndrome is caused by loss of the same area of the paternally derived chromosome. The syndromes are distinct but both are associated with mental retardation. It is of note that genomic imprinting (i.e. the inactivation of one parent's copy of a gene) does occur naturally without harmful effect. Both Fragile-X syndrome and Friedreich ataxia are examples of trinucleotide repeat disorders. Patau's syndrome is caused by trisomy of chromosome 13.

79. C Oxytocin

As well as transporting molecules between the mother and the fetus, the placenta functions as an important endocrine organ during pregnancy. It synthesises and secretes many hormones which function to maintain and support the pregnancy.

It synthesises and secretes two major types of hormones: steroid hormones (progesterone and oestrogen) and protein hormones [human chorionic gonadotropin (hCG), relaxin and human placental lactogen].

The syncytiotrophoblast cells of the placenta secrete hCG, progesterone and oestrogen. The placental lactogens are thought to be involved in mobilising energy stores for the fetus. Relaxin works synergistically with progesterone in maintaining the pregnancy.

Oxytocin is secreted by the posterior pituitary gland and is not produced by the placenta.

80. D Umbilical arteries arise from the internal iliac artery

The umbilical cord contains three vessels: two arteries and one vein. These vessels are contained in Wharton's jelly. The cord is formed at 5 weeks' gestation and at term has a mean length of 50 cm and width of 2 cm. The umbilical arteries arise from the internal iliac artery and the veins drain mainly into the inferior vena cava (80%) via the ductus venosus and 20% into the hepatic vein. One per cent of umbilical cords have a single artery and of this 1%, 20% will have a cardiovascular abnormality. Other abnormalities of the cord include knots which may be false or true. False knots are unusual vascular structures and true knots are more common in longer cords. Velamentous cord insertion describes the situation, where the umbilical cord inserts into the chorioamniotic membranes rather than the mass of the placenta. These vessels are therefore not protected in part by Wharton's jelly. This is associated with vasa praevia.

81. A Active transport: amino acids

The placenta supplies the growing fetus with both oxygen and nutrients, as well as providing a means for the removal of carbon dioxide and other waste products and metabolites. The movement of these substances is largely dictated by their size and occurs through passive diffusion, active transport and facilitated diffusion, in addition to exocytosis and endocytosis.

Transport across the placenta:

- **Passive diffusion**: oxygen, carbon dioxide, free fatty acids, urea
- **Active transport**: amino acids
- **Facilitated diffusion**: glucose
- **Receptor mediated endocytosis**: IgG

82. E Vasodilation

Oestrogen exerts a series of effects, both at local and systemic levels. Oestrogen promotes vascular tone, leading to vasodilation, with both rapid and chronic effect. There are two oestrogen receptors: α and β. The α-receptor is found on the endothelial cell membrane and directly activates nitric oxide. Oestrogen is involved in other systemic changes, e.g. it helps maintain bone density levels, increases clotting and decreases cholesterol and low-density lipoprotein levels. Other properties include protection against atherosclerosis.

83. B It contains 154 mmol/L sodium chloride

Normal saline is a commonly used for intravenous fluid replacement; however, the physiology associated with its use is important.

0.9% normal saline is a crystalloid solution and contains 154 mmol/L sodium chloride. It has an osmolarity of 308 mOsmol/L and does not contain any potassium chloride. There is, however, the capacity to add potassium chloride to the fluid if there is an indication to replace these electrolytes, e.g. gastric loss. It mainly replaces the extracellular fluid component of body water and only a quarter of the volume replaced will make it into the plasma.

Colloids are better volume expanders than crystalloid fluids as they remain in the intravascular compartment for a longer period.

Postoperatively, there is a sympathoadrenal stress response. This may lead to an increase in the retention of sodium and water as a result of increased antidiuretic hormone secretion and therefore the use of saline may not be the most appropriate fluid to use.

84. B The fetus loses metabolites to the mother

The Bohr effect describes a situation where an increase in carbon dioxide in the blood and a decrease in pH leads to a reduction in the affinity for oxygen.

The double Bohr effect refers to the situation in the maternal–fetal circulation where the Bohr effect is operative on both sides. This improves the oxygen transfer between mother and fetus.

Maternal:

- Reduced maternal pH
- Oxygen curve shift to right
- Reduced affinity to oxygen
- Uptake of fetal metabolites

Fetal:

- Increased fetal pH
- Oxygen curve shift to left
- Increased affinity to oxygen
- Loss of metabolites to maternal circulation

Heining M. Chapter 7: Fluid and Acid-Base Balance. In: Fiander A, Thilganathan B (eds). Your Essential Revision Guide MRCOG Part 1. London: RCOG Press, 2010.

85. C Two alpha chains and two gamma chains ($\alpha_2\gamma_2$)

Fetal haemoglobin (HbF) is the predominant form of haemoglobin present in fetal life and consists of four chains, α_2 and γ_2. HbF replaces embryonic haemoglobin after around 10 weeks' gestation and is present in high levels throughout gestation. Adult haemoglobin (HbA) has α_2 chains and two β_2 chains. HbA is also present in small amounts from the first trimester, but production starts to increase in the third trimester in preparation of ex-utero life. At birth HbF represents at least 50% of the haemoglobin present, but by 6 months of age this has been replaced by adult haemoglobin. Unlike adult haemoglobin, HbF does not bind with 2,3-diphosphoglycerate (2,3-DPG). As a consequence HbF has a higher affinity for oxygen than adult haemoglobin, allowing oxygen to dissociate from maternal haemoglobin and be transferred to the fetal circulation across the placenta. With a higher affinity for oxygen than adult haemoglobin, the dissociation curve for HbF sits to the left of that of adult haemoglobin. The dissociation curve illustrates that with its higher affinity for oxygen HbF becomes saturated with oxygen at lower partial pressures than HbA.

86. B Luteinising hormone

The luteinising hormone surge (LH) instigates the series of steps that lead to ovulation. During the follicular phase of the menstrual cycle the level of LH slowly increases. The dominant follicle expresses LH receptors leading to increasing amounts of oestradiol production by the theca cells (due to the conversion of cholesterol). This elevated level of oestrogen instigates a positive feedback response by LH with a subsequent surge at around day 14. This surge leads to the extrusion of the oocyte from the follicle. After release of the oocyte LH supports the corpus luteum, formed from the disrupted granulosa and thecal cells, to produce progesterone and oestradiol.

87. D At fertilisation

Oogenesis is the process where an ovum is formed in females from primordial germ cells. The primordial germ cells develop in the fetal gonadal tissue which eventually becomes the fetal ovary. Here these primordial germ cells become oogonia. The oogonia undergo division by mitosis, rapidly increasing in number to form several million oogonia by the second trimester of fetal life. Oogonia then become primary oocytes through mitosis. Surrounded by primordial follicles the primary oocytes are diploid; they begin meiosis 1 during the third trimester of pregnancy, and this is arrested at prophase. They remain in this state until ovulation many years later. At ovulation, meiosis 1 recommences leading to the production of the secondary oocyte and the first polar body. The secondary oocyte is haploid and immediately after meiosis 1 is completed enters meiosis 2. This second meiotic division becomes halted at metaphase II. The second meiotic division, leading to the production of a mature ovum and the second polar body, is only completed should fertilisation occur.

88. B Inferior vena cava

The ductus venosus acts as one of the three fetal circulatory shunts, in addition to the ductus arteriosus and the foramen ovale. The ductus venosus is the blood vessel that runs from the umbilical vein and communicates with the inferior vena cava (IVC). This shunt allows much of the fetal oxygenated blood supply to bypass the liver, with preferential distribution to the brain. The ductus venosus starts to close soon after birth. In adults the remnant of the ductus venosus is known as the ligamentum venosum. The fetal umbilical vein eventually becomes the ligamentum teres. The passage between the fetal left and right atria is known as the foramen ovale. Blood passes through the foramen ovale from the right atria to the left atria. The foramen ovale closes soon after birth and eventually becomes the fossa ovalis. Failure of the foramen ovale to close is not uncommon and in the majority of individuals the persistence of this shunt remains undiagnosed. It has been suggested that a patent foramen ovale may be associated with unexplained transient ischaemic events and migraines.

89. D Superior gluteal artery

The internal iliac artery is the main artery of the pelvic organs and also the perineum. The internal iliac artery begins at the bifurcation of the common iliac artery. It then divides into anterior and posterior branches. The branches of the anterior division of the internal iliac artery predominantly supply the pelvic organs, i.e. the uterus, vagina, bladder, lower part of the rectum as well as several muscles of the buttocks. The superior gluteal artery is a branch of the posterior division of the internal iliac artery (**Tables 15.2** and **15.3**). Note the ovaries are supplied by the ovarian artery which is a branch of the abdominal aorta.

Table 15.2 Major branches of the internal iliac artery	
Artery	**Female organs and muscles supplied**
Umbilical	Superior part of urinary bladder
Obturator	Femoral head, ilium, muscles of medial thigh, pelvic muscles
Uterine	Uterus, fallopian tubes, vagina, uterine ligaments
Internal pudendal	Perineum, anal canal, external genitalia
Middle rectal	Lower part of rectum
Inferior gluteal	Pelvic diaphragm

Table 15.3 Major branches of the posterior iliac artery

Artery	Organ
Iliolumbar	Muscles of posterior abdominal walls, i.e. quadrates lumborum, iliacus and psoas major
	Cauda equina
Lateral sacral arteries (superior and inferior)	Piriformis, erector spinae, sacral canal
Superior gluteal	Gluteus minimus
	Gluteus maximus
	Gluteus medius
	Tensor fascia lata
	Piriformis

90. B Iliacus

The iliacus muscle does not form part of the anterior abdominal wall and is innervated by the femoral nerve.

The anterior abdominal wall provides support for the internal structures. The muscles of the anterior abdominal wall are:

- Rectus abdominis – from costal cartilages to the pubic crest
- Pyramidalis – may be absent (1 in 5 individuals), lies anterior to lower fibres of rectus abdominis
- External oblique – runs downwards and forwards from large insertion from lower 8th ribs
- Internal oblique – runs opposite to the external oblique, upwards and forwards from anterior iliac crest and inguinal ligament

Mock paper 2

The 30 multiple choice questions and 60 single best answers presented in this chapter should be worked through under exam conditions, and completed in two and a half hours.

Questions: MCQs

Answer each stem 'True' or 'False'.

1. **Heparin:**
   A Low-molecular weight heparin has a shorter half-life than unfractionated heparin
   B Action is measured using the activated partial thromboplastin time
   C Is reversed with protamine
   D Can cause bleeding in the fetus
   E Can cause hypoaldosteronism

2. **Placenta and drugs:**
   A Insulin crosses the placenta
   B The rate of diffusion is dependent on the thickness of the membrane
   C Lipophilic molecules readily diffuse across the placenta
   D Pethidine is freely diffusible across the membrane
   E Benzodiazepines consumed by the mother do not pass into fetal circulation

3. **Danazol:**
   A Is used as a treatment for endometriosis
   B Is a gonadotrophin agonist
   C Can cause osteoporosis
   D Inhibits ovarian steroidogenesis
   E Can cause clitoral hypertrophy

4. **The following are antimetabolites:**
   A Cisplatin
   B Cyclophosphamide
   C 5-fluorouracil
   D Methotrexate
   E Mercaptopurine

5. **The following are probe movements used in transabdominal ultrasound scanning:**
   A Angle
   B Dip

    C   Rotate

    D   Slide

    E   Tilt and tip

6. **Concerning magnetic resonance imaging (MRI):**

    A   MRI uses ionising radiation

    B   In T1-weighted MRI water-containing tissues appear bright

    C   In T2-weighted MRI bone appears dark

    D   The Tesla is the international system unit used to denote magnetic field strength

    E   The presence of cardiac pacemaker is a relative contraindication to MRI

7. **Dual energy X-ray absorptiometry:**

    A   Is used to estimate bone density

    B   Uses ultrasound

    C   Osteoporosis is diagnosed with a Z score of less than –2.5

    D   Can be used to detect malignancy

    E   Can be used in children

8. **Risk factors for placenta praevia include:**

    A   Smoking

    B   Previous caesarean section

    C   Past history of endometriosis

    D   Assisted conception

    E   Multiple pregnancy

9. **Laparoscopic injuries:**

    A   Serious complications occur in 1 in 1000 cases

    B   Usually occur before visualisation of the peritoneal cavity

    C   It is easier to diagnose bowel injury than bladder injury

    D   Intra-abdominal pressures of 5–10 mmHg should be used for gas insufflation for insertion of the primary trochar

    E   Direct trochar insertion is an acceptable technique

10. **Causes of a severe headache in pregnancy include:**

    A   Subarachnoid haemorrhage

    B   Pre-eclampsia

    C   Sagittal venous thrombosis

    D   Migraine

    E   Meningitis

11. **Regarding chickenpox exposure in pregnancy:**

    A   Children with chickenpox are only infectious once the rash appears

    B   The majority of women in the UK should be vaccinated at the time of their first midwife's appointment

    C   Shingles in the thoracolumbar region is highly contagious

    D   Varicella zoster immune globulin administration is safe in the first trimester of pregnancy

    E   There is increased risk of respiratory sequelae

12. **With regard to polycystic ovary syndrome:**
    A   Sex hormone binding globulin decreases
    B   Insulin increases
    C   Testosterone decreases
    D   Follicle-stimulating hormone:luteinising hormone ratio increases
    E   Oestradiol increases

13. **With regard to thyroid disease in pregnancy:**
    A   Human chorionic gonadotrophin is thyrotropic
    B   Thyrotoxicosis occurs in approximately 1 in 200 pregnancies
    C   Altered thyroid function can be present with hyperemesis gravidarum
    D   Thyroid-stimulating hormone levels increase in third trimester
    E   The presence of thyroid autoantibodies confirms hypothyroidism

14. **Regarding parvovirus B19:**
    A   Seropositivity for parvovirus B19 IgG antibodies suggests immunity
    B   Incubation period is 4–20 days
    C   The virus mainly affects lymphocytes
    D   Diagnosis is via virus-specific IgA in the serum
    E   Can result in hydrops fetalis

15. **Regarding type I hypersensitivity reactions:**
    A   The antigen is presented by major histocompatibility complex class I
        molecules
    B   CD4$^+$ Th2 cells induce class switching of antigen specific B cells
    C   IgE antibodies are produced on first contact with the antigen
    D   Prostaglandins cause bronchial relaxation
    E   Histamine contracts smooth muscle

16. **Regarding human leucocyte antigen (HLA) class 1 antigen:**
    A   They are expressed on most nucleated cells
    B   They are composed of two light chains
    C   They are essential for viral antigen recognition by cytotoxic cells
    D   The genes for HLA class 1 molecules are located on chromosome 6 and 15
    E   CD8$^+$ cells only recognise antigen presented with HLA class II molecules

17. **Concerning cytokines:**
    A   Interferons inhibit viral replication
    B   IL-2 is produced by B cells
    C   Tumour necrosis factor (TNF)-α inhibits macrophages
    D   TNF induces production of nitric oxide
    E   IL-4 has an active role in B cell class switch to IgE

18. *Actinomyces israelii*:
    A   Is a Gram-positive rod
    B   Is a mouth commensal
    C   Is an obligate aerobe

    D   Produces sulphur granules

    E   Can lead to granuloma formation

19. **The following are risk factors for the transmission of Group B streptococcal infection to the neonate:**

    A   Artificial rupture of membranes

    B   Birth prior to 37 weeks' gestation

    C   Fetal blood sampling

    D   Instrumental delivery

    E   Rupture of membranes for longer than 12 hours

20. **Necrotising fasciitis:**

    A   Is an infection of subcutaneous tissue

    B   Is unresponsive to broad-spectrum antimicrobials

    C   Can lead to toxic shock syndrome

    D   Type 1 has polymicrobial origins

    E   Type 2 is caused by Group B streptococcal infection

21. **Regarding viruses:**

    A   HIV is a lentivirus

    B   Hepatitis B is a hepadnavirus

    C   Parvovirus B19 is an RNA virus

    D   The Epstein–Barr virus is a member of the herpes family

    E   The HIV virus consists of double-stranded RNA

22. **Regarding varicella zoster and pregnancy:**

    A   An episode of maternal shingles at the time of delivery does not cause neonatal infection

    B   Exposure is a risk factor for first trimester miscarriage

    C   Fetal varicella syndrome is the result of acute infection

    D   Fetal varicella syndrome can cause chorioretinitis

    E   Diagnosis of fetal infection should be made by amniocentesis

23. **Regarding the rubella virus:**

    A   Is a herpes virus

    B   Is single-stranded RNA virus

    C   Has an incubation period of 2–3 weeks

    D   Is successfully treated with antiviral drugs

    E   Vaccination is recommended in pregnancy if no immunity is detected

24. **Regarding the presence of an imperforate hymen:**

    A   It has a familial inheritance

    B   It can present with amenorrhoea

    C   It can present with an abdominal mass

    D   It occurs in up to 1% of infant girls

    E   The hymen originates embryologically from the urogenital sinus

25. **Placenta accreta:**

   A   Is a risk factor for postpartum haemorrhage
   B   Is invasion by the placenta through the myometrium
   C   Can be caused by Asherman's syndrome
   D   Can be easily diagnosed by ultrasound
   E   Occurs in approximately 1 in 25,000 pregnancies

26. **Regarding the occurrence of a single umbilical artery:**

   A   Congenital abnormalities are present in 80% of cases
   B   Maternal diabetes is a risk factor
   C   It can be present in syringomyelia
   D   Occurs in 1% of cords
   E   Indicates the presence of two vessels

27. **Atrophic vaginitis:**

   A   Is caused by a reduction in oestrogen levels before menopause
   B   The normal pH of the vagina is 3.5–4.5
   C   Can be caused by chemotherapy
   D   Is rarely the sole cause of urinary symptoms
   E   Topical progesterone is an effective treatment

28. **The following tumour markers are associated with these tumours:**

   A   CA-125: ovarian cancer
   B   Carcinoembryonic antigen: breast cancer
   C   CA 19-9: pancreatic cancer
   D   Human chorionic gonadotropin: testicular seminomas
   E   Alpha-fetoprotein: colorectal cancer

29. **Sarcomas:**

   A   Are tumours of the connective tissue
   B   Contain spindle cells on microscopy
   C   Are benign tumours
   D   Are formed from mesenchymal tissue
   E   Kaposi's sarcoma is a form of sarcoma

30. **Risk factors for umbilical cord prolapse include:**

   A   Twin pregnancy
   B   Oligohydramnios
   C   Unengaged presenting part
   D   Nulliparity
   E   Artificial rupture of membranes

Questions: SBAs

For each question, select the single most appropriate answer from the five options listed.

31. What is the range of wave frequencies used in ultrasonography?

    A   0.5–1 MHz
    B   1–20 MHz
    C   30–50 MHz
    D   50–100 MHz
    E   100 MHz

32. A 32-year-old woman is para one and is seen in the antenatal clinic at 36 weeks' gestation to discuss the mode of delivery. Her last labour ended in an emergency caesarean section at 8 cm dilatation for a fetal bradycardia. You are counselling her about the risks of vaginal birth after caesarean section (VBAC).

What risk of uterine rupture should be quoted to patients when counselling about VBAC?

    A   1 in 100
    B   1 in 200
    C   1 in 500
    D   1 in 1000
    E   1 in 2000

33. A 28-year-old multiparous woman attends for a dating scan in early pregnancy. She is unsure of the first day of her last menstrual period and reports that her periods are irregular. Fetal heart activity is detected on the transvaginal scan.

What is the earliest gestation that fetal heart action can be detected on a transvaginal ultrasound scan?

    A   3–4 weeks
    B   4–5 weeks
    C   5–6 weeks
    D   6–7 weeks
    E   7–8 weeks

34. A 40-year-old multiparous woman is 32 weeks pregnant. She reports recurrent palpitations. Her general practitioner arranges for her to have an electrocardiogram (ECG).

Which of the following features of a standard ECG represents ventricular depolarisation?

    A   P-wave
    B   PR interval
    C   QRS complex

    D QT interval

    E T wave

35. A 33-year-old woman with known HIV is seen in a genitourinary clinic. She has not commenced antiretroviral therapy. She describes deep dyspareunia, bilateral pelvic pain and increased vaginal discharge. She is otherwise well and is apyrexial. Serum inflammatory markers are normal. She is treated for suspected pelvic inflammatory disease.

What is the most appropriate treatment?

    A An extended course of oral antibiotics for 1 month

    B Initiation of antiretrovirals

    C Inpatient treatment for intravenous antibiotics

    D Standard 2 weeks of antibiotic treatment

    E None of the above

36. A 27-year-old woman presents at 26 weeks' gestation with a 2-day history of painful genital lesions. She does not recall having had any previous episodes. On examination, she has labial vesicles which are tender to touch. She is diagnosed with genital herpes.

What is the most appropriate management?

    A Arrange for an elective caesarean section at 37 weeks' gestation

    B Counsel the woman regarding termination of pregnancy

    C Organise ultrasound scans every 4 weeks for the remainder of the pregnancy

    D Referral to a genitourinary physician for treatment in line with her condition

    E None of the above

37. A 32-year-old woman presents with a 7-year history of painful periods, and a 3-year history of primary subfertility. Her serum follicular-stimulating hormone level is 6.8 IU/mL and luteinising hormone is 6.7 IU/mL. Pelvic ultrasound was unremarkable and her partner's semen analysis was normal.

What is the most appropriate investigation in this woman?

    A Laparoscopy and dye test

    B Brain MRI to exclude a prolactinoma

    C Postcoital test

    D Serum anti-müllerian hormone levels

    E Serum testosterone level

38. A 40-year-old woman at 28 weeks' gestation presents to the delivery suit with a 4-hour history of absent fetal movements and abdominal pain. On examination, she is pale and has a hard tender abdomen. There is no fetal heart audible.

What is the most appropriate immediate plan of management?

    A Administer corticosteroids

    B Category one caesarean section

    C Induction of labour with prostaglandins
    D Intravenous access and resuscitation
    E Magnesium sulphate infusion

39. A 41-year-old grand multiparous woman has a vaginal delivery. The midwife reports that she felt dizzy and has now collapsed in a pool of blood while walking to the toilet.

What is the most appropriate initial management?

    A Call for immediate help
    B Cannulate the patient and send blood for a cross match
    C Ensure her placenta is complete
    D Prescribe 40 IU oxytocin over 4 hours
    E Catheterise the patient as her bladder is palpable

40. A 25-year-old primiparous woman who is currently 35 weeks' gestation is seen at a routine antenatal clinic. Her body mass index at booking was 23. Her blood pressure is 110/62. She has moderate ankle oedema and is worried she has pre-eclampsia.

Which action is the most appropriate?

    A Admit to hospital
    B Assess serum transaminase levels
    C Re-check her blood pressure in 30 minutes
    D Perform a urine dipstick to assess for proteinuria
    E Start antihypertensives immediately

41. A 32-year-old woman is admitted to hospital 10 days after a first trimester miscarriage. She complains of abdominal pain, increased vaginal bleeding and offensive smelling discharge. An ultrasound scan reveals evidence of retained products of conception of 45 × 50 × 37 mm.

What is the most appropriate management?

    A Evacuation of retained products of conception (ERPC)
    B Intravenous antibiotics
    C Intravenous antibiotics and ERPC
    D Oral antibiotics and repeat ultrasound scan in 2 days
    E Repeat ultrasound scan in 2 weeks

42. A 39-year-old woman attends the gynaecology clinic complaining of increasingly irregular menstrual cycles and mood swings with weight gain. Hormone profile shows the following:

Follicle-stimulating hormone	32 IU/L
Luteinising hormone	4 IU/L
Oestradiol	52 IU/L
Prolactin	215 mIU/L
Thyroid function tests	Normal

What is the most likely diagnosis?

A   Asherman's syndrome
B   Addison's disease
C   Polycystic ovarian syndrome
D   Pregnancy
E   Premature ovarian failure

43. A 33-year-old woman attends the gynaecology clinic for investigation of her recurrent first trimester miscarriages. A thrombophilia screen has been performed as part of routine investigation.

Which of the following positive results would most likely suggest an acquired thrombophilia, rather than an inherited one?

A   Activated protein C resistance
B   Anticardiolipin antibodies
C   Antithrombin III deficiency
D   Protein C deficiency
E   Protein S deficiency

44. A 32-year-old woman attends for a review at 28 weeks' gestation. She complains of a circular rash on her legs and mild shortness of breath. Chest X-ray reveals bilateral hilar lymphadenopathy. Her blood tests show a mildly elevated serum angiotensin-converting enzyme level.

What is the most likely diagnosis?

A   Crohn's disease
B   Polyarteritis nodosa
C   Sarcoidosis
D   Tuberculosis
E   Wegener's granulomatosis

45. A multiparous woman is in spontaneous labour at 40 weeks' gestation. She has had one previous caesarean section. She is being continuously monitored in labour using cardiotocography (CTG). Her midwife is concerned that the CTG shows reduced beat-to-beat variability.

Regarding CTG analysis, what is considered the normal range for beat-to-beat variability?

A   1–5 beats per minute
B   2–8 beats per minute
C   5–10 beats per minute
D   5–15 beats per minute
E   10–25 beats per minute

46. A 23-year-old woman attends her 16 week antenatal appointment. Her booking blood tests for hepatitis serology are as follows:

HBsAg	Positive
Anti-HBc	Positive
Anti-HBs	Negative
Anti-HBc IgM	Negative

What is the patient's most likely hepatitis B status?

A   Acutely infected
B   Chronically infected
C   Previous immunisation
D   Resolving acute infection
E   Susceptible to hepatitis B infection

47. A 29-year-old hirsute woman attends the gynaecology outpatient clinic. She has oligomenorrhea and secondary subfertility. Her ultrasound scan shows ovaries with multiple peripheral cysts.

What is her anti-Müllerian hormone profile most likely to be?

A   Undetectable
B   3.7 pmol/L
C   10 pmol/L
D   17.3 pmol/L
E   65 pmol/L

48. A nulliparous woman has an early pregnancy ultrasound scan and her serum human chorionic gonadotropin (hCG) level taken as part of a study looking at the correlation between gestational age and serum hCG levels. The scan shows a single ongoing intrauterine pregnancy at 7 weeks' gestation.

Which is the most likely serum hCG level to correspond with this pregnancy?

A   5000 IU/L
B   300,000 IU/L
C   120 IU/L
D   50 IU/L
E   300 IU/L

49. Type III hypersensitivity reactions occur in which of the following conditions?

A   Goodpasture syndrome
B   Multiple sclerosis
C   Rheumatoid arthritis
D   Streptococcal nephritis
E   Tuberculosis

50. Which of the following immunoglobulin isotopes crosses the placenta to give the fetus passive immunity?

A   IgA
B   IgD

C   IgE
D   IgG
E   IgM

51. Which of the following is a major function of the complement system?

A   Acquisition of fetal immunity
B   Hypersensitivity
C   Opsonisation
D   Pyknosis
E   Sensitisation

52. A 37-year-old woman is seen in the gynaecology outpatient clinic complaining of a profuse, fishy-smelling, thin grey vaginal discharge; microscopy shows the presence of clue cells; the whiff test is positive.

Which is the most likely causative agent?

A   *Candida albicans*
B   *Chlamydia trachomatis*
C   *Gardnerella vaginalis*
D   *Escherichia coli*
E   *Trichomonas vaginalis*

53. A 35-year-old nulliparous woman is 14 weeks pregnant. She has recently arrived in the United Kingdom from a South American country. She is under the care of the infectious diseases team who are concerned she has yaws.

Which of the following is the cause of yaws?

A   *Treponema pallidum carateum*
B   *Treponema pallidum endemicum*
C   *Treponema pallidum pallidum*
D   *Treponema pallidum pertenue*
E   *Treponema paraluis cuniculi*

54. A 25-year-old nulliparous woman is being seen in a fetal medicine clinic following the detection of hydrops fetalis at a routine anomaly scan. Following investigation primary maternal cytomegalovirus infection is suspected.

Which of the options below gives the genome structure for cytomegalovirus (CMV)?

A   dsDNA
B   ssDNA
C   dsRNA
D   dsDNA-RT
E   ssRNA-RT

55. A 53-year-old woman undergoes a total abdominal hysterectomy and bilateral salpingo-oophorectomy after an ovarian mass was discovered on MRI. Her body

mass index is 38 and postoperative recovery is delayed by a suspected wound infection. Three days postoperatively, she has a temperature of 38.1°C, heart rate of 110 beats per minute and blood pressure of 94/56 mmHg. On examination, her wound is erythematous with serosanguineous exudate.

What is the most likely cause?

A   *Escherichia coli*
B   *Proteus*
C   *Pseudomonas aeruginosa*
D   *Staphylococcus aureus*
E   *Streptococcus pyogenes*

56. A 26-year-old woman undergoes a grade one emergency caesarean section for fetal bradycardia. She has diabetes and is obese. Ten days after the operation, she is readmitted with a wound infection. The wound is erythematous and discharging pus. There were no intraoperative complications.

What is the most likely operative factor contributing to the infection?

A   Length of operation
B   Presence of foreign material at operative site
C   Sterilisation of instruments
D   Surgical technique
E   Underlying medical disorder

57. A 19-year-old woman has attended her local genitourinary medicine clinic for a sexual health screening. Routine vaginal and endocervical swabs are taken and show the presence of a Gram-negative bacterium. A diagnosis of *N. gonorrhoeae* is made. The presence of which bacterial cell component is detected by the Gram stain?

A   Glycocalyx
B   Mycolic acid
C   N-acetyl glucosamine
D   N-acetyl muramic acid
E   Peptidoglycan

58. A woman attends the emergency department with severe left iliac fossa pain and a small amount of vaginal bleeding. On examination, her abdomen is distended with guarding and rebound tenderness. A urine pregnancy test is positive. An urgent transvaginal scan shows a left tubal ectopic pregnancy.

Which of the following is a recognised risk factor for ectopic pregnancy?

A   Combined oral contraceptive pill usage
B   Multiparity
C   Obesity
D   Smoking
E   Young maternal age

59. Which of the following is typical of acute inflammation?

   A   Angiogenesis
   B   Centralisation of leucocytes
   C   Decreased capillary hydrostatic pressure
   D   Increased efficiency of axial blood flow
   E   Increased endothelial permeability

60. Which of the following is a site of primary choriocarcinoma occurrence?

   A   Liver
   B   Lungs
   C   Testicles
   D   Thyroid
   E   Urinary bladder

61. A 40-year-old woman primiparous woman has an emergency caesarean section at 36 weeks' gestation following the onset of severe pre-eclampsia. After delivery the placenta is sent for histological analysis.

Which of the following is a histological change seen in the placenta in pre-eclampsia?

   A   Decreased syncytial knots
   B   Fibrosed villi
   C   Mass of small capillaries
   D   Non-specific trophoblast hyperplasia
   E   Villous hypovascularity with evidence of infarctions

62. A 26-year-old nulliparous woman attends a colposcopy clinic following an abnormal smear test. A biopsy taken at colposcopy shows dysplasic changes typical of cervical intraepithelial neoplasia.

Which of the following is a histological change seen in dysplasia?

   A   Increased nuclear size
   B   Increased number of cells
   C   Hyperchromatism
   D   Presence of meiotic figures
   E   Reduction in cell size

63. Which of the following is a cause of pregnancy-related microangiopathic haemolytic anaemia?

   A   Disseminated intravascular coagulopathy
   B   Gestational diabetes
   C   Polymorphic eruption of pregnancy
   D   Pregnancy-induced hypertension
   E   Pregnancy-induced idiopathic thrombocytopaenic purpura

64. A 53-year-old woman is brought to the emergency department by ambulance. She had a total abdominal hysterectomy and bilateral salpingo-oophorectomy 7 days ago and is in extremis. She is clearly unwell and the doctors treating her suspect she has systemic inflammatory response syndrome.

     Which of the following is one of the diagnostic criteria of SIRS?

     A   Heart rate: >75 beats per minute
     B $PaCO_2$: >6.3 kPa
     C   Respiratory rate: >15 breaths per minute
     D   Temperature: >37.5 °C
     E   White cell count: <4 × 10^9 cells/L

65. Which of the following hormones is secreted by the acidophils of the anterior pituitary gland?

     A   Adrenocorticotrophic hormone
     B   Follicle-stimulating hormone
     C   Growth hormone
     D   Oxytocin
     E   Thyroid-stimulating hormone

66. What is the most common type of pituitary adenoma?

     A   Adrenocorticotrophic hormone-secreting adenoma
     B   Growth hormone-secreting adenoma
     C   Prolactin-secreting adenoma
     D   Mammosomatotroph adenoma
     E   Mixed growth hormone/prolactin-secreting adenoma

67. Which of the following is a premalignant condition?

     A   Erythroplakia
     B   Herpes simplex infection
     C   Lichen sclerosus
     D   Lichen planus
     E   Pemphigus vulgaris

68. Which of the following is a recognised risk factor for the development of cervical cancer?

     A   Early menarche
     B   Higher socioeconomic status
     C   Late age of first sexual intercourse
     D   Having a male partner who has been circumcised
     E   Use of the oral contraceptive pill

69. A 56-year-old woman attends the gynaecology outpatient clinic with a history of postmenopausal bleeding. A pelvic ultrasound shows an endometrial thickness of 6 mm. Following an endometrial Pipelle biopsy and an MRI, a diagnosis of stage 1a endometrial cancer is made.

Which of the following is a risk factor for the development of endometrial cancer?

A   History of endometriosis
B   Multiparity
C   Non-hormonal intrauterine device (IUD) usage
D   Obesity
E   Premature menopause

70. A 27-year-old woman has a smear test as part of the UK screening programme. Following an abnormal result she attends a colposcopy clinic. On colposcopy, the whitened appearance of her cervix on application of acetic acid is suggestive of a human papilloma virus (HPV) infection.

Which of the following HPV subtypes is high-risk for the development of cervical intraepithelial neoplasia?

A   HPV 2
B   HPV 6
C   HPV 11
D   HPV 16
E   HPV 63

71. Which receptor is responsible for the analgesic effect of morphine?

A   Acetylcholine
B   δ
C   κ
D   μ
E   N-methyl-D-aspartate (NMDA) receptor

72. A 42-year-old woman delivers a baby at term weighing 2.5 kg. The baby is found to have abnormalities including chondrodysplasia and hypoplasia of the nasal bridge.

Which medication is most likely to have caused these abnormalities?

A   Azathioprine
B   Chloramphenicol
C   Gentamicin
D   Sodium valproate
E   Warfarin

73. What is the mechanism of action of warfarin?

A   Activation of antithrombin III
B   Increases action of factor Xa
C   Increases production of factors II, VII, IX and X
D   Increases production of vitamin K
E   Inhibits enzymic reduction of vitamin K

74. A 24-year-old woman undergoes a grade I caesarean section under general anaesthetic.

What is the most appropriate induction agent that should be used?

A   Etomidate
B   Ketamine
C   Midazolam
D   Propofol
E   Thiopental

75. A 16-year-old primiparous woman is seen on the postnatal ward round, 3 days after delivery. She wishes to discuss contraception as this pregnancy was unplanned. She is breastfeeding.

What is the most appropriate contraception?

A   Condoms
B   Copper coil
C   Combined oral contraceptive pill
D   Diaphragm
E   Progesterone-only contraceptive pill

76. A 19-year-old woman who is 28 weeks pregnant requests treatment for acne and is prescribed an antibiotic by her general practitioner (GP). She goes on to deliver a healthy baby girl at term. Two years later her daughter is noted to have unusually grey teeth.

Which treatment for acne did her GP prescribed for acne?

A   Chloramphenicol
B   Cefalexin
C   Co-trimoxazole
D   Erythromycin
E   Oxytetracycline

77. A 36-year-old woman with essential hypertension is 5 weeks pregnant. Prior to pregnancy she was taking an antihypertensive that has been associated with the development of fetal renal defects and oligohydramnios.

Which antihypertensive was she taking?

A   Atenolol
B   Labetalol
C   Methyldopa
D   Nifedipine
E   Ramipril

78. A 25-year-old nulliparous woman with a lifelong history of tonic-clonic seizures sees her neurologist for advice as she is wishes to start a family.

Which anticonvulsant drug is the most potentially teratogenic?

A   Carbamazepine
B   Lamotrigine

    C   Levetiracetam
    D   Phenytoin
    E   Sodium valproate

79. A 21-year-old woman presents to the emergency department with vaginal spotting and lower abdominal pain. She has a positive pregnancy test and serum human chorionic gonadotrophin is 2562 IU/L. She is found to have evidence of a left tubal ectopic pregnancy on pelvic ultrasound scan. After counselling she chooses to have medical treatment for the ectopic pregnancy.

    Which is the most appropriate treatment?

    A   Methotrexate 75 mg IM once
    B   Methotrexate 5 mg PO daily for 14 days
    C   Mifepristone 600 mg PO once
    D   Misoprostol 400 µg PO once
    E   No treatment

80. What is the greatest risk factor for placental abruption?

    A   Breech presentation
    B   Fibroid uterus
    C   Placental abruption in previous pregnancy
    D   Pre-eclampsia
    E   Previous caesarean section

81. Which of the following statements describes the action of calcitonin?

    A   It acts in the renal tubule to promote calcium reabsorption
    B   It acts in the renal tubule to reduce phosphate reabsorption
    C   It increases osteoclast activity
    D   It inhibits osteoblast activity
    E   It promotes vitamin D activation

82. Which of the following is an inhibitor of lactation?

    A   A fall in oestrogen levels
    B   Cabergoline therapy
    C   Infant suckling
    D   Prolactin
    E   Reduced progesterone levels after delivery

83. Which of the following ovarian tumours is responsible for the majority of ovarian malignancies?

    A   Brenner's tumour
    B   Dermoid cyst
    C   Ovarian fibroma
    D   Serous cystadenocarcinoma
    E   Sertoli–Leydig cell tumour

84. What percentage of teratomas of the ovary are bilateral:

   A   1%
   B   5%
   C   10%
   D   15%
   E   20%

85. Which of the following primary bone tumours is malignant in nature?

   A   Chondroma
   B   Haemangioma
   C   Fibroma
   D   Osteoid osteoma
   E   Osteosarcoma

86. Which of the following is the most common form of cervical cancer?

   A   Adenocarcinoma
   B   Adenosquamous carcinoma
   C   Clear cell carcinoma
   D   Squamous cell carcinoma
   E   Villoglandular adenocarcinoma

87. Which of the following cytological changes is characteristic of cervical intraepithelial neoplasia?

   A   Decreased nuclear/cytoplasmic ratio
   B   Decreased mitotic activity
   C   Increased meiotic activity
   D   Koilocytosis
   E   Mononuclear cells

88. A 72-year-old woman has a sudden onset loss of speech and hemiparesis. On arrival in hospital her symptoms and neurological examination is suggestive of a cerebrovascular incident. Subsequent imaging supports the diagnosis of an ischaemic stroke, affecting her left cerebral hemisphere.

   Which of the following forms of tissue necrosis is associated with her loss of function?

   A   Caseous necrosis
   B   Coagulative necrosis
   C   Colliquative necrosis
   D   Fat necrosis
   E   Gangrenous necrosis

89. A 24-year-old primiparous woman is 10 weeks pregnant. She is known to have a form of thrombophilia, as do members of her immediate family. She is referred for obstetric-led care by her booking midwife.

Which of the following is a congenital thrombophilia?

A   Antiphospholipid syndrome
B   Heparin induced thrombocytopaenia
C   Nephrotic syndrome
D   Paroxysmal nocturnal haemoglobinuria
E   Protein C deficiency

90. A 33-year-old nulliparous woman is referred to a recurrent miscarriage clinic by her general practitioner. She has had four consecutive first trimester miscarriages. She would like preconception advice and investigation.

Which of the following is an acquired thrombophilia?

A   Antiphospholipid syndrome
B   Antithrombin III deficiency
C   Dysfibrinogenemia
D   Factor V Leiden
E   Protein S deficiency

Answers

1. A False

    B True

    C True

    D False

    E True

    Low-molecular weight heparin (LMWH) has a longer half life than unfractionated heparins with more predictable effects, allowing for less frequent dosing. The action of unfractionated heparin is monitored using the activated partial thromboplastin time (APTT). The APTT is a measure of both the intrinsic and common coagulation pathways.

2. A False

    B True

    C True

    D True

    E False

    There are two drugs, commonly used in obstetric practice, which do not cross the placenta into the fetal circulation: heparin and insulin.

    Pethidine is 50% protein bound and is nearly totally freely diffusible across the placenta. Maximum fetal uptake occurs approximately 2 hours after administration.

    The rate of transfer across the placental membrane is dependent on factors including thickness of the membrane, the diffusion coefficient and the area of diffusion.

    Factors affecting transfer include:

    - Lipid solubility: lipophilic molecules transfer more readily
    - Ionisation: non-ionised molecules transfer
    - pH: pH of maternal blood affects the degree of ionisation of drug
    - Protein binding: unbound fraction diffuses
    - Molecular weight: smaller molecules diffuse more easily

3. A True

    B False

    C False

    D True

    E True

    Danazol is a derivative of ethisterone which is a form of modified testosterone. Originally used for the treatment of endometriosis it is also used to treat menorrhagia, fibrocystic breast disease and hereditary angioedema. Danazol works by inhibiting ovarian steroidogenesis by directly inhibiting the release of the pituitary gonadotrophins. Side effects reflect the androgenic nature of this drug and include weight gain, mild hirsutism, voice change, acne and decreased breast size; rarely, it can cause clitoral hypertrophy. It is not associated with the development of osteoporosis, but may be linked to the development of liver disease such as benign hepatic adenomata. Exposure to Danazol during pregnancy may lead to the masculinisation of the female fetus and therefore it is contraindicated.

4. A False

    B False

    C True

    D True

    E True

Antimetabolites are a group of substances that inhibit the action of normal cellular metabolic pathways. Through the interruption of normal metabolic processes they are able to interfere with events such as cell division and DNA replication. The ability to interfere with events such as cell division and DNA replication means they play a valuable role in the treatment of malignancy.

The action of antimetabolites is the interruption of nucleic acid synthesis through the inhibition of its key components, i.e. purine, pyrimidine and folate, and therefore interruption of the S phase of the cell cycle. Methotrexate is a folic acid antagonist which acts by competitively binding to dihydrofolate reductase, preventing the formation of tetrahydrofolate, an essential component needed for purine and pyrimidine synthesis. Through this action methotrexate is used as a form of chemotherapy in the treatment of malignancies such as Burkitt's lymphoma. Mercaptopurine is a purine analogue and interferes with purine synthesis, making it useful in the treatment of leukaemias. 5-fluorouracil prevents synthesis of pyrimidine and hence blocks DNA synthesis, via inhibition of thymidylate synthase; it is widely used in the treatment of malignancies such as breast cancer and colorectal cancer.

5. A True

    B True

    C True

    D True

    E False

Sonographers use a series of standard basic probe movements. Sliding, also known as alignment, involves moving the ultrasound probe up and down the area being scanned. Dipping uses pressure to press one end of the probe into the tissue, whilst rotation involves moving the probe from the longitudinal to transverse plane. Angling, also known as tilting, involves positioning the probe at different angles to the area of interest.

Timor-Tritsch IE, Goldstein SR. Ultrasound in Gynecology. Churchill Livingstone, 2006.

6. A False

    B False

    C True

    D True

    E False

Magnetic resonance imaging (MRI) is a modality which uses magnetic fields and non-ionising radiation to induce movement of atomic nuclei (specifically protons) within tissues. The excitation and subsequent relaxation of these protons can be recorded and used to produce images. The Tesla is the international system unit used to denote magnetic field strength. Absolute contraindications to MRI include cardiac pacemakers, intracerebral aneurysm clips and automatic defibrillators. Relative contraindications to MRI include pregnancy, cochlear implants and prosthetic heart valves. T1-weighted images show tissues containing water and fluid as dark, whereas fat appears bright. In T2-weighted images tissues containing water and fluid appear as bright, and fat and bone appear dark.

7. A True

    B False

    C False

    D False

    E True

Dual energy X-ray absorptiometry (DEXA) is used to assess bone density.

DEXA uses two beams of X-rays, each with varying levels of radiation, which are directed over bone. Bone mineral density (BMD) is calculated by subtracting soft tissue absorption from the beam that is passed through the bone. The results of the bone mineral density calculation can be used to give the patient a bone density Z and T score. The T score compares the patient's bone density to that of young person with a normal bone mass. A T score of more than −1 is normal, a score of −1 to −2.5 is suggestive of osteopenia, whereas a score of less than −2.5 is required for a diagnosis of osteoporosis. The Z score provides a measure of bone density using age-matching by comparing the patient's BMD with that of other individuals of the same sex and same age.

8. A True

    B True

    C False

    D True

    E True

Placenta praevia is the partial or complete insertion of the placenta into the lower segment of the uterus. It is associated with an increased risk of antepartum haemorrhage, which can be life-threatening. It is usually diagnosed on ultrasound and is present in around 0.5% of term pregnancies. Risk factors for the occurrence of placenta praevia include previous caesarean section, assisted conception, multiple pregnancy, uterine structural anomalies and smoking.

Royal College of Obstetricians and Gynaecologists. Placenta praevia, Placenta Praevia Accreta and Vasa Praevia: Diagnosis and Management. Green-top Guideline 27. London: RCOG, 2011.

9. A True

    B True

    C False

    D False

    E True

Laparoscopic surgery is now widely used, with around 1 in 1000 cases being associated with serious complications. The risk of injury is highest before the peritoneal cavity has been clearly visualised. Recognised entry techniques include the closed entry technique using a Veress needle that is widely practised in gynaecological surgery and also the open Hasson technique which is more commonly used by general surgeons. Palmer's point entry may also be used. The Hasson technique involves direct insertion of a blunt-ended trochar. This technique can be used in very thin or obese women or those with multiple previous surgical scars. Intra abdominal pressures of 20–25 mmHg should be obtained using gas insufflation prior to insertion of the primary trochar. This can then be reduced to allow easier ventilation of the patient. See **Figure 16.1** for images of female pelvis obtained using laparoscopy.

Royal College of Obstetricians and Gynaecologists. Preventing entry related gynaecological laparoscopic injuries. Green-top Guideline 49. London: RCOG, 2008.

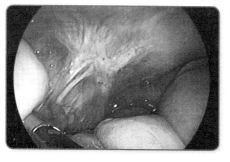

Figure 16.1 Laparoscopy (showing endometriosis).

10. A True

    B True

    C True

    D True

    E True

A severe headache in pregnancy may be due to any of the differential diagnoses listed. It is important that a careful history is taken to exclude life-threatening disease processes. Migraine and headache are common in pregnancy and can occur in women with no previous history of them. Cerebral vein thrombosis (CVT) may present with signs of raised intracranial pressure, in addition to headache. Vomiting, seizures and focal neurology may also be present. CVT may be associated with the procoagulant state of pregnancy and the postnatal period. Neurological input and further imaging is important in women who, at presentation, have any concerning features. In women who are critically unwell CT and MRI should not be delayed, and women should be reassured with regards to any potential harmful effects to the fetus.

11. A False

    B False

    C False

    D True

    E True

The majority of women within the UK have previously had chickenpox and are therefore immune to the varicella zoster virus (VZV). It may be appropriate to arrange vaccination for women who have no history of contact with chickenpox prior to pregnancy or in the postnatal period. Vaccination is not suitable during pregnancy. The VZV is infectious for 48 hours prior to the appearance of any vesicles and remains so until they have crusted over. Any VZV non-immune pregnant woman who has come into contact with chickenpox should be tested for the presence of VZV IgG antibodies, which indicate previous infection. Any woman who is non-immune should be given varicella zoster immunoglobulin. In addition to the risks of fetal varicella syndrome, pregnant women with varicella have increased morbidity, in particular 10% will develop pneumonia.

Royal College of Obstetricians and Gynaecologists. Chickenpox in Pregnancy. Green-top Guideline 13. London: RCOG, 2007.

12. A True

    B True

    C False

    D False

    E True

Polycystic ovary syndrome (PCOS) is a common endocrine condition affecting women which may lead to anovulatory subfertility. The Rotterdam criteria for diagnosing PCOS are:

- Irregular or absent ovulation
- Clinical or biochemical signs of hyperandrogenism
- Polycystic ovaries on ultrasound (**Figure 16.2**)

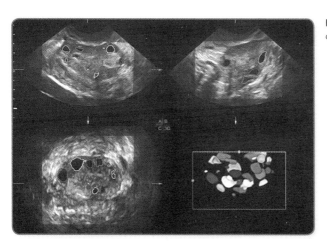

Figure 16.2 Polycystic ovaries on ultrasound.

In PCOS, there is increased secretion of luteinising hormone (LH) and an elevated LH:follicle-stimulating hormone (FSH) ratio, usually 3:1, however this is not included in the diagnosis. The elevated LH levels cause stimulation of androgen secretion. There is usually also a decrease in sex hormone-binding-globulin (SHBG). Insulin resistance is common and there is a strong association with diabetes mellitus type II. Treatment includes lifestyle modification, controlling the symptoms of hyperandrogenism and managing subfertility.

13. A True

   B False

   C True

   D True

   E False

Thyroid disease is common in the general population and is more common in women than men. Thyrotoxicosis complicates approximately 1 in 500 pregnancies. There are natural changes in the thyroid hormones in pregnancy including raised levels of T3 and T4. Thyroid-stimulating hormone (TSH) levels may rise or fall in early pregnancy, however the level of TSH generally rises in the third trimester. As human chorionic gonadotrophin rises in the first trimester, it can lead to a reduction in serum TSH as it may mimic T4 hormone. Hyperemesis gravidarum may be associated with a raised T4 level and low TSH.

14. A True

   B True

   C False

   D False

   E True

Parvovirus B19 is a single stranded DNA virus which is most commonly found in children, when it is known as slapped cheek syndrome. Up to 60% of the adult population are thought to be immune to parvovirus B19, having formed IgG antibodies from a previous infection. The incubation period is between 4 and 20 days, with the infectious period being from 5–10 days after the exposure to just before the onset of the rash. Parvovirus B19 affects rapidly dividing cells, especially erythroblasts. This can lead to severe anaemia in the fetus and hydrops fetalis. Diagnosis is confirmed by identifying the presence of IgM antibodies to the virus, even though the person infected with the virus may be asymptomatic. In the presence of hydrops fetalis, parvovirus should always be investigated.

15. A False

    B True

    C False

    D False

    E True

Type I hypersensitivity reactions are the most common and potentially life-threatening of the hypersensitivity reactions. Immunoglobin E (IgE) antibodies are produced as a result of previous contact with the antigen. The sensitisation process occurs through CD4+ Th2 cells, inducing class switching of antigen specific B cells. When exposure reoccurs, the allergenic substance becomes bound to IgE antibodies which are already bound to mast cells. This binding causes the mast cells to degranulate with the rapid release of histamine. The release of histamine is associated with systemic effects such as the contraction of smooth muscle (by acting on H1 receptors), including that of the bronchi, leading to breathing difficulties.

16. A False

    B False

    C True

    D True

    E False

Human leucocyte antigen (HLA) is another term for the major histocompatibility complex (MHC). The MHC is located on the cell surface and presents protein chains (peptides or antigens) to T cells. MHC class I molecules are expressed on the surface of all nucleated cells, whereas MHC class II molecules are present only on specialised antigen-presenting cells. The MHC class I molecule presents CD8+ T cells with endogenous (cytoplasmically derived) antigen in the form of a short protein chain, for example a peptide from an intracellular virus. It is made up of a heavy chain and a β_2-microglobulin. HLAs of the MHC class II type present CD4+ T cells with exogenous antigens (derived from intracellular vesicles).

17. A True

    B False

C False

D True

E True

Cytokines are small molecules that act as signals between cells. The different types of cytokines are listed below:

- Interferons: inhibit viral replication
- Lymphokines: IL-2 made by T cells, IL-4 produced by Th2 cells and mast cells
- Monokines: IL-1, IL-6, IL-8, IL-12 and tumour necrosis factor-α
- Chemokines: activate and direct appropriate cells to sites of tissue damage or trauma

18. A True

B True

C False

D True

E True

Actinomyces israelii is a Gram-positive anaerobic rod-shaped non-sporing bacterium which is a commensal of the colon, mouth and vagina. It is the commonest cause of actinomycosis, a chronic, suppurative and granulomatous inflammatory infection. The presence of sulphur granules is characteristic of actinomyces infection. The majority of cases of actinomycosis affect the cervicofacial area, classically presenting as painless facial lumps; however thoracic, abdominal and pelvic forms do rarely occur. Pelvic infection may be associated with long-term usage of an intrauterine contraceptive device. Treatment of actinomycosis requires a long course of penicillin.

19. A False

B True

C False

D False

E False

In addition to the incidental finding of maternal vaginal carriage of Group B streptococcal (GBS) a series of risk factors have been identified which increase the likelihood of transmission to the fetus as it makes its way through the birth canal. These risk factors include prolonged rupture of membranes of more than 18 hours, maternal pyrexia in labour of >38°C and gestation of < 37 weeks. The current RCOG guidance advises that routine administration of antibiotics when these risk factors are present is appropriate. Having had a child previously affected by neonatal GBS disease is also an indication for antibiotic therapy; however, the known carriage of GBS in a previous pregnancy is not an indication for administration.

Royal College of Obstetricians and Gynaecologists. Prevention of Early Onset Group B Streptococcal Disease. Green-top Guideline 36. London: RCOG, 2003.

20. A True

    B False

    C True

    D True

    E False

Necrotising fasciitis is an infection of subcutaneous tissue and may be caused by either group A streptococcal infection (type 2 necrotising fasciitis) or by the colonisation of a series of bacteria including *Enterobacter* species, streptococci and staphylococci (type 1 necrotising fasciitis). Toxic shock syndrome may be caused by the exotoxins released by Group A *Streptococcus* (*Streptococcus pyogenes*) and *Staphylococcus aureus*; it may occur as a sequelae of necrotising fasciitis. The mainstay of the medical emergency is immediate resuscitation, surgical debridement of the affected tissue and the speedy administration of intravenous broad-spectrum antimicrobials.

21. A True

    B True

    C False

    D True

    E False

The main types of human herpesviruses are:

- Herpes simplex virus type I and type II
- Epstein–Barr virus
- Cytomegalovirus
- Varicella zoster virus

Herpes type I and type II viruses have double-stranded DNA. Cytomegalovirus rarely causes diseases unless patients are immunocompromised. About half of the population has antibodies to this virus without ever having had symptoms. Epstein–Barr virus infection is very common, with most of the population having been exposed by adulthood.

Parvovirus B19 is a single-stranded DNA virus. Hepatitis B virus contains double-stranded DNA and replicates using reverse transcriptase. Hepatitis A, C and E all have the positive-sense, single-stranded RNA genome.

HIV is lentivirus, and a member of the retrovirus family, with a single-stranded RNA genome.

22. A True

    B False

    C False

D **True**

E **False**

Fetal varicella syndrome (FVS) is caused by reactivation of the varicella zoster virus (VZV) in utero. FVS is associated with a series of fetal abnormalities such as limb hypoplasia and microcephaly and dermatomal skin scarring. Amniocentesis is not used for diagnosis as the risk of infection is low even in the presence of VZV DNA in the amniotic fluid.

Royal College of Obstetricians and Gynaecologists. Chickenpox in Pregnancy. Green-top Guideline 13. London: RCOG, 2007.

23. A **False**

B **True**

C **True**

D **False**

E **False**

Rubella virus is a single stranded RNA togavirus. It is spread by droplet transmission and is not treatable by antivirals. It is a live, attenuated vaccine and is therefore not suitable to be given during pregnancy. If no immunity is found at the first midwife (booking) appointment, vaccination should be offered after birth, prior to leaving hospital. The prevalence of rubella is low in the UK due to the vaccination programme. African countries, India and Pakistan have a prevalence rate of up to 17%. Congenital defects follow rubella infection which has occurred during the first 16 weeks of pregnancy; after that it point does not seem to cause fetal abnormalities. The main defects associated with infection are cataracts, deafness, and cardiac abnormalities. Maternal rubella can also increase the risk of miscarriage and stillbirths.

Health Protection Agency. Guidance on Viral Rash in Pregnancy: Investigation, Diagnosis and Management of Viral Illness Rash, or Exposure to Viral Rash Illness, in Pregnancy. London: HPA, 2011.

24. A **False**

B **True**

C **True**

D **False**

E **True**

The presence of an imperforate hymen is often diagnosed in teenage girls presenting with amenorrhoae and abdominal pain. The hymen develops from the urogenital sinus and by menarche the central portion is open. An imperforate hymen acts as a solid membrane between proximal uterovaginal tract and the introitus. An imperforate hymen is surgically easily resolved. It does not have a familial inheritance.

Balen AH, Creighton SM, Davies MC, MacDougall J, Stanhope R. Paediatric and Adolescent Gynecology: A Multidisciplinary Approach. Cambridge: Cambridge University Press, 2004.

25. A True

    B False

    C True

    D False

    E False

Placenta accreta is a relatively rare condition occurring in approximately 1 in 2500 pregnancies and complicates 5–10% of cases of placenta praevia. It is defined as the invasion of the placental chorionic villi into the myometrium and predisposes to postpartum haemorrhage (PPH). Causes of placenta accreta include Asherman's syndrome, as well as previous caesarean section and increased maternal age. It is difficult to diagnose antenatally, however it may cause antepartum bleeding.

Royal College of Obstetricians and Gynaecologists. Placenta Praevia, Placenta Praevia Accreta and Vasa Praevia: Diagnosis and Management. Green-top Guideline 27. London: RCOG, 2011.

26. A False

    B True

    C True

    D True

    E True

The presence of a single umbilical artery is associated with congenital abnormality in 30% of cases, including renal, musculoskeletal and cardiac conditions. It also has an association with maternal diabetes and epilepsy. In patients with a single umbilical artery, there are usually two vessels present: one artery and one vein, instead of the usual two arteries.

Cunningham FG, Leveno KJ, Bloom SL, Hauth JC, Rouse DJ, Spong CY. William's Obstetrics, 23rd edn. MacGraw-Hill, 2010.

27. A False

    B True

    C True

    D False

    E False

Atrophic vaginitis is a common condition in postmenopausal women. It is caused by reduced oestrogen levels, which leads to a change in tissue composition of the vaginal wall. These changes include a proliferation of connective tissue and hyalinisation of collagen. Symptoms include dryness, itchiness and urinary symptoms. Treatment usually consists of replacing the deficient oestrogen with topical preparations.

Chapter 16: Genital Tract Infections. In: Collins S, Arulkumaran S, Hayes K, et al. Oxford Handbook of Obstetrics and Gynaecology, 2nd edn. Oxford: Oxford University Press, 2010: 521.

28. A True

    B False

    C True

    D True

    E False

Tumour markers are often useful in the monitoring of cancers; however, as they may also be raised in numerous non-malignant conditions, they should be used cautiously in the diagnosis of malignancy.

29. A True

    B True

    C False

    D True

    E False

Sarcomas are malignant tumours of connective tissues, i.e. bone, muscle and cartilage. These mesenchymal tumours form from tissue that was originally embryonic mesoderm. They are highly vascular tumours, which grow quickly and can metastasise via the bloodstream to the lungs and other sites. On microscopy they consist of spindle cells. Sarcomas may be treated using radiotherapy, chemotherapy or surgical excision. Patients with conditions such as Li–Fraumeni syndrome, neurofibromatosis and carriers of the retinoblastoma gene have a higher likelihood of developing sarcomas. Kaposi's sarcoma is not, in fact, a form of sarcoma but is actually a cancer of lymphatic endothelium which is associated with human herpesvirus 8 and is also considered an AIDs-defining illness.

National Institute for Health and Clinical Excellence. Improving Outcomes for People with Sarcoma: The Manual. London: NICE, 2006.

30. A True

    B False

    C True

    D False

    E True

Umbilical cord prolapse is the descent of the cord past the presenting part of the fetus, when the membranes are no longer intact. Cord prolapse is an obstetric emergency with a high rate of perinatal mortality, predominantly due to fetal asphyxia. Many of the risk factors for cord prolapse are related to common interventions and therefore can be pre-empted. These include artificial rupture of membranes, external cephalic version, stabilising inductions of labour and vaginal manipulation of the presenting part after membranes have ruptured, either artificially or spontaneously. Risk factors relating to the mother or pregnancy itself include multi-parity, prematurity, low birth weight, polyhydramnios, unstable or abnormal lie, an unengaged presenting part and prior to the delivery of a second twin.

On recognition of umbilical cord prolapse, delivery should be expedited by emergency grade one Caesarean section if delivery is not imminent vaginally.

Royal College of Obstetricians and Gynaecologists. Umbilical Cord Prolapse. Green-top Guideline 50. London: RCOG, 2008.

31. B 1–20 MHz

Ultrasound is a non-ionising imaging modality that uses very high frequency sound waves. The frequencies typically used in modern ultrasonography range from 1–10 MHz, however ultrasonography can sometimes use frequencies of up to 20 MHz. An abdominal ultrasound typically uses wave frequencies of 2–3 MHz, whereas transvaginal ultrasound uses a higher frequency of around 5 MHz. In addition to producing images, ultrasound can be used to provide therapeutic interventions. For example, lithotripsy is a modality of treatment for renal stones using ultrasound technology. **Figure 16.3** shows an ultrasound image of a uterine fibroid.

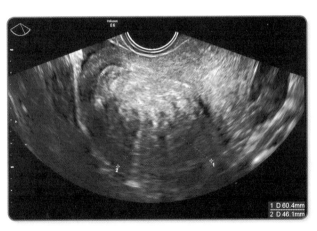

Figure 16.3 Ultrasound image showing uterine fibroid.

32. B 1 in 200

Women who have undergone delivery by previous caesarean section need adequate counselling early in the antenatal period in order to ensure that the subsequent delivery proceeds safely. Women who have had a previous uncomplicated lower segment caesarean section at term are usually able to be offered a vaginal birth after a caesarean (VBAC), providing there are no contraindications to a vaginal delivery. One specific risk that women should be counselled about is the risk of uterine rupture through the previous scar. This is frequently quoted as 1 in 200 and it should be explained to women that this is one of the reasons for continuous monitoring via cardiotocograph. Other risks for patients undergoing VBAC include a 1% additional risk of requiring a blood transfusion, increased risk of endometritis and increased birth-related risk of perinatal death and morbidity, such as hypoxic ischaemic encephalopathy.

Royal College of Obstetricians and Gynaecologists. Birth After Previous Caesarean Birth. Green-top Guideline 45. London: RCOG, 2007.

33. C 5–6 weeks

Evidence of fetal heart action depends on the mode of ultrasound and the gestation. Transvaginal ultrasound provides earlier visualisation of the fetal heart, which should be evident from 5–6 weeks' gestation. If transabdominal ultrasound is used, fetal heart action may not be seen until 6–7 weeks' gestation. Transvaginal ultrasound doesn't need the urinary bladder to be full, contrary to transabdominal ultrasound where an empty bladder leads to very poor visualisation of intrauterine pregnancy.

34. C QRS complex

The electrocardiogram (ECG) pictorially represents electrical activity in the heart, with the resultant waveforms signifying both the location in the heart where the electrical activity is taking place and also the direction of electrical conduction. In the standard 12-lead ECG the P wave represents the passage of electricity from the sinoatrial node through the atria, causing atrial depolarisation. The PR interval represents the time it takes for the electrical signal to pass from the sinoatrial node, through the atria and then to the atrioventricular node ready to begin ventricular depolarisation. It is the QRS complex which represents the depolarisation of the ventricles. The T wave represents repolarisation of the ventricles, whereas the QT interval signifies the time taken for the sequential ventricular depolarisation, followed by repolarisation, to occur.

35. D Standard 2 weeks of antibiotic treatment

Women who have HIV and are diagnosed with pelvic inflammatory disease should be treated with the same antibiotic regimens as non-HIV positive women. They may present with more clinically severe symptoms but should respond just as well to treatment. Hospital admission should be considered based on individual clinical findings and is not mandatory. Women who are on antiretroviral drugs should be managed in conjunction with their HIV specialist doctor to prevent drug interactions.

Royal College of Obstetricians and Gynaecologists. Management of Acute Pelvic Inflammatory Disease. Green-top Guideline 32. London: RCOG, 2008.

36. D Referral to a genitourinary physician for treatment in line with her condition

If a woman presents with primary genital herpes during her pregnancy she should be referred to a genitourinary unit. She is likely to need antivirals such as acyclovir in oral or intravenous form, depending on the severity of her symptoms.

As there is the risk of vertical transmission at delivery, any woman who presents towards the end of her pregnancy (within 6 weeks of likely delivery) needs investigation to establish whether there is primary or secondary infection. Type-specific herpes simplex virus antibody testing differentiates between primary and secondary herpes. Detection of IgG antibodies matching those from genital swabs confirms secondary herpes.

Caesarean section is the recommended mode of delivery for women who have primary genital herpes confirmed within 6 weeks of their anticipated delivery date. Women with recurrent genital herpes infection should not routinely be offered a caesarean section as there is a much smaller risk of vertical transmission.

Royal College of Obstetricians and Gynaecologists. Management of Genital Herpes in Pregnancy. Green-top Guideline 30. London: RCOG, 2007.

37. A Laparoscopy and dye test

Primary subfertility with painful periods for a long duration raises the suspicion of chronic conditions like endometriosis, fibroids and chronic pelvic inflammatory disease (PID). Ultrasound and clinical examination may help in diagnosis, but definitive diagnosis of endometriosis and adhesions can only be made effectively with laparoscopy. Additionally, performing a dye test allows for the assessment of tubal patency. Postcoital test, brain MRI and serum anti-müllerian hormone along with serum testosterone should not be the initial investigations in this case and can be performed later if need be.

National Institute for Health and Clinical Excellence. Fertility Assessment and Management for People with Fertility Problems. Clinical Guideline CG11. London: NICE, 2004.

38. D Intravenous access and resuscitation

This patient has had a placental abruption. The finding of a hard, tender abdomen is suggestive of a major abruption which may have led to fetal demise. Not all women with placental abruption will present with revealed vaginal bleeding. Risk factors for placental abruption include previous abruption, advanced maternal age, pre-eclampsia, polyhydramnios, intrauterine infection, pregnancy following assisted reproduction, fetal growth restriction drug use and smoking.

Maternal resuscitation and multi-disciplinary care is paramount. Blood and clotting factors will need to be requested and transfused as necessary. Ultrasound should be carried out to establish if there has been intrauterine death. If there is fetal demise a vaginal delivery is generally aimed for. Women who have abruption in one pregnancy are more likely to have a recurrence in future pregnancies.

Royal College of Obstetricians and Gynaecologists. Antepartum Haemorrhage. Green-top Guideline 63. London: RCOG, 2011.

39. A Call for immediate help

When faced with any collapsed patient, you must always ask for help immediately. The patient should be actively resuscitated and treatment for a postpartum haemorrhage (PPH) initiated. The causes of PPH are often referred to as the four Ts; Tone, Trauma, Tissue and Thrombin (**Table 16.1**).

Royal College of Obstetricians and Gynaecologists. Prevention and management of postpartum haemorrhage. Green-top Guideline 52. London: RCOG, 2009.

Table 16.1 Causes of postpartum haemorrhage

Causes of postpartum haemorrhage	Risk factors
Tone	Placenta praevia
	Grand multiparity
	Multiple pregnancy
	Obesity
	Increasing age
	History of postpartum haemorrhage
Thrombin	Pre-eclampsia
	Placental abruption
	Pyrexia in labour
Tissue	Retained placenta
Trauma	Caesarean section
	Operative vaginal delivery
	Big baby

40. D Perform a urine dipstick to assess for proteinuria

Pregnant women should have their urine checked for protein at every antenatal visit. If protein is detected, a urine tract infection and pre-eclampsia should be excluded. Ankle oedema is very common in pregnancy, and is in itself not a worrying sign. A diagnosis of hypertension cannot be made on a single blood pressure reading. Recognised risk factors for pre-eclampsia in pregnancy are advanced maternal age, obesity, multiple pregnancy, chronic hypertension and pre-existing diabetes. See **Table 16.2** for classification of hypertension in pregnancy.

National Institute of Health and Clinical Excellence. Hypertension in Pregnancy. Clinical Guideline CG107. London: NICE, 2010.

Table 16.2 Classification of hypertension in pregnancy

Classification of hypertension in pregnancy	Blood pressure ranges (systolic/diastolic)
Mild	140/90–149/99 mmHg
Moderate	150/100–159/109 mmHg
Severe	≥160/110 mmHg

41. C Intravenous antibiotics and ERPC

Retained products of conception may persist after a spontaneous miscarriage and occasionally even after an evacuation of the retained products of conception (ERPC). In this case there is evidence of infection and prior to any surgical intervention it would be appropriate to administer intravenous antibiotics to reduce the chance of infection and uterine perforation.

42. E Premature ovarian failure

Premature ovarian failure, or premature menopause, is defined as the onset of menopause before the age of 40 years. The most common presentation is amenorrhoea or oligomenorrhoea and there may be coexisting medical conditions.

Causes

Primary: genetic, autoimmune disease, Turner's syndrome, enzyme deficiencies
Secondary: chemotherapy, infection, hysterectomy +/– oophorectomy

Investigations

Follicle-stimulating hormone level is high, usually above >30 IU/L
Levels of oestradiol, luteinising hormone and progesterone are of limited value

Treatment

Management of infertility if conception is desired
Women usually need oestrogen replacement until the age of approximately 52 years

43. B Anticardiolipin antibodies

Thrombophilia may be acquired or inherited and results in a high-risk of thromboembolic events. Thrombophilia in pregnancy results in an even higher risk. Inherited thrombophilias include protein C and S deficiency, antithrombin III deficiency and activated protein C resistance (Factor V Leiden). Activated protein C resistance is autosomal dominant and in individuals heterozygous for the condition, there is up to a 10 times greater lifetime risk of thrombosis.

Antiphospholipid syndrome is an acquired thrombophilia and is found in approximately 15% of women presenting with recurrent miscarriage. Antiphospholipid syndrome can be diagnosed when there are anticardiolipin antibodies or lupus anticoagulant with three or more consecutive miscarriages before 10/40 with or without thrombosis. Some of these conditions may not be revealed until a precipitating event occurs, such as pregnancy. All women with thrombophilia are classed as high-risk.

Royal College of Obstetricians and Gynaecologists. The Investigation and Treatment of Couples with Recurrent First-trimester and Second-trimester Miscarriage. Green-top Guideline 17. London: RCOG, 2011.

44. C Sarcoidosis

Sarcoidosis is a granulomatous disease that affects many body systems. The granulomata are non-caseating, unlike in tuberculosis. It mainly affects adults aged 20–40 years, however prevalence during pregnancy is uncommon, affecting only 0.05% of all pregnancies. It is often asymptomatic and may be discovered incidentally. Symptoms of pulmonary disease include a dry cough, shortness of breath and chest pain. Extrapulmonary signs and symptoms include erythema nodosum, uveitis, fever and hypercalcaemia. Erythema nodosum usually manifests as painful, red lesions on the arms and legs and may occur spontaneously in pregnancy without any underlying pathology. The most common feature on chest X-ray is bilateral hilar lymphadenopathy, but there may also be evidence of fibrosis. Serum levels of serum angiotensin-converting enzyme may be altered in pregnancy and therefore are not a useful marker of disease. Pregnancy can often lead to an improvement in the disease which is thought to occur as a result of increased levels of cortisol.

45. D 5–15 beats per minute

Beat-to-beat variability is normal and should be between 5–15 beats per minute. Variability increases as the gestational age increases. The variability in heart rate will be affected by sleep patterns, movement and periods of accelerations and decelerations. It may be normal for the fetus to have a sleep pattern for up to 90 minutes; however, this only becomes evident on a cardiotocography trace after 28 weeks' gestation.

National Institute for Health and Clinical Excellence. Intrapartum Care. Clinical Guideline CG55. London: NICE, 2007.

46. B Chronically infected

Hepatitis B serology screening forms part of the standard booking blood tests. During an acute infection, hepatitis B surface antigen is found in the serum and is positive. Presence of hepatitis B core antibody indicates previous infection and would usually be detected in the blood 6 weeks after the initial infection. The surface antigen disappears if the infection becomes inactive and the surface antibody is then formed. Chronic infection is indicated in this case as the patient is positive for hepatitis surface antigen and core antibody. If the acute infection is not cleared from the bloodstream, then there is a risk of developing liver cirrhosis in the future. Hepatitis infection during pregnancy poses a risk of vertical transmission. All babies born to mothers with hepatitis B infection are vaccinated at birth, with the addition of immunoglobulin if the mother is highly infectious.

47. E 65 pmol/L

Hirsutism is characterised by coarse hairs with a male-like distribution. It may affect up to 15% of women. Polycystic ovary syndrome (PCOS) is the most common cause of hirsutism. This patient's hormone profile is suggestive of PCOS. Her anti-müllerian hormone level is raised, both of which are consistent with this diagnosis.

It can be difficult to make a diagnosis of PCOS and therefore the Rotterdam criteria are used once other causes have been excluded. The Rotterdam criteria make a diagnosis on the basis of the presence at least two out of three of features of (1) polycystic ovaries on ultrasound scan, (2) oligo/anovulation and (3) hyperandrogenism (clinical or biochemical). On presentation this patient meets two of the criteria.

Hirsutism is distressing to many women. A standardised scoring system such as Ferriman–Gallwey score may be useful to evaluate efficacy of treatment which may be cosmetic, medical or a combination of both. Medical treatment may include a combination of oestrogen and antiandrogen-cyproterone acetate.

Weight reduction of 5–10% can induce an improvement in hirsutism by 40–55% within 6 months of weight loss. In obese women with PCOS, a weight loss programme should be the first line of intervention.

Swingler R, Awala A, Gordon U. Hirsutism in young women. The Obstetrician & Gynaecologist 2009; 11:101–107.

48. A 5000 IU/L

In early pregnancy, an expert transvaginal ultrasound combined with serum human chorionic gonadotropin (hCG) have a very high positive predictive for diagnosing an ectopic pregnancy. A singleton intrauterine pregnancy should be visible with hCG from 1000–2400 IU/L. Multiple pregnancies may be visible with higher hCG values.

The diagnosis of ectopic pregnancy should be based on the identification of an extrauterine sac and indirect signs such as a complex adnexal mass or free fluid.

Progesterone levels >25 nmol/L are likely to indicate, and >60 nmol/L are strongly associated with, pregnancies subsequently shown to be intrauterine, although a small proportion of ectopic pregnancies have been reported with a serum progesterone concentration of >60 nmol/L.

Sagili H, Mohamed K. Pregnancy of unknown location: an evidence-based approach to management . The Obstetrician & Gynaecologist 2008; 10:224–230.

49. D Streptococcal nephritis

Streptococcal nephritis is an example of type III reaction where there is immune complex deposition. In Goodpasture syndrome type II hypersensitivity reactions occur. Blood transfusion reactions are another example of a form of type II hypersensitivity. In this reaction antibodies are directed against antigen on the individual's cells. Type I reactions are caused by immediate activation of IgE antibody and can also be described as anaphylactic hypersensitivity. Type IV reactions are associated with activation of T-lymphocytes. Type IV hypersensitivity reactions occur in conditions such as tuberculosis, rheumatoid arthritis and multiple sclerosis (**Table 16.3**).

Table 16.3 Hypersensitivity reactions

Timing	Type	Mechanism
Immediate	I	IgE antibodies
5–8 hours	II	Antibody and complement
2–8 hours	III	Immune complex
>24 hours	IV	T-cell mediated
> 12 hours	V	Antibody mediated

50. D IgG

Immunoglobin (IgG) is the most plentiful of the immunoglobulin isotopes and is fundamental to the secondary immune response. It is also the only form of antibody that is able to cross the placenta and by doing so confers the growing fetus with passive immunity. Maternal IgA is found in large quantities in breast milk and therefore confers passive immunity to the newborn. The immune system of the fetus starts to develop early on in the first trimester and includes the production of complement and the antibody IgM. IgA has been detected in fetal serum during the third trimester.

51. C Opsonisation

The complement system forms part of both the innate and acquired immune systems. The complement proteins produced by the liver are activated in the form of a cascade, via three different pathways (classical, alternative and lectin). The different products of each stage of the complement cascade have different roles. Opsonisation is one of the major functions of the complement system. Complement proteins cover the surfaces of pathogens, such as bacteria, which then attract cells such as macrophages, which phagocytose the pathogen. The complement protein C3b is the main protein involved in opsonisation. Other functions of the complement system include cell lysis, chemotaxis, increasing vascular permeability by stimulating histamine release and activation of the lipoxygenase pathway.

52. C *Gardnerella vaginalis*

Bacterial vaginosis (BV) is caused by overgrowth of the anaerobic bacterium *Gardnerella vaginalis* together with other bacteria such as *Prevotella* species, *Mobiluncus* species and *Mycoplasma hominis*. Amsel's criteria can be used to aid diagnosis when three of the following are present: (1) thin white homogenous discharge, (2) clue cells on microscopy, (3) pH of vaginal secretions >4.5 and (4) fishy odour on adding alkali (the whiff test). Women may be asymptomatic or may notice increased foul-smelling vaginal discharge. Although not a sexually transmitted infection, there is a higher prevalence of BV in sexually active women. In pregnant women with BV there is an increase incidence of premature rupture of membranes, late miscarriage and preterm delivery. Treatment with antibiotic therapy such as metronidazole may provide relief, although it may self-resolve.

British Association for Sexual Health and HIV. National Guideline for the Management of Bacterial Vaginosis. London: BASHH, 2006. www.bashh.org

53. D *Treponema pallidum pertenue*

Human syphilis, yaws, pinta and bejel are all caused by different sub-species of the Gram-negative spirochaeta *Treponema pallidum*. Yaws is caused by *Treponema pallidum pertenue* and is a disease found in tropical areas of the world, where it manifests as an infection of skin, bones and joints. It may form infective cutaneous lesions and can be transmitted by skin to skin contact. Bejel is caused by *Treponema pallidum endemicum*, pinta by *Treponema pallidum carateum* and finally syphilis by *Treponema pallidum pallidum*. It is important to remember that infection with the non-venereal forms of treponema will also cause a positive result on tests for syphilis, such as the fluorescent treponemal antibody–absorption (FTA–abs) test.

54. A dsDNA

Cytomegalovirus, also known as human herpesvirus 5, belongs to the herpes family of viruses and its genome consists of double-stranded DNA. The majority of adults will have been exposed to the virus and are seropositive if tested. Concern regarding the timing of exposure occurs during pregnancy, as fetal infection may be associated with an array of defects including microcephaly, hepatitis, cerebral palsy and sensorineural hearing loss. The answer stems given for this question derive from the Baltimore classification system. The system classifies viruses according to their genome, i.e. whether their nucleic acid is RNA or DNA, whether they are double-stranded (ds) or single-stranded (ss), their sense (+ or –) and whether their replication uses reverse transcriptase (RT).

Health Protection Agency. Guidance on Viral Rash in Pregnancy: Investigation, Diagnosis and Management of Viral Illness Rash, or Exposure to Viral Rash Illness, in Pregnancy. London: HPA, 2011. www. hpa.org.uk

55. D *Staphylococcus aureus*

Surgical wound infections are a common postoperative complication and standard policies are in place to try and minimise them. Examples of attempts to minimise wound infections include stringent hand hygiene, aseptic technique and in certain situations prophylactic antibiotics given at the time of procedure. Organisms enter the area of the wound from normal skin commensals, droplet spread and, more specific to obstetric and gynaecology, may be spread from the perineum or anal region. Common pathogens implicated in wound infections are Gram-positive cocci, such as *Staphylococcus aureus*, which causes up to 20% of wound infections. Other common causes of infection include *Streptococcus pyogenes* and *Escherichia coli*. Management would include appropriate resuscitative treatment including intravenous fluids, oxygen and prompt broad spectrum antibiotics. Blood culture and a wound swab should also be taken prior to antibiotics.

56. E Underlying medical disorder

All of the above are potential operative risk factors. In this case, we know that there were no intraoperative complications and therefore the length of operation is unlikely to be a cause. Sterility of the instruments should be confirmed prior to operation and there should be no foreign material present after the operation.

Factors associated with an increased risk of wound infection are as follows.

Operative factors:

- Length of operation
- Ventilation of theatre
- Sterility of instruments

- Contaminated or dirty surgery
- Foreign material at operation site
- Preoperative skin preparation

Patient factors:

- Age
- Body mass index
- Smoker
- Diabetes mellitus
- Impaired immunity

57. E Peptidoglycan

Gram-staining detects the presence of peptidoglycan in bacterial cell walls. The Gram-stain is therefore used to differentiate between Gram-positive and Gram-negative bacteria and it is the composition of the cell wall which gives them these properties. Gram-positive bacteria have a thicker peptidoglycan layer than Gram-negative bacteria. Gram-positive bacteria stain blue/black; Gram-negative stain pink/red. The bacterial cell wall is made up of N-acetyl glucosamine and N-acetyl muramic acid linked to peptidoglycan. It is this lipid, sugar and polypeptide structure which is responsible for maintaining the rigidity of the cell wall. The presence of a slimy glycocalyx on the surface of the bacteria is protective against destruction, e.g. by antimicrobials. Mycolic acid is found in high concentrations in the cell walls of organisms that are classified as 'acid-fast', such as *Mycoplasma*.

58. D Smoking

An ectopic pregnancy is a pregnancy that occurs when the embryo implants outside the uterine cavity. The most common site for an ectopic pregnancy is within the fallopian tubes; however, they may also occur in the ovaries, the cornua of the uterus, the cervix and rarely the abdominal cavity. Smoking is known to have an association with ectopic pregnancy, however obesity is not a recognised risk factor.

Any form of previous pelvic surgery raises the risk of a subsequent ectopic pregnancy, e.g. appendicectomy, due to the occurrence of adhesions. Other risk factors include pelvic inflammatory disease (genital infection), previous ectopic pregnancy, tubal surgery, endometriosis, use of the coil and usage of the progesterone-only contraceptive pill.

59. E Increased endothelial permeability

Acute inflammation describes the initial changes in the process of inflammation which are designed to neutralise or eliminate the cause of injury. Within the vasculature there is vasodilatation secondary to the action of histamine and nitric oxide and increased capillary permeability. Marginalisation of leucocytes occurs in the capillaries and is enhanced by the action of adhesion molecules. The rouleau effect may be seen as a result of erythrocytes collecting centrally. The usual axial blood flow is slowed with the subsequent development of stasis. Angiogenesis and fibrosis occur as part of chronic inflammation.

60. C Testicles

Choriocarcinoma is classified as both a form of gestational trophoblastic disease and also as a form of primary germ cell tumour. Rarely choriocarcinoma can be found as a germ cell tumour in the testicles and in the ovaries. When present in the testes choriocarcinoma is classified as an non-seminomatous germ cell tumour and is known to be the most aggressive and rapidly metastasising form of this type of tumour. More commonly, choriocarcinoma is described as a malignancy of trophoblastic cells and usually occurs following the development of a partial or complete molar pregnancy, although it can occur after normal pregnancy, ectopic pregnancy or following termination of pregnancy. This form of tumour macroscopically has a fleshy appearance, whereas microscopically there is an abundance of cytotrophoblasts and syncytiotrophoblasts with an absence of chorionic villi. Typically there is also evidence of haemorrhage.

61. E Villous hypovascularity with evidence of infarction

Pre-eclampsia is a multisystem disorder associated with abnormal placentation. Its sequelae occur as a consequence of widespread endothelial dysfunction, increased vascular permeability and vasoconstriction. In pregnancies affected by pre-eclampsia the placenta is found to have a series of histological changes including placental infarcts, increased syncytial knots and villous hypovascularity. Retroplacental haematomas are also more common. These changes reflect earlier placental implantation inadequate to stand up to the demands of the growing fetus. The histological appearance of a mass of small capillaries and non-specific trophoblast hyperplasia is associated with choriocarcinoma, not pre-eclampsia.

62. C Hyperchromatism

The histological term dysplasia is used to describe abnormal changes, both architectural and cytological, in the development of a cell type.

Dysplasia is characterised by the following:

- Anisocytosis: cells of varying size
- Hyperchromatism: excessive pigmentation due to abnormal chromatin
- Poikilocytosis: abnormally shaped cells
- Presence of mitotic figures: indicative of high cell turnover
- Loss of cell orientation

Dysplasia typically occurs in response to an environmental stimulus, e.g. the dysplastic changes seen in Barrett's oesophagus occur in response to chronic exposure to stomach acid. These changes may be an indicator of malignant potential, but they may be reversible. The cervical intraepithelial neoplasia (CIN) grading system refers to the severity of dysplastic changes in the cervix, where CIN I refers to mild dysplasia, CIN II to moderate dysplasia and CIN III severe dysplasia.

63. E Pregnancy-induced idiopathic thrombocytopaenic purpura

In haemolytic anaemia there is premature destruction of red cells, together with the reduced lifespan of circulating red cells. In pregnancy this form of anaemia may be caused by pre-eclampsia, haemolysis, elevated liver enzymes, low platelet count syndrome, haemolytic uraemic syndrome (HUS) and disseminated intravascular coagulopathy.

Chronic idiopathic thrombocytopaenic purpura (ITP) is a platelet disorder, not a haemolytic disorder. It caused by the development of IgG autoantibodies to platelets. It may be secondary to a variety of conditions such as systemic lupus erythematosus (SLE) and HIV. The condition manifests with peripheral thrombocytopaenia, however examination of the bone marrow may reveal the presence of megakaryocytes.

Primary ITP is a diagnosis of exclusion and can only be made after secondary causes have been excluded. Treatment is supportive and may include the administration of corticosteroids.

Thrombotic thrombocytopaenic purpura (TTP) shares similarities with HUS, and in both conditions there is microvascular platelet aggregation. In HUS there is predominantly renal involvement. HUS typically presents in the postnatal period. Polymorphic eruption of pregnancy (PEP) is an itchy erythematous rash that has no known cause, although it usually occurs during a first pregnancy. The distinguishing feature is sparing of the umbilical region and both PEP and gestational diabetes are not associated with microangiopathic haemolytic anaemia.

64. E White cell count: $< 4 \times 10^9$ cells/L

Systemic inflammatory response syndrome (SIRS) refers to the multisystem response seen in adults following a non-specific insult. It can be caused by infection but may also be a response to causes such as trauma, burns, pancreatitis, haemorrhage or inflammation. SIRS can be diagnosed when there are two of the following:

- Heart rate > 90 beats per minute
- Temperature >38°C or <36°C
- Respiratory rate of >20 breaths per minute or a PCO_2<4.3 kPa (32 mmHg)
- White cell count <4 × 10^9 cells/L or >12 × 10^9 cells/L

SIRS should not be confused with sepsis, a term which should only be used when there is SIRS alongside sepsis. The International Surviving Sepsis Campaign has developed guidelines to ensure that patients with SIRS are quickly and effectively managed. Rapid intravenous fluid resuscitation, alongside the use of broad-spectrum intravenous antibiotics provide first-line treatment approaches. Additional management may include the administration of corticosteroids and inotropes. Untreated SIRS may result in end-organ damage and multiorgan failure and, in severe cases, may be fatal.

Dellinger RP, Levy MM, Carlet, JM, et al. Surviving Sepsis Campaign: International guidelines for management of severe sepsis and septic shock: 2008. Crit Care Med 2008; 36:296 –327.

65. E Thyroid-stimulating hormone

The pituitary gland sits in a bony fossa at the base of the cranium. The adenohypophysis (also known as the anterior pituitary) is derived from oral ectoderm. The adenohypophysis can be further divided into the pars distalis, the pars intermedia and the pars tuberalis. The neurohypophysis (also known as the posterior pituitary) is derived from neural ectoderm and is in fact an extension of the hypothalamus.

Histological staining identifies three types of cells in the adenohypophysis: acidophils, basophils and chromophobes. Acidophils produce both growth hormone and prolactin. Basophils produce thyroid-stimulating hormone, adrenocorticotrophic hormone, follicle-stimulating hormone and luteinising hormone. The neurohypophysis produces oxytocin and antidiuretic hormone, also known as vasopressin.

66. C Prolactin-secreting adenoma

The pituitary gland is composed of a single anterior lobe and a posterior lobe, with the anterior lobe forming the majority of the gland. Prolactin-secreting adenomas, known as prolactinomas, are the commonest form of pituitary adenomas, which in themselves are the most common form of pituitary tumours. The most common site of a pituitary adenoma is the anterior lobe. Only one-third of adenomas infiltrate the brain. These tumours may be functional or non-functional and are typically found in adults of 30–60 years of age. Affected individuals may present with subfertility, amenorrhoea and galactorrhoea.

67. A Erythroplakia

Premalignant diseases are conditions that, if untreated, have a high likelihood of becoming malignant. Erythroplakia (and leukoplakia) are both precancerous conditions of the oropharynx. Other examples of premalignant conditions include Crohn's disease, ulcerative colitis and Barrett's oesophagus where there is chronic inflammation leading to increased risk of bowel and oesophageal cancers respectively. Actinic keratosis, if left untreated, may develop into squamous cell carcinoma. Cervical intraepithelial neoplasia has the potential to change into cervical cancer if not monitored and appropriately treated. Lichen sclerosus is not a premalignant condition, however it thought around 5% of women with the condition go on to develop vulval cancer. Neither lichen planus nor herpes simplex infection are associated with the subsequent development of malignant conditions.

68. E Use of the oral contraceptive pill

The main risk factors for the development of cervical cancer include: early age for first sexual intercourse, overall number of sexual partners, smoking and use of the oral contraceptive. Unsurprisingly woman who are immune-compromised, i.e. have HIV/AIDs or are on immunosuppressant drugs following an organ transplant, are more likely to develop cervical cancer. Cervical cancer is more common in women in deprived areas and therefore in those women with a lower socioeconomic status. Having a male partner who has been circumcised is associated with a lower risk for the development of cervical cancer. Early menarche is not a risk factor for cervical cancer.

69. D Obesity

The incidence of endometrial cancer in United Kingdom is around 20 per 100,000 women, the majority of which are postmenopausal. The combined oral contraceptive, especially in users of more than 10 years, halves the risk of this form of cancer. Endometrial hyperplasia is recognised as being a premalignant condition. Simple hyperplasia is likely to be treated with progesterone. Atypical hyperplasia on the other hand may indicate that cancer is already present on other parts of the uterus and, if not, will lead to endometrial cancer in 30% of cases. Invasion of endometrial cancer is local, through the myometrium and into the peritoneal cavity. An MRI is performed to assess the extent of myometrial invasion and stage the disease. Stage 1a and 1b disease is treated by performing a total abdominal hysterectomy (TAH) and bilateral oophorectomy (BSO). Stage 1c and 2a disease are treated by TAH and BSO, followed by radiotherapy. Risk factors for the disease are related to high levels of oestrogen (i.e. obesity) or many menses, i.e. nulliparous women and those of who have had a late menopause.

70. D HPV 16

Human papilloma virus (HPV) is a double-stranded DNA virus. There are many subtypes of the virus, 30 of which are present in the human genital tract. Most lead to focal epithelial proliferation. High-risk virus types commonly detected in women with CIN II and CIN III are HPV16, HPV18 and HPV31. However, the prevalence of HPV in sexually active women under 30 years old is as high as 40%, but most will clear it within 6–8 months. Being older and smoking decreases the chance of the virus being cleared. HPV2 and 63 are associated with the presence of common warts. HPV6 and 11 are commonly associated with anogenital warts.

71. D μ

There are three main opioid receptors: μ, δ and κ. It is now widely accepted that most of the analgesic effects of opioids are achieved through the μ receptor. All opioid receptors are G-protein coupled receptors and act through the inhibition of adenylate cyclase. Action at these receptors also leads to opening of potassium channels causing hyperpolarisation. There is also inhibition of release of neurotransmitter via inhibition of calcium release at the calcium channels. Other effects of opioids include dysphoria (κ receptor), reduced gastrointestinal motility (all receptors), respiratory depression (μ and δ receptor) and physical dependence (μ and κ receptor).

72. E Warfarin

Warfarin, a coumarin, is a teratogen and should be avoided during pregnancy. Alternative therapy with a low-molecular weight heparin is more appropriate in women who require anticoagulation during pregnancy.

The most teratogenic effects occur if given during the first trimester and can lead to fetal warfarin syndrome. Warfarin given in the second and third trimesters is thought to be associated with a lower level of birth defects. Fetal warfarin syndrome, or embryopathy, includes low birth weight, nasal hypoplasia and chondrodysplasia punctata. It can also lead to more global central nervous system abnormalities such as learning difficulties and neurodevelopmental delay.

73. E Inhibits enzymic reduction of vitamin K

Warfarin is an oral anticoagulant and inhibits the vitamin K dependent synthesis of various clotting factors (II, VII, IX and X). It reduces the post-translational gamma carboxylation of glutamic acid in clotting factors II, VII, IX and X and this is achieved via enzymic reduction of vitamin K. As the process of this enzymic reduction is competitive with vitamin K, ingestion of vitamin K will affect the efficacy of the drug. The onset of action of warfarin is delayed until the clotting factors have been eliminated from the blood.

Heparin and low-molecular weight heparin (LMWH) act in a different way. They activate antithrombin III which in turn inhibits thrombin. LMWHs increase the action of antithrombin III on factor Xa, but do not change the effect on thrombin. Heparin is safe to use during pregnancy.

74. E Thiopental

To reduce the risk of gastric aspiration, rapid sequence induction with cricoid pressure is used for these women. To minimize the placental transfer of anaesthetic agent to the fetus, catheterisation, cleaning and draping should be performed prior to administration of anaesthetic in order that the surgeon can begin the procedure immediately. Intravenous anaesthetic agents:

- **Thiopental:** barbiturate, very high lipid solubility
- **Etomidate:** involuntary movements during induction
- **Propofol:** rapidly metabolised and recovery with no hangover, used especially for day-case surgery
- **Ketamine:** causes profound analgesia, blocks NMDA receptor
- **Midazolam:** benzodiazepine, used for preoperative sedation.

75. E Progesterone only contraceptive pill

Patients are potentially fertile 3 weeks postpartum. Women who are exclusively breastfeeding are unlikely to ovulate and can therefore rely on this lactational amenorrhoea as long as they are exclusively breastfeeding, they are 6 months or less postpartum and the baby is not receiving supplementary feeds.

There are several options for this patient. As she is breastfeeding, the combined oral contraceptive (COC) pill is contraindicated. As the pregnancy was unplanned, condoms may not be reliable enough. The copper coil is a suitable choice for postpartum patients, but is not usually inserted until at least 6 weeks postpartum. A progesterone-only pill can be initiated immediately in this patient. She will need to remember to take the pill every day at the same time, as there is only a 3-hour window.

76. E Oxytetracycline

Tetracyclines, such as doxycycline and oxytetracycline, are broad-spectrum bacteriostatic antibiotics giving them a wide variety of uses, including the treatment of acne. They are known to chelate calcium leading to tetracycline deposition in growing teeth and bone. Given in the second and third trimester of pregnancy may cause maternal hepatotoxicity and fetal teeth discolouration in addition to skeletal deformities. These effects can also theoretically occur with breastfeeding, although it has been speculated that the calcium in milk may help prevent teeth discolouration. Because of these risks all tetracyclines should be avoided in pregnant women, those breastfeeding and in children under the age of 12 years.

77. E Ramipril

Ramipril is an angiotensin-converting enzyme (ACE) inhibitor and is used for the treatment of conditions such as hypertension and heart failure. They act on the renin–angiotensin–aldosterone system, preventing the conversion of angiotensin I to angiotensin II and therefore reduce arterial pressure and cardiac load. Unfortunately the use of ACE inhibitors in pregnancy, particularly in the first trimester, is associated with problems such as fetal skull defects, cardiovascular malformation, fetal renal problems and oligohydramnios. Alternatives treatments for hypertension in pregnancy include labetalol, a first line treatment choice and nifedipine and methyldopa as a second-line therapy.

Cunningham FG, Leveno KJ, Bloom SL et al (eds). William' s Obstetrics, 23rd edn. The MacGraw-Hill, 2010.

78. E Sodium valproate

All of the antiepileptic drugs (AEDs) are associated with an increased incidence of teratogenesis, which increases with the number of agents used. Sodium valproate, as a single agent, is associated with the greatest incidence of fetal malformation in comparison to other AEDs and is associated with abnormalities such as neural tube defects, cardiac defects, fetal growth restriction and craniofacial defects. Current NICE guidance recommends that sodium valproate should be avoided in pregnant women and cites data from the UK Epilepsy and Pregnancy Register from 2002. This found a 7.2% incidence of teratogenesis in pregnancies when the woman used sodium valproate, in comparison with incidences of 3% for lamotrigine and 2.3% for carbamazepine. There is limited data regarding the teratogenic risks of levetiracetam in pregnancy, however current evidence suggests this is less than the older antiepileptic drugs. Counselling of pregnant women with epilepsy is essential and should always include a discussion regarding the risks to both the mother and fetus if AEDs are discontinued.

National Institute for Health and Clinical Excellence. Newer drugs for epilepsy in adults. NICE: Technology Appraisal, 2004.

79. A Methotrexate 75 mg IM once

The administration of methotrexate intramuscularly may be a suitable treatment for ectopic pregnancy in certain circumstances. Methotrexate is an antimetabolite which inhibits folate reductase. Current RCOG guidance advises that the administering a single 75 mg intramuscular injection of methotrexate is a suitable treatment for ectopic pregnancy in cases where β-human chorionic gonadotropin (β-hCG) is < 3000 IU/mL. Mifepristone and misoprostol both have a role in termination of pregnancy and the medical management of miscarriage but are not suitable for the management of tubal ectopic pregnancy.

Royal College of Obstetrics and Gynaecology. The Management of Tubal Pregnancy. Green-top Guideline 24. London: RCOG, 2010.

80. C Placental abruption in previous pregnancy

Placental abruption is where the placenta separates from the uterus prior to the delivery of the fetus. It is one of the most common causes of antepartum haemorrhage (bleeding from the vagina or genital tract after 24 weeks of pregnancy). There are several known risk factors for placental abruption, including pre-eclampsia, polyhydramnios, advanced maternal age and smoking. The greatest risk factor for placental abruption is an abruption in a previous pregnancy. Abruption complicates up to 25% of pregnancies where abruption has occurred in two previous pregnancies. Prevention of abruption is via the limitation of risk factors. In women who have had a pregnancy complicated by previous abruption, there may be an indication for antithrombotic therapy.

Royal College of Obstetricians and Gynaecologists. Antepartum Haemorrhage, Green-top Guideline 63. London: RCOG, 2012.

81. B It acts in the renal tubule to reduce phosphate reabsorption

Calcitonin is an amino acid that is synthesised by the parafollicular cells of the thyroid gland. Parafollicular cells are neuroendocrine in origin and are derived from the neural crest. These neuroendocrine cells make up only 0.2% of the total thyroid gland cells. Calcitonin is regulated by circulating levels of calcium. When there are high levels of calcium, the level of calcitonin increases and vice versa. The primary organ of action is in the bone where it reduces the activity of osteoclasts. In the renal tubules, calcitonin acts to reduce the reabsorption of phosphate and calcium.

82. B Cabergoline therapy

Prolactin is produced from the anterior pituitary gland. Its production and release is increased by thyrotrophin-releasing hormone and inhibited by dopamine. Cabergoline is a dopamine antagonist and is used to suppress lactation postpartum in cases of mothers with HIV or who have suffered from a stillbirth.

High levels of oestrogen and progesterone during pregnancy inhibit lactation, but a drop in the level of these hormones after delivery and suckling lead to ongoing production of prolactin.

83. D Serous cystadenocarcinoma

Ovarian cancer is the most common gynaecological malignancy and over 50% of cases present in women aged 45–65 years. They are classified into different groups according to their cell type: epithelial, sex cord stromal or germ cell. They may be benign, borderline or malignant. The most common ovarian cancers are serous cystadenocarcinomas; these malignant tumours account for around 75% of primary ovarian cancers.

Serous cystadenoma is the most common benign epithelial tumour. They are bilateral in 10% of cases. Mucinous cystadenoma are typically unilateral and larger in comparison to serous cystadenoma. The majority of Brenner tumours are benign with 10–15% being bilateral. They are generally small in size. Some Brenner tumours secrete oestrogen so may cause irregular vaginal bleeding.

Most common ovarian tumours in young women are benign germ cell tumours. They contain elements of all three layers of embryonic tissue.

84. C 10%

Teratomas are germ cell tumours of the ovary. They are typically benign, occurring in women under the age of 30 years. Only 10% of teratomas are bilateral. They rarely rupture and in most cases patients are asymptomatic, however up to 10% result in torsion and patients may present with an acute abdomen. They are mostly unilocular and thin-walled. The vast majority of ovarian teratomas are mature and cystic and are known as dermoid cysts. They usually measure < 20 cm.

85. E Osteosarcoma

Osteosarcomas are the most common malignant primary bone tumour and are a form of mesenchymal tumour. Most commonly they are found at the metaphysis of long bones. Chondromas are benign tumours of hyaline cartilage. Haemangiomas are not a type of bone tumour and actually describe benign tumours characterised by blood vessels filled with blood. They are typically seen in infancy and often spontaneously resolve. Fibromas are benign tumours of fibrous connective tissue. Osteoid osteomas are small benign bone tumours that are most commonly arise in young adults.

86. D Squamous cell carcinoma

Around 80% of cervical cancers are squamous cell carcinomas. Adenocarcinomas are thought to be increasing in incidence and are present in around 10% of cases. Clear cell carcinoma of the cervix occurs in 1% of cases. This form of cervical cancer is historically associated with in utero exposure to diethylstilbestrol. Glassy cell carcinomas of the cervix are very rare and associated with <1% of cases and typically present with vaginal bleeding in the absence of an abnormal smear. Other rare forms of cervical cancer include neuroendocrine tumours. By far the majority of cervical cancers are caused by HPV infection. Unfortunately some cervical tumour types are less effectively detected by national screening programmes and typically present at a more advanced stage, e.g. adenocarcinomas and neuroendocrine tumours.

87. D Koilocytosis

Cervical intraepithelial neoplasia (CIN) is a premalignant condition that if left untreated has the potential to become cervical cancer. CIN is divided into three grades depending on the epithelial depth of the dysplastic changes occurring in the cells of the transformation zone of the cervix.

CIN is caused by chronic human papillomavirus infection, predominantly virus types 16 and 18. Liquid cytology now provides the method used for screening for CIN in the UK.

Cytological changes characteristic of CIN of dysplasia include poikilocytosis (abnormally shaped cells), an increased nuclear:cytoplasmic ratio, nuclear hyperchromasia, multinucleated cells and evidence of increased mitoses, suggesting a high cell turnover.

Koilocytosis refers to presence of cells infected with HPV which have abnormally large and irregularly shaped nuclei. See **Table 16.4** for classification of CIN.

Table 16.4 Histology, management and malignant potential of cervical intraepithelial neoplasia (CIN)

Grade	Thickness of squamous epithelium affected	Current monitoring and treatment	Malignant potential
CIN I	Basal 1/3	Conservative: 6 monthly colposcopy and repeat cytology Or LLETZ	Low malignant potential (around 1%); spontaneous regression common
CIN II	Bottom 2/3	LLETZ treatment required	Approx. 5% in 10 years
CIN III	>2/3 to full thickness affected	LLETZ treatment required	20–30% in 10 years

LLETZ, large loop excision of transformation zone.

88. C Colliquative necrosis

Necrosis describes the death of living cells following an insult. It is associated with cell shrinkage, and the breakdown of cellular contents. During necrosis there is pyknosis, karyolysis and karyorrhexis of the nucleus and its contents and enzymatic degradation with the release of inflammatory mediators. The form of necrosis that occurs is secondary to the form of insult and the tissues involved. In cerebral infarction there is colliquative necrosis whereby enzymatic degradation of cellular material may lead to affected tissue turning into a fluid form. Myocardial infarction typifies coagulative necrosis caused by hypoxic damage. Caseous necrosis is seen in tuberculosis where foci of infected necrotic tissue have a soft cheese-like appearance. Fat necrosis occurs in and around peritoneal tissue; it is associated with pancreatic damage and breast tissue whereby trauma to adipocytes leads to an inflammatory reaction with subsequent scarring and sometimes with calcium deposition leading to calcium soap formation. Gangrenous necrosis is not a distinct form of necrosis; however, it describes the appearance of black, dead tissue. Gangrene usually occurs in the absence of an adequate blood supply. Gangrene can be described as dry (for example, in an ischaemic limb), wet (for example, in the presence of Gram-negative bacterial infection), and finally as gas gangrene (in the presence of gas-producing bacteria such as *Clostridium perfringens*).

89. E Protein C deficiency

Thrombophilias may be inherited or acquired. These hypercoagulable states all increase the risk of thrombus formation. Protein C deficiency is an autosomal dominant condition. Protein C acts against activated factor V and VIII which are coagulation factors, as well as augmenting fibrinolysis. Hence, in the presence of protein C deficiency there is an increased risk of venous thrombosis. Other inherited thrombophilias include factor V Leiden, protein S deficiency, antithrombin deficiency and hyperhomocystinaemia.

90. A Antiphospholipid syndrome

Antiphospholipid syndrome is an acquired thrombophilia associated with increased risk of thrombosis, recurrent miscarriage, stillbirth and pre-eclampsia in the presence of persistent antiphospholipid antibodies such as anticardiolipin antibodies and lupus anticoagulant. Other forms of acquired thrombophilias include heparin-induced thrombocytopaenia (HIT) and paroxysmal nocturnal haemoglobinuria. HIT occurs when administration of heparin and subsequent binding to platelets leads to antibody production which goes on to cause platelet activation and subsequent thrombosis. Paroxysmal nocturnal haemoglobinuria is a rare disorder of bone marrow associated with anaemia and thrombosis. Antithrombin III deficiency, dysfibrinogenemia, factor V Leiden and protein S are all inherited thrombophilias.

Index

Note: Page numbers in **bold** or *italic* refer to tables or figures respectively.